D1703256

Congenital Heart Disease in Adolescents and Adults

Endorsed by

The ESC Working Group on Grown-up Congenital Heart Disease
AEPC Adult with Congenital Heart Disease Working Group

Series Editors

M. Chessa
San Donato Milanese, Italy

H. Baumgartner
Münster, Germany

A. Eicken
Munich, Germany

A. Giamberti
San Donato Milanese, Italy

The aim of this series is to cast light on the most significant aspects – whether still debated or already established – of congenital heart disease in adolescents and adults and its management. Advances in the medical and surgical management of congenital heart disease have revolutionized the prognosis of infants and children with cardiac defects, so that an increasing number of patients, including those with complex problems, can reach adolescence and adult life. The profile of the adult population with congenital heart disease (ACHD) is consequently changing, and in future many adult patients will present different hemodynamic and cardiac problems from those currently seen. A cure is rarely achieved, and provision of optimal care is therefore dependent on ongoing surveillance and management in conjunction with experts in this highly specialized field. Specialists in ACHD management need to have a deep knowledge not only of congenital cardiac malformations and their treatment in infancy and childhood, but of general medicine, too. A training in adult cardiology, including coronary artery disease, is also essential. Similarly, surgeons need to acquire expertise and good training in both adult and pediatric cardiosurgery. Readers will find this series to be a rich source of information highly relevant to daily clinical practice.

More information about this series at http://www.springer.com/series/13454

Jolien W. Roos-Hesselink
Mark R. Johnson
Editors

Pregnancy and Congenital Heart Disease

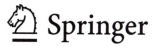
Springer

Editors
Jolien W. Roos-Hesselink
Erasmus MC University Medical Center
Rotterdam
Gelderland
The Netherlands

Mark R. Johnson
Imperial College London
Chelsea and Westminster Hospital
London
UK

ISSN 2364-6659 ISSN 2364-6667 (electronic)
Congenital Heart Disease in Adolescents and Adults
ISBN 978-3-319-38911-0 ISBN 978-3-319-38913-4 (eBook)
DOI 10.1007/978-3-319-38913-4

Library of Congress Control Number: 2016955961

© Springer International Publishing Switzerland 2017
This work is subject to copyright. All rights are reserved by the Publisher, whether the whole or part of the material is concerned, specifically the rights of translation, reprinting, reuse of illustrations, recitation, broadcasting, reproduction on microfilms or in any other physical way, and transmission or information storage and retrieval, electronic adaptation, computer software, or by similar or dissimilar methodology now known or hereafter developed.
The use of general descriptive names, registered names, trademarks, service marks, etc. in this publication does not imply, even in the absence of a specific statement, that such names are exempt from the relevant protective laws and regulations and therefore free for general use.
The publisher, the authors and the editors are safe to assume that the advice and information in this book are believed to be true and accurate at the date of publication. Neither the publisher nor the authors or the editors give a warranty, express or implied, with respect to the material contained herein or for any errors or omissions that may have been made.

Printed on acid-free paper

This Springer imprint is published by Springer Nature
The registered company is Springer International Publishing AG
The registered company address is: Gewerbestrasse 11, 6330 Cham, Switzerland

Preface to the Series

In Europe, we are currently faced with an estimated ACHD population of 4.2 million; adults with congenital heart disease now outnumber children (approximately 2.3 million). The vast majority cannot be considered cured but rather having a chronic heart condition that requires further surveillance and timely re-intervention for residual or consequent anatomical and/or functional abnormalities. ACHD patients have very special needs and the physicians taking care of them need expert training. Special health care organization and training programs for those involved in ACHD care are therefore required to meet the needs of this special population.

ACHD problems remain a small part of general cardiology training curricula around the world, and pediatric cardiologists are trained to manage children with CHD and may, out of necessity, continue to look after these patients when they outgrow pediatric age.

There are clearly other health issues concerning the adult with CHD, beyond the scope of pediatric medicine, that our patients now routinely face. Adult physicians with a non-CHD background are therefore increasingly involved in the day-to-day management of patients with CHD.

Experts in congenital heart disease should work to improve the health care system, so that teens and young adults have an easier time making the transition from receiving health care in pediatric cardiology centers to receiving care from specialists in adult cardiology.

The aim of this series is to cast light on the most significant aspects of congenital heart disease in adolescents and adults and its management, such as transition from pediatric to adulthood, pregnancy and contraception, sport and physical activities, pulmonary hypertension, burning issues related to surgery, interventional catheterization, electrophysiology, intensive care management, and heart failure.

This series wishes to attract the interest of cardiologists, anesthesiologists, cardiac surgeons, electrophysiologists, psychologists, GPs, undergraduate and postgraduate students, and residents, and would like to become relevant for courses of cardiology, pediatric cardiology, cardiothoracic surgery, and anesthesiology.

We thank both the wonderful groups of leading cardiovascular experts from around the world, for donating their precious time, producing excellent textbooks and making this book series a reality, and the members of the two Working Groups (ESC and AEPC ACHD/GUCH Working Group) for the invaluable suggestions and support without which this work would not be possible.

San Donato, Italy	Massimo Chessa
Münster, Germany	Helmut Baumgartner
Munich, Germany	Andreas Eicken
San Donato, Italy	Alessandro Giamberti

Preface

Advances in diagnostic modalities and treatment options for children born with a congenital heart defect have changed the landscape of patients with congenital heart disease considerably. Advanced cardiac surgery and intensive care have dramatically improved the outcome for these patients: before the introduction of the heart-lung machine, survival was about 15 %; now more than 90 % of patients reach adulthood. Half are women, and most of them want to start a family and raise children. However, pregnancy has a major impact on the cardiovascular system. It not only leads to an increase in cardiac output of up to 50 % but also increases the risk of thromboembolic complications and the development of arrhythmias. Further, pregnancy appears to affect vessel structure, increasing the risk of aortic dissection. Delivery is the period of dramatic fluid shifts predisposing to the development of pulmonary oedema.

Most patients with congenital heart disease are diagnosed when young and have undergone corrective cardiac surgery. However, some still have residual lesions, and, in others, the diagnosis was missed or the condition was found to be inoperable. As a group, women with CHD are at higher risk of developing complications during pregnancy and after delivery. Cardiovascular mortality and morbidity are higher in patients with heart disease; heart failure and arrhythmias are especially common. Therefore, timely counselling and risk stratification are of great importance. In addition, the mother's life expectancy and the impact of the pregnancy on her condition should be discussed openly. Some women may need treatment before embarking on a pregnancy, and others may need to have existing treatment optimized. Follow-up during pregnancy and the timing, place and mode of delivery are also important and sometimes difficult issues.

Specific knowledge is not available from large randomized trials in this field, and therefore, many decisions are made based on "expert knowledge". This book is an extremely valuable resource for all those looking after women with congenital heart disease especially when they are pregnant. It provides up-to-date information on specific topics and gives detailed, lesion-specific information from well-known experts in this field. We hope this book will be the definitive resource for cardiologists, obstetricians, anaesthetists and other members of the team providing care and support to women with congenital heart disease.

Rotterdam, The Netherlands Jolien W. Roos-Hesselink
London, UK Mark R. Johnson

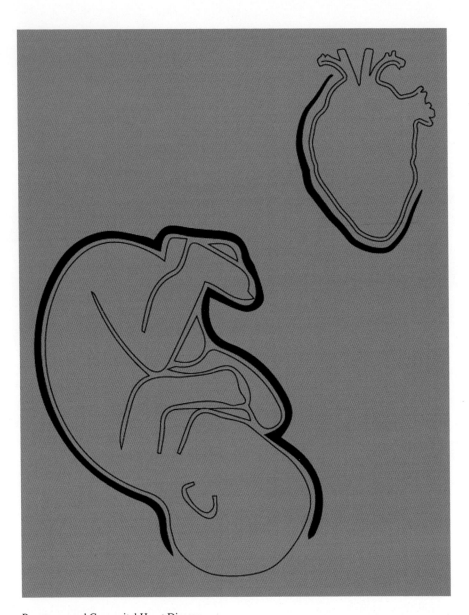

Pregnancy and Congenital Heart Disease

Contents

Part I General Issues

1. **Fetal Heart Disease** 3
   Julene S. Carvalho and Olus Api

2. **Contraception and Cardiovascular Disease** 23
   Jan S. Erkamp and Jérôme Cornette

3. **Preconception Counseling** 35
   M.A.M. Kampman and P.G. Pieper

4. **Inheritance of Congenital Heart Disease** 51
   Ingrid van de Laar and Marja Wessels

5. **Care During Pregnancy** 67
   Iris M. van Hagen and Jolien W. Roos-Hesselink

6. **The Management of Labour and the Post-partum Period in CHD** ... 83
   Matt Cauldwell, Mark Cox, Roisin Monteiro, and Mark R. Johnson

Part II Specific Lesions

7. **Pregnancy in Repaired Tetralogy of Fallot** 99
   Sonya V. Babu-Narayan, Wei Li, and Anselm Uebing

8. **Transposition of the Great Arteries** 113
   Daniel Tobler and Matthias Greutmann

9. **Shunt Lesions** 129
   Antonia Pijuan-Domenech and Maria Goya

10. **Aortic Stenosis** 141
    Stefan Orwat and Helmut Baumgartner

11. **Pregnancy in Hypertrophic Cardiomyopathy** 155
    Michelle Michels

12	**Aortopathy**..	165
	Julie De Backer, Laura Muiño-Mosquera, and Laurent Demulier	
13	**Aortic Coarctation**	195
	Margarita Brida and Gerhard-Paul Diller	
14	**Ebstein Anomaly**...	207
	Andrea Girnius, Gruschen Veldtman, Carri R. Warshak, and Markus Schwerzmann	
15	**Fontan**	225
	Margherita Ministeri and Michael A. Gatzoulis	
16	**Cyanotic Lesions**...	243
	Matthias Greutmann and Daniel Tobler	
17	**Pulmonary Hypertension**..................................	257
	Werner Budts	
18	**Pulmonary Stenosis**..	271
	Marianna Stamatelatou and Lorna Swann	

Part I
General Issues

Fetal Heart Disease

Julene S. Carvalho and Olus Api

Abbreviations

3VTV	Three vessels and trachea view
3VV	Three-vessel view
CHD	Congenital heart disease
ISUOG	International Society of Ultrasound in Obstetrics and Gynecology
LA	Left atrium
LV	Left ventricle
NHS FASP	National Health Service Fetal Anomaly Screening Programme
NT	Nuchal translucency
PA	Pulmonary artery
RA	Right atrium
RV	Right ventricle
SSA	Sequential segmental analysis
SVC	Superior vena cava
VMax	Maximal velocity

J.S. Carvalho, MD, PhD, FRCPCH (✉)
Brompton Centre for Fetal Cardiology, Royal Brompton Hospital and St. George's University Hospitals NHS Foundation Trust, Reader in Fetal Cardiology, Molecular and Sciences Research Institute, St. George's University of London, London, UK
e-mail: j.carvalho@rbht.nhs.uk

O. Api, MD, PhD
Department of Obstetrics and Gynecology, Yeditepe University Hospital, Istanbul, Turkey
e-mail: olusapi@gmail.com

© Springer International Publishing Switzerland 2017
J.W. Roos-Hesselink, M.R. Johnson (eds.), *Pregnancy and Congenital Heart Disease*, Congenital Heart Disease in Adolescents and Adults,
DOI 10.1007/978-3-319-38913-4_1

1.1 Introduction

Imaging of the fetal heart started in the 1980s but was mainly targeted at high-risk pregnancies [1–3], such as those with previous family history of congenital heart disease (CHD). The introduction of the four-chamber view into routine obstetric scans of low-risk pregnancies was first reported by Fermont et al. in 1985 [4] and initiated the pathway for antenatal screening. However, based on this view alone, antenatal detection remained low, being 23 % in the UK in the mid-1990s [5]. The importance of adding outflow tract views as well as training professionals at the forefront of screening cannot be underestimated, but over the years, improvements in detection rates have been slow. More recently however, dissemination of clinical guidelines and national protocols have had a positive impact on screening.

1.2 Birth Prevalence of CHD

Congenital heart defects are the most common cause of major congenital anomalies. In the EUROCAT study, they accounted for 28 % of major defects [6]. Whilst a birth prevalence of 8 per 1000 live births is generally accepted, there seems to be variation worldwide and over time [7–9]. According to a recent systematic review and meta-analysis, which included eight common types of major CHD, total CHD birth prevalence was found to increase substantially over time. It changed from 0.6 per 1000 live births in 1930 to 1934 to 9.1 per 1000 live births after 1995 but has remained stable over the last 15 years to 2010 [8]. Ventricular septal defects were the most commonly encountered CHD. Significant geographical differences also occurred, being highest in Asia (birth prevalence of 9.3 per 1000 live births) and significantly higher in Europe (8.2 per 1000) than in North America (6.9 per 1000) [8].

Limited access to health care and diagnostic facilities such as echocardiography may be responsible for some of the differences in reported birth prevalence. On the other hand, observed variations may also be of ethnic, genetic and environmental origin. In part, however, some of the differences are due to inclusion of a milder form of CHD such as small ventricular septal defects, mild pulmonary stenosis and bicuspid aortic valves [7, 9]. From the fetal cardiologist's perspective, the more significant forms of CHD are the ones most likely to be suspected on routine screening. These are also more likely to have an impact on fetal and neonatal outcome. Hoffman and Kaplan [9] reported an incidence for moderate to severe forms of CHD of 6 per 1000 live births. In general, approximately half of defects are considered major, i.e. with a prevalence of about 4 per 1000 live births [10].

1.3 Risk Factors for CHD

Inheritance of CHD is multifactorial. Various risk factors, from genetic or genome variations to teratogen exposure, trigger molecular responses during cardiac development that may lead to CHD [11]. However, the vast majority of fetuses with heart defects are seen in families without a known risk factor, which highlights the importance of having an effective screening programme for the detection of fetal heart disease.

In Chap. 4, inheritance of CHD is discussed at length. Briefly, recurrence is low for most forms of structural defects. In a population-based study, previous history of any CHD in first-degree relatives accounted for 2.2 % of the heart defects [12]. The risk associated with a previous child with a non-syndromic defect is around 2–3 %, rising to 10 % with two previously affected pregnancies [13, 14]. If one of the parents has CHD, the overall risk is increased to about 2–4 % [14, 15] but higher in the presence of maternal CHD (~6 %) [15]. A higher risk is also seen in association with left-sided obstructive lesions [16]. Risks other than family history can be of maternal or fetal origin. They also constitute an indication for fetal echocardiography and are summarized below.

1.3.1 Maternal Risk Factors

1.3.1.1 Autoantibodies

The risk associated with maternal autoantibodies (anti-Ro/SSA, anti-La/SSB) is mainly related to development of fetal heart block rather than structural CHD. With no previously affected child, the risk is around 4 % but significantly higher (19 %) if a previous child has developed heart block [17]. Serial scans are often performed, aiming to capture the development of first- and second-degree block, even though there is no effective evidence-based therapy to prevent progression to complete heart block. Recent evidence also suggests that the individual risk of heart block is affected by the level of maternal antibodies and that serial scans should be restricted to pregnant women with high levels [18]. Currently however, antibody levels are not widely available at the time women are referred for fetal echocardiography.

Autoantibodies have also been linked to myocardial dysfunction and endocardial fibroelastosis [19] and, rarely, rupture of mitral valve subvalvar apparatus leading to important mitral regurgitation [20].

1.3.1.2 Pre-gestational Diabetes

The risk associated with maternal diabetes is five times greater than the general population [21] and up to 8.5 per 100 live births in one study [22]. Common defects include double-outlet right ventricle, truncus arteriosus, transposition of the great arteries and ventricular septal defect [23, 24]. A link with isomerism has also been established [25]. Hyperglycaemia is known to modify multiple biochemical and signal transduction pathways; thus high maternal levels of haemoglobin A1c during early pregnancy are associated with increased risk of malformations [26, 27]. However, maternal diabetes continues to influence the fetal heart through the second and third trimesters. Reversible hypertrophic cardiomyopathy has long been described in infants of the diabetic mothers [28]. It may be observed whether or not there is reasonable metabolic control [26, 29], although there is some evidence that fetal insulin levels are related to myocardial wall thickness [30].

1.3.1.3 Phenylketonuria

Maternal phenylketonuria also increases the risk of CHD significantly, being 15-fold above the general population in untreated pregnancies [31]. High maternal levels of phenylalanine (>30 mg/dL) increase the risk significantly. Preconception or early pregnancy low phenylalanine diet to achieve a basal maternal level <15 mg/dL especially in the first 8 weeks of pregnancy may be effective in preventing CHD. Tetralogy of Fallot, aortic coarctation and hypoplastic left heart syndrome have been reported in the offspring [31, 32].

1.3.1.4 Maternal Obesity

There is some evidence that obese women are at increased risk of having a child with CHD [33, 34]. In a population-based study, the odds ratio of women with BMI >30 having an affected child was 1.15 (95 % CI 1.07–1.23) compared to normal weight women. The risk was even higher for women with BMI >40 compared to BMI >30 (Odds ratio = 1.33 95 % CI 1.15–1.54). A significant trend existed between increasing obesity and the odds ratio of having a child with CHD [33]. There is additional evidence that risks remain high, after excluding women with pregestational diabetes and controlling for oral glucose tolerance test, suggesting that factors other than abnormal glucose metabolism may be involved [34].

1.3.1.5 Folic Acid

There is some evidence that preconceptual folic acid supplementation protects against the development of CHD [35, 36], similar to the known risk reduction for neural tube defects [35–37]. This finding was first identified from a Hungarian randomized trial on birth defects where the use of multivitamins containing folic acid was associated with an approximate 60 % overall reduction in risk for CHD [38, 39]. A similar population-based case-control study done in Atlanta revealed an approximate 25 % overall reduction in risk for CHD [40]. Although folic acid-containing multivitamin supplements seem to have a possible protective effect for CHD, the results are still inconclusive due to the limited number of studies and the multifactorial nature of CHD.

1.3.1.6 Teratogenic Drugs

Exposure to teratogenic drugs during pregnancy may be unavoidable, including anticonvulsants (e.g. phenytoin, carbamazepine and valproic acid) and antidepressants (e.g. lithium carbonate). Other examples include retinoids, ethanol and ACE inhibitors [37].

1.3.2 Fetal Risk Factors

1.3.2.1 Increased Nuchal Translucency

An increased nuchal translucency (NT) thickness measured by ultrasound in the fetus at 10–14 weeks of gestation is a recognized marker for chromosomal abnormalities and is also an independent risk factor for CHD [41]. The reason for this association is unclear but may be related to the lymphatic system [42]. In chromosomally normal fetuses, the risk of CHD increases with increasing NT measurement [42, 43]. Thus, in a proportion of affected pregnancies, CHD can potentially be identified in the late first/early second trimester. In a pooled analysis of CHD diagnosed in four major centres, increased NT was associated with earlier diagnosis by approximately 6 weeks [44]. However, despite this strong association, the NT measurement alone is only modestly effective as a screening tool as most fetuses with major CHD have normal measurements [45]. It has been shown that NT>95th centile (~2.5 mm but value varies with fetal crown-rump-length) and NT >99th centile (> 3.5 mm) may predict 37 % and 31 % of major CHD, respectively [46]. The presence of increased NT in combination with tricuspid regurgitation and abnormal ductus venosus Doppler flow profile in the first trimester is a stronger marker for CHD [47].

It is currently recommended that all women with a fetal NT measurement greater than 3.5 mm be referred for detailed fetal cardiac assessment. Depending on local resources and expertise, fetuses with NT >4 mm may be evaluated in early pregnancy, at 13–16 weeks of gestation.

1.3.2.2 Extra-Cardiac and Chromosomal Abnormalities

Certain extra-cardiac and chromosomal abnormalities should prompt referral to fetal cardiology. Conversely, in the presence of a major CHD, fetal medicine assessment is also indicated. Important examples include abdominal wall defects (e.g. exomphalos), gastrointestinal obstruction (e.g. duodenal atresia) and diaphragmatic hernia [48–50]. In the latter, the fetal heart may also show features of left heart hypoplasia, even in the absence of a structural defect, which may represent functional alterations due to external compression [51]. Fetal cardiac abnormalities may also occur in association with central nervous, genitourinary and skeletal systems.

The most common examples of chromosomal defects associated with CHD are trisomy 21 (Down syndrome) and micro-deletion of chromosome 22q11 (Di George syndrome), with a high prevalence of atrioventricular septal defects and conotruncal malformations, respectively.

1.3.2.3 Suspected CHD

It is long known that the most important factor to detect fetal CHD is to suspect an abnormality during routine screening. About 80 % of abnormal cases in Alan's series were cases of suspected CHD [1]. Many other reports have echoed these findings and as outflow tract views are gradually incorporated into routine screening, the detection rate of CHD is expected to increase.

1.4 Screening for CHD

Following the French initiative to introduce the four-chamber view to routine obstetric scans and subsequent introduction of outflow tract views, in utero detection of major CHD still remains around 50 % according to most recent studies [52–55]. Cardiac lesions that require intervention in the first 28 days of life are defined as critical CHD, and without prenatal diagnosis, some may not be identified until after neonatal discharge, leading to increased morbidity and mortality [56–58]. Some reports have shown that prenatal diagnosis of specific types of CHD has a positive impact on outcome [59–61]. Thus, every effort should be made to improve antenatal detection of CHD.

1.4.1 Screening Guidelines and UK Cardiac Protocol

Over the years, the importance of assessing outflow tracts when screening for CHD in pregnancy has been stressed – but with the caveat 'when technically feasible' [62–64]. In 2008, the UK National Institute for Health and Care Excellence [65] also recommended that outflow tracts should be included to screening. However, this was only implemented in 2010 when the National Health Service Fetal Anomaly Screening Programme (NHS FASP), now part of NHS England, published a national cardiac protocol. The FASP protocol included assessment of (1) situs, (2) four-chamber view, (3) left ventricular outflow tract and (4) right ventricular outflow tract or three-vessel view.

In 2013, the International Society of Ultrasound in Obstetrics and Gynecology (ISUOG) also published revised guidelines whereby a comprehensive assessment of the fetal heart is recommended and achieved through five axial planes of the fetal chest [66, 67] (Fig. 1.1). The 2010 FASP protocol did not include the fifth plane (three-vessel and trachea view), which is to be incorporated in the UK screening programme in 2016 [68]. Both ISUOG and FASP recommended that fetal laterality and visceral situs be part of screening. This was first suggested in 1997 [69]. Its screening value should not be underestimated as many complex forms of CHD are associated with atrial isomerism/heterotaxy.

In practice, it is difficult to ensure that guidelines are followed at national and international level in order to deliver equal care to all pregnant women worldwide. It is well accepted that the effectiveness of any screening programme is highly dependent on training, so that professionals responsible for screening can deliver such care [70–72]. Data from the UK National Institute for Cardiovascular Outcomes Research [73] shows that the percentage of infants requiring surgery or catheter intervention for CHD has increased over the years since 2003. A steeper increase around 2010 suggests this may be related to introduction of the FASP cardiac protocol.

1.5 Fetal Cardiology Assessment

The role of a fetal cardiologist, beyond making an accurate diagnosis, is to provide the parents with a comprehensive, evidence-based picture of the outcome possibilities, starting with pregnancy, through childhood, and into adult life [74]. This is not an easy task. Surgical results and outcomes are constantly changing and naturally, counselling is lesion specific (e.g. tetralogy of Fallot) and within each lesion, it is further tailored to the scan findings in each individual fetus (e.g. tetralogy of Fallot with pulmonary stenosis versus pulmonary atresia).

Ideally, fetal cardiac assessment happens within a fetal medicine unit or in close collaboration with a fetal medicine specialist to facilitate a multidisciplinary approach. In the fetus with a cardiac abnormality, risk of extra-cardiac, chromosomal or genetic abnormalities and the option of invasive tests (amniocentesis or cordocentesis) need to be discussed. The first step, however, is to establish an accurate diagnosis. Similarly to postnatal cardiology, it is important to adopt a structured approach, often based on a sequential segmental analysis (SSA) of the heart [75–77].

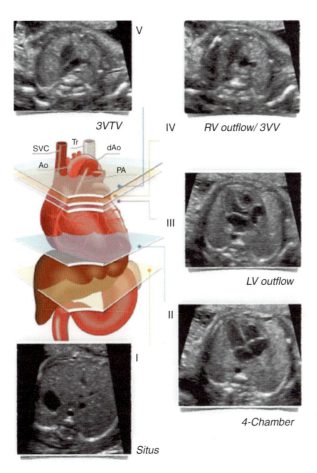

Fig. 1.1 (a) The five axial views for optimal fetal heart screening. The colour image shows the trachea, heart and great vessels, liver and stomach, with the five planes of insonation indicated by polygons corresponding to the grey-scale images, as indicated. (*I*) Most caudal plane, showing abdominal situs. (*II*) Four-chamber view. (*III*) Left ventricular (*LV*) outflow tract. (*IV*) Right ventricular (*RV*) outflow tract/three-vessel view (*3VV*). (*V*) Three vessels and trachea view (*3VTV*). *Ao* aorta, *dAo* descending aorta, *PA* pulmonary artery, *SVC* superior vena cava, *Tr* trachea (Modified with permission from Carvalho et al. and Yagel et al. © ISUOG [66, 67]). (**b**) Increase in number referrals for suspected cardiac abnormalities, 2003–2013, Fetal Medicine Unit, St George's Hospital, London, UK

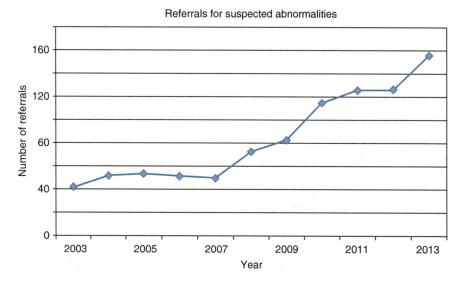

Fig. 1.1 (continued)

1.5.1 Structural Fetal CHD

Being able to confirm normality of the fetal heart is as important as making the diagnosis of CHD, simple or complex. For the pregnant woman who is aware of the increased risk of cardiac malformation in her unborn child, reassurance is of paramount importance. For those referred because of a suspected abnormality, accuracy of diagnosis forms the platform for subsequent pregnancy management. Neither scenario can be underestimated. In both instances, it is important to approach the fetal heart in a logical manner. The SSA offers a step-by-step approach to describing the cardiac anatomy in normal and malformed fetal hearts. Determination of situs, cardiac connections and associated defects facilitates understanding of the pathophysiology of abnormalities, which is essential for counselling families.

When applied to the fetus, the SSA differs, in that prior to ascertaining abdominal situs and by inference, atrial arrangement, it is imperative to determine fetal laterality [69, 77]. This is achieved by assessing fetal lie within the maternal abdomen so that the right and left sides of the fetus can be established. Subsequently, the same 7postnatal rules and definitions used in the SSA apply.

The diagnosis of major CHD involving abnormalities of cardiac connections is often straightforward, such as in tricuspid atresia and complete transposition of the great arteries (Fig. 1.2). More complex lesions, including those seen in the setting of atrial isomerism, can also be identified accurately but are also more challenging.

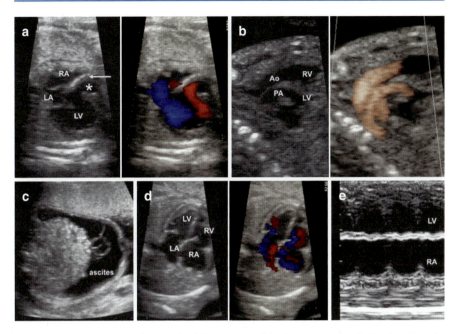

Fig. 1.2 (**a**) Four-chamber view obtained from a fetus with tricuspid atresia, obtained at 32 weeks of gestation. *Left* panel, 2D and *right* panel, with colour Doppler. The *arrow* points to the absent right atrioventricular connection. (**b**) Images obtained from a fetus at 23 weeks of gestation, with complete transposition. *Left* panel (2D) and *right* panel (e-flow mapping) are sagittal views of the fetus showing the parallel arrangement of the two vessels with an anterior aorta and posterior pulmonary artery. (**c–e**) Images obtained from a hydropic fetus at 25 weeks of gestation, with supraventricular tachycardia, partially controlled on dual maternal therapy. (**c**) Shows fetal ascites, (**d**) four-chamber view shows cardiomegaly and mitral and tricuspid regurgitation, (**e**) M-mode recoding shows 1:1 atrioventricular conduction with heart rate=215 bpm. Pretreatment rate was 270 bpm. The rhythm was sinus a few days afterward. *Ao* aorta, *LA* left atrium, *LV* left ventricle, *RA* right atrium, *RV* right ventricle, *PA* pulmonary artery, * rudimentary RV

It can be more difficult to exclude relatively minor defects, e.g. a small to moderate perimembranous ventricular septal defect, than to diagnose a complex abnormality. If images are suboptimal, additional scans may be needed.

An important consideration in fetal heart disease relates to potential progression of obstructive lesions as pregnancy advances [78–80]. A classical example is seen in critical aortic stenosis in mid-pregnancy that is likely to progress to hypoplastic left heart syndrome (Fig. 1.3). Also to be taken into account in predicting postnatal presentation of CHD are the physiological perinatal circulatory changes. In addition to closure of the foramen ovale, ductus arteriosus and ductus venosus, changes in right and left ventricular preload and afterload may alter the appearances of the normal and abnormal heart. This is particularly relevant in cases of borderline left ventricle when trying to predict if it will be able to sustain a biventricular circulation after birth.

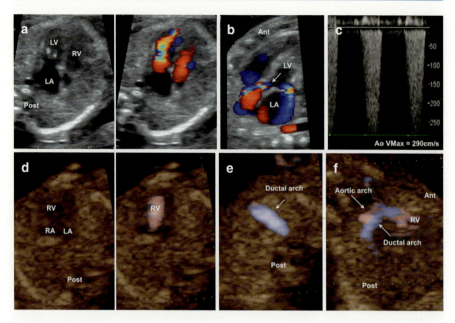

Fig. 1.3 (**a–c**) Images obtained from a fetus at 21 weeks of gestation with critical aortic stenosis. (**a**) Four-chamber view in diastole on 2D (*left* panel) and colour flow (*right* panel) shows a dilated left atrium. The left ventricle reaches the cardiac apex and shows areas of hyperechogenicity. (**b**) Left ventricular outflow tract view in systole. Note the presence of important mitral regurgitation and a narrow jet (*arrow*) of forward flow across the aortic valve. (**c**) Pulsed wave Doppler shows high aortic velocity (290 cm/s, normal for gestation ~60–70 cm/s). (**d–f**) Images obtained from a fetus at 14 weeks of gestation with hypoplastic left heart syndrome. (**d**) Four-chamber view in diastole, on 2D (*left* panel) and e-flow mapping (*right* panel). Note filling of the right ventricle only. (**e**) Transverse view through upper mediastinum at the level of the three-vessel view. E-flow mapping shows a large ductal arch only. No aortic flow seen at this level. (**f**) Sagittal view demonstrates forward flow across the ductal arch and reversed flow in the transverse aortic arch. *Ant* anterior, *LA* left atrium, *LV* left ventricle, *Post* posterior, *RA* right atrium, *RV* right ventricle, *VMax* maximal velocity

1.5.2 Fetal Arrhythmias

Fetal cardiac rhythm should be regular and heart rate roughly ranges from 120 to 160 beats per minute (bpm). M-mode echocardiography and pulsed-wave Doppler are the most commonly used methods to assess rhythm in the fetus, based on simultaneous recording of atrial and ventricular activities [81]. The most common rhythm disturbances are intermittent extrasystoles, which are of little clinical relevance. Arrhythmias that potentially affect fetal well-being or have postnatal implications for the newborn and child are relatively uncommon. Less than 10 % of referrals are due to sustained tachy- or bradyarrhythmias [81].

Intermittent extrasystoles are frequently encountered, usually of atrial origin and generally considered to be 'benign'. They are often described as 'skipped' or 'missed' beats, which can cause a lot of anxiety, even if the vast majority resolve spontaneously and require no treatment. In about 2% of cases, skipped beats may represent incomplete heart block [82] or be associated with intermittent tachycardia. Therefore, it is important that these possibilities be excluded. A scan performed locally by the sonographer or obstetrician usually suffices. If heart rate is within normal range, with no fluid accumulation in any fetal compartment and the cardiac screening views are normal, the pregnant woman can be reassured. Urgent referral to a specialist is only warranted in a few selected cases when either heart rate and/or the scan findings are abnormal [83]. If the ectopic beats occur 'very frequently' (i.e. the rhythm is irregular most of the time), there is a slightly higher risk of fetus developing a tachyarrhythmia [84] and a referral is also warranted, after the initial assessment in the local hospital.

Tachycardia is defined as rate ≥ 180 bpm. If persistent, it may lead to congestive heart failure and hydrops fetalis (Fig. 1.3). If it is intermittent or not, urgent referral to the fetal cardiologist is required. However, not all cases need treatment as sometimes the arrhythmia resolves spontaneously. Thus, if the fetus is stable, close monitoring of fetal heart rate for 24 h or so to determine if the arrhythmia persists may be appropriate, before initiating therapy. If there is sustained tachycardia or it persists for >50% of the time, or the fetus is compromised, fetal treatment or delivery of the baby (if gestational age ≥ 37 weeks) is indicated. Choice of medication varies from centre to centre and with experience. Maternal transplacental transfer is the preferred option to deliver the chosen drug to the fetus. Currently, a randomized controlled trial for treatment of fetal tachyarrhythmia is on its early implementation phase [85].

Traditionally, fetal bradycardia has been defined as rates <100 bpm but current obstetric threshold is 110 bpm [86]. More recently, gestational age-specific heart rates have been developed and centile charts are available [87]. Transient periods of sinus bradycardia during scanning are common and benign. Persistent sinus bradycardia is relatively rare and may be a manifestation of long QT syndrome [87]. More commonly however, fetal bradycardia is due to blocked atrial bigeminy, which typically presents with heart rate around 70–80 bpm. This can be transient or last for days or weeks. Whilst it is well tolerated by the fetus and of no hemodynamic consequence, it is important to differentiate blocked bigeminy from second-degree atrioventricular block with 2:1 conduction [82]. Heart block is often caused by transplacental passage of circulating maternal IgG antibodies (anti-Ro/ SSA and anti-La/SSB), which causes injury to the conduction tissue with subsequent fibrous replacement. Certain forms of CHD can also lead to fetal heart block, notably cases which are associated with left isomerism, but it can also occur in the presence of atrioventricular discordance. The prognosis for autoimmune-mediated complete atrioventricular block is better than if associated with CHD but there still is significant mortality and morbidity. Most survivors require pacemaker implantation in the first year of life [88].

1.5.3 Inherited Cardiac Conditions

Despite recent advances in genetics and better understanding of inherited cardiac conditions that may confer a 50% risk to the fetus, little has been reported in fetal life. Inherited cardiomyopathies are relatively uncommon in the fetus [89]. Hypertrophic cardiomyopathy rarely manifests prenatally, but can be associated with Noonan syndrome. Among channelopathies, recent data on prenatal manifestation of long QT syndrome, bradycardia with rates below the 3rd centile for gestational age, has increased interest in identifying affected fetuses [87]. Among aortopathies and related conditions, there are scarce fetal reports, mainly related to the infantile type of Marfan syndrome [90].

1.5.4 Early Fetal Echocardiography

Initial observations of CHD diagnosed in the first trimester of pregnancy were made by obstetricians utilizing a transvaginal approach [91, 92]. Subsequently, it became clear that the transabdominal route could also be used in clinical practice to image the fetal heart at less than 14 weeks gestation [93]. Over the years, this practice has become more common. The number of fetal cardiologists offering a detailed assessment of the fetal heart at 15–16 weeks has increased but it is not yet universally available. Early scans can be challenging due to the small fetal heart size and additional technical limitations sometimes imposed by fetal position and maternal characteristics. Nevertheless, its clinical utility in high-risk pregnancies has been shown by a number of investigators [94–97]. Similarly to mid-gestation, it is very important that the fetus with CHD identified early in pregnancy be assessed by a multidisciplinary team, especially in cases referred because of increased NT measurements. Figure 1.3 illustrates a case of hypoplastic left heart syndrome diagnosed at 14 weeks in a woman referred with family history of CHD.

1.6 Counselling and Pregnancy Options

Counselling a woman who attends for a fetal echocardiogram should start before the scan is performed. For each family, the perceived risks of encountering an abnormality during the scan and/or the likelihood of the scan being normal should be discussed. Limitations posed by early scans (<16 weeks) should be highlighted. This prepares the woman for what to expect, especially when she is referred due to a suspected abnormality.

Following the diagnosis of any form of CHD, the ultrasound findings are explained to the family, often with the help of diagrams to help them understand the anatomy and pathophysiological implications of the defect. An account of the likely postnatal manifestations of the disease, surgical options, risks and need for long-term follow-up is provided. In cases where progression is expected to occur during pregnancy, the need for serial fetal scans is reinforced. Family consultation is often in the presence of a fetal cardiac nurse specialist who provides the family with ongoing support. An obstetric/fetal medicine assessment should also be arranged on the same day or shortly afterwards to exclude or document extra-cardiac abnormalities and review pregnancy risks for chromosomal abnormalities and genetic syndromes.

The option of an invasive procedure (amniocentesis or cordocentesis) to check fetal karyotype is discussed, often jointly between the fetal cardiac and fetal medicine specialists. Depending on the type of CHD, associated abnormalities and gestational age, the option of TOP, if legally possible, is also discussed. Interrupting the pregnancy often involves induction of labour and may require fetocide, depending on gestational age. In the UK, the Royal College of Obstetricians and Gynecologists recommend this be performed at >22 completed weeks of gestation. Spontaneous fetal demise in the absence of heart failure/ hydrops is uncommon, but the risk is increased if there is an associated chromosomal abnormality (e.g. trisomy 21).

There is growing literature – summarized in a recent meta-analysis, indicating that, in the absence of known chromosomal or genetic abnormalities, the child with major CHD is at increased risk of brain abnormalities (detected on neuroimaging) and neurodevelopmental delay [98, 99]. Most of the reported cases are examples of hypoplastic left heart syndrome and complete transposition. In this analysis, the findings were independent of surgical risk, but it did not provide data to indicate if the origin was fetal or postnatal. On a more recent meta-analysis, there is some evidence to suggest that at least in part, some of these changes occur before birth [100]. However, a survey of experts' attitudes towards counselling families regarding risks of development delay in CHD advises caution [101]. Any information provided needs to be accurate but is inevitably based on current knowledge, which is limited by the retrospective nature of the published studies and lack of correlation between individual neuroimaging abnormalities and developmental outcome. Further research is required in this important area.

1.7 Perinatal Plan for the Fetus with CHD

One of the strengths of prenatal diagnosis is optimization of perinatal care. Fetuses expected to have neonatal intervention require delivery in a hospital with facilities to stabilize the neonate. In some instances, this needs to be at or close to a cardiac unit. However, local delivery is also possible, depending on the abnormality and available local human and medical resources [102–105].

Ideally, babies with CHD will be delivered at term. For those with critical defects, retrospective data suggest that mortality is lower if delivery occurs at 39–40 completed weeks. Delivery before 39 weeks is also associated with increased morbidity. However, premature delivery may be unavoidable, for example, if there is spontaneous labour or obstetric concern about fetal growth.

The neonatal team will be aware that a child with major or critical CHD is to be delivered and should be aware of the initial postnatal management.

1.8 Changing Pattern of Fetal CHD

Traditionally, fetal CHD meant complex CHD. The defects were often associated with worse prognosis, with many abnormalities leading to a univentricular circulation. For many years, abnormal hearts showing a normal four-chamber view were unlikely to be recognized on routine screening. In the mid-1990s only 3% of infants with complete transposition undergoing surgery were antenatally diagnosed [5]. With improvements in screening and especially the introduction of outflow tract views, fetal diagnosis of less complex abnormalities with potential for biventricular repair has increased. However, there has also been an increase in detection of CHD that may not require intervention or may be considered variants of normal. This new, emerging pattern of fetal CHD will enhance our understanding of natural history. For example, it is clear that many children with an isolated right aortic arch are asymptomatic [106] and would have not been diagnosed had it not been for prenatal screening. It also seems that persistence of a left superior vena draining into the coronary sinus as an isolated finding is not uncommon. Nevertheless, when a pregnant woman is referred for fetal cardiology assessment, the anxiety generated is not insignificant and prompt evaluation is required in order to clarify if fetal CHD is present and the potential impact it may have on the child and family.

References

1. Allan LD, Crawford DC, Chita SK, Tynan MJ (1986) Prenatal screening for congenital heart disease. Br Med J 292(6537):1717–1719
2. Lange LW, Sahn DJ, Allen HD, Goldberg SJ, Anderson C, Giles H (1980) Qualitative real-time cross-sectional echocardiographic imaging of the human fetus during the second half of pregnancy. Circulation 62(4):799–806
3. Kleinman CS, Hobbins JC, Jaffe CC, Lynch DC, Talner NS (1980) Echocardiographic studies of the human fetus: prenatal diagnosis of congenital heart disease and cardiac dysrhythmias. Pediatrics 65(6):1059–1067
4. Fermont L, De Geeter B, Aubry MC, Kachener J, Sidi D (1986) A close collaboration between obstetricians and pediatric cardiologists allows antenatal detection of severe cardiac malformations by two-dimensional echocardiography. In: Doyle EF, Engle MA, Gersony WM, Rashkind WJ, Talner NS (ed). Pediatric cardiology. Proceedings of the second world congress, New York
5. Bull C (1999) Current and potential impact of fetal diagnosis on prevalence and spectrum of serious congenital heart disease at term in the UK. Lancet 354(9186):1242–1247
6. Dolk H, Loane M, Garne E (2011) European Surveillance of Congenital Anomalies Working G. Congenital heart defects in Europe: prevalence and perinatal mortality, 2000 to 2005. Circulation 123(8):841–849
7. Bernier PL, Stefanescu A, Samoukovic G, Tchervenkov CI (2010) The challenge of congenital heart disease worldwide: epidemiologic and demographic facts. Semin Thorac Cardiovasc Surg Pediatr Card Surg Annu 13(1):26–34
8. van der Linde D, Konings EE, Slager MA, Witsenburg M, Helbing WA, Takkenberg JJ et al (2011) Birth prevalence of congenital heart disease worldwide: a systematic review and meta-analysis. J Am Coll Cardiol 58(21):2241–2247
9. Hoffman JI, Kaplan S (2002) The incidence of congenital heart disease. J Am Coll Cardiol 39(12):1890–1900
10. Buskens E, Grobbee DE, Frohn-Mulder IM, Stewart PA, Juttmann RE, Wladimiroff JW et al (1996) Efficacy of routine fetal ultrasound screening for congenital heart disease in normal pregnancy. Circulation 94(1):67–72
11. Lage K, Greenway SC, Rosenfeld JA, Wakimoto H, Gorham JM, Segre AV et al (2012) Genetic and environmental risk factors in congenital heart disease functionally converge in protein networks driving heart development. Proc Natl Acad Sci U S A 109(35):14035–14040

12. Oyen N, Poulsen G, Boyd HA, Wohlfahrt J, Jensen PK, Melbye M (2009) Recurrence of congenital heart defects in families. Circulation 120(4):295–301
13. Allan LD, Crawford DC, Chita SK, Anderson RH, Tynan MJ (1986) Familial recurrence of congenital heart disease in a prospective series of mothers referred for fetal echocardiography. Am J Cardiol 58(3):334–337
14. Gill HK, Splitt M, Sharland GK, Simpson JM (2003) Patterns of recurrence of congenital heart disease: an analysis of 6,640 consecutive pregnancies evaluated by detailed fetal echocardiography. J Am Coll Cardiol 42(5):923–929
15. Burn J, Brennan P, Little J, Holloway S, Coffey R, Somerville J et al (1998) Recurrence risks in offspring of adults with major heart defects: results from first cohort of British collaborative study. Lancet 351(9099):311–316
16. Blue GM, Kirk EP, Sholler GF, Harvey RP, Winlaw DS (2012) Congenital heart disease: current knowledge about causes and inheritance. Med J Aust 197(3):155–159
17. Friedman DM, Kim MY, Copel JA, Davis C, Phoon CKL, Glickstein JS et al (2008) Utility of cardiac monitoring in fetuses at risk for congenital heart block. The PR Interval and Dexamethasone Evaluation (PRIDE) Prospective Study. Circulation 117:485–493
18. Jaeggi E, Laskin C, Hamilton R, Kingdom J, Silverman E (2010) The importance of the level of maternal anti-Ro/SSA antibodies as a prognostic marker of the development of cardiac neonatal lupus erythematosus a prospective study of 186 antibody-exposed fetuses and infants. J Am Coll Cardiol 55(24):2778–2784
19. Nield LE, Silverman ED, Taylor GP, Smallhorn JF, Mullen JB, Silverman NH et al (2002) Maternal anti-Ro and anti-La antibody-associated endocardial fibroelastosis. Circulation 105(7):843–848
20. Cuneo BF, Fruitman D, Benson DW, Ngan BY, Liske MR, Wahren-Herlineus M et al (2011) Spontaneous rupture of atrioventricular valve tensor apparatus as late manifestation of anti-Ro/SSA antibody-mediated cardiac disease. Am J Cardiol 107(5):761–766
21. Wren C, Birrell G, Hawthorne G (2003) Cardiovascular malformations in infants of diabetic mothers. Heart 89(10):1217–1220
22. Becerra JE, Khoury MJ, Cordero JF, Erickson JD (1990) Diabetes mellitus during pregnancy and the risks for specific birth defects: a population-based case-control study. Pediatrics 85(1):1–9
23. Ferencz C, Rubin JD, McCarter RJ, Clark EB (1990) Maternal diabetes and cardiovascular malformations: predominance of double outlet right ventricle and truncus arteriosus. Teratology 41(3):319–326
24. Kitzmiller JL, Gavin LA, Gin GD, Jovanovic-Peterson L, Main EK, Zigrang WD (1991) Preconception care of diabetes. Glycemic control prevents congenital anomalies. JAMA 265(6):731–736
25. Splitt M, Wright C, Sen D, Goodship J (1999) Left-isomerism sequence and maternal type-1 diabetes. Lancet 354(9175):305–306
26. Hornberger LK (2006) The effect of diabetes on the fetal heart. Heart 92:1019–1021
27. Greene MF, Hare JW, Cloherty JP, Benacerraf BR, Soeldner JS (1989) First-trimester hemoglobin A1 and risk for major malformation and spontaneous abortion in diabetic pregnancy. Teratology 39(3):225–231
28. Gutgesell HP, Speer ME, Rosenberg HS (1980) Characterization of the cardiomyopathy in infants of diabetic mothers. Circulation 61(2):441–450
29. Weber HS, Copel JA, Reece EA, Green J, Kleinman CS (1991) Cardiac growth in fetuses of diabetic mothers with good metabolic control. J Pediatr 118(1):103–107
30. Hagemann LL, Zielinsky P (1996) Prenatal study of hypertrophic cardiomyopathy and its association with insulin levels in fetuses of diabetic mothers. Arq Bras Cardiol 66(4):193–198
31. Levy HL, Guldberg P, Guttler F, Hanley WB, Matalon R, Rouse BM et al (2001) Congenital heart disease in maternal phenylketonuria: report from the Maternal PKU Collaborative Study. Pediatr Res 49(5):636–642
32. Pierpont MEM, Sletten LJ, Smith CF, Berry H, Berry SA, Fisch RO (1995) Congenital cardiac malformations in offspring of mothers with phenylketonuria and hyperphenylalaninemia. Intern Pediatr 10:242

33. Mills JL, Troendle J, Conley MR, Carter T, Druschel CM (2010) Maternal obesity and congenital heart defects: a population-based study. Am J Clin Nutr 91(6):1543–1549
34. Brite J, Laughon SK, Troendle J, Mills J (2014) Maternal overweight and obesity and risk of congenital heart defects in offspring. Int J Obes 38(6):878–882. doi:10.1038/ijo.2013.244
35. Ionescu-Ittu R, Marelli AJ, Mackie AS, Pilote L (2009) Prevalence of severe congenital heart disease after folic acid fortification of grain products: time trend analysis in Quebec, Canada. BMJ 338:b1673
36. Bailey LB, Berry RJ (2005) Folic acid supplementation and the occurrence of congenital heart defects, orofacial clefts, multiple births, and miscarriage. Am J Clin Nutr 81(5):1213S–1217S
37. Jenkins KJ, Correa A, Feinstein JA, Botto L, Britt AE, Daniels SR et al (2007) Noninherited risk factors and congenital cardiovascular defects: current knowledge: a scientific statement from the American Heart Association Council on Cardiovascular Disease in the Young: endorsed by the American Academy of Pediatrics. Circulation 115(23):2995–3014
38. Czeizel AE (1998) Periconceptional folic acid containing multivitamin supplementation. Eur J Obstet Gynecol Reprod Biol 78(2):151–161
39. Botto LD, Mulinare J, Erickson JD (2000) Occurrence of congenital heart defects in relation to maternal mulitivitamin use. Am J Epidemiol 151(9):878–884
40. Scanlon KS, Ferencz C, Loffredo CA, Wilson PD, Correa-Villasenor A, Khoury MJ et al (1998) Preconceptional folate intake and malformations of the cardiac outflow tract. Baltimore-Washington Infant Study Group. Epidemiology 9(1):95–98
41. Nicolaides KH, Heath V, Cicero S (2002) Increased fetal nuchal translucency at 11–14 weeks. Prenat Diagn 22(4):308–315
42. Carvalho JS (2005) The fetal heart or the lymphatic system or …? The quest for the etiology of increased nuchal translucency. Ultrasound Obstet Gynecol 25(3):215–220
43. Hyett J, Perdu M, Sharland G, Snijders R, Nicolaides KH (1999) Using fetal nuchal translucency to screen for major congenital cardiac defects at 10–14 weeks of gestation: population based cohort study. BMJ 318(7176):81–85
44. Makrydimas G, Sotiriadis A, Huggon IC, Simpson J, Sharland G, Carvalho JS et al (2005) Nuchal translucency and fetal cardiac defects: a pooled analysis of major fetal echocardiography centers. Am J Obstet Gynecol 192(1):89–95
45. Mavrides E, Cobian-Sanchez F, Tekay A, Moscoso G, Campbell S, Thilaganathan B et al (2001) Limitations of using first-trimester nuchal translucency measurement in routine screening for major congenital heart defects. Ultrasound Obstet Gynecol 17(2):106–110
46. Makrydimas G, Sotiriadis A, Ioannidis JP (2003) Screening performance of first-trimester nuchal translucency for major cardiac defects: a meta-analysis. Am J Obstet Gynecol 189(5):1330–1335
47. Clur SA, Ottenkamp J, Bilardo CM (2009) The nuchal translucency and the fetal heart: a literature review. Prenat Diagn 29(8):739–748
48. Copel JA, Pilu G, Kleinman CS (1986) Congenital heart disease and extracardiac anomalies: associations and indications for fetal echocardiography. Am J Obstet Gynecol 154(5):1121–1132
49. Greenwood RD, Rosenthal A, Nadas AS (1976) Cardiovascular abnormalities associated with congenital diaphragmatic hernia. Pediatrics 57(1):92–97
50. Mlczoch E, Carvalho JS (2014) Interrupted inferior vena cava in fetuses with omphalocele. Case series of fetuses referred for fetal echocardiography and review of the literature. Early Hum Dev 91(1):1–6
51. Vogel M, McElhinney DB, Marcus E, Morash D, Jennings RW, Tworetzky W (2010) Significance and outcome of left heart hypoplasia in fetal congenital diaphragmatic hernia. Ultrasound Obstet Gynecol 35(3):310–317
52. Oster ME, Kim CH, Kusano AS, Cragan JD, Dressler P, Hales AR et al (2014) A population-based study of the association of prenatal diagnosis with survival rate for infants with congenital heart defects. Am J Cardiol 113(6):1036–1040
53. Marek J, Tomek V, Skovranek J, Povysilova V, Samanek M (2011) Prenatal ultrasound screening of congenital heart disease in an unselected national population: a 21-year experience. Heart 97(2):124–130

54. Trines J, Fruitman D, Zuo KJ, Smallhorn JF, Hornberger LK, Mackie AS (2013) Effectiveness of prenatal screening for congenital heart disease: assessment in a jurisdiction with universal access to health care. Can J Cardiol 29(7):879–885
55. Escobar-Diaz MC, Freud LR, Bueno A, Brown DW, Friedman KG, Schidlow D et al (2015) Prenatal diagnosis of transposition of the great arteries over a 20-year period: improved but imperfect. Ultrasound Obstet Gynecol 45(6):678–682
56. Schultz AH, Localio AR, Clark BJ, Ravishankar C, Videon N, Kimmel SE (2008) Epidemiologic features of the presentation of critical congenital heart disease: implications for screening. Pediatrics 121(4):751–757
57. Brown KL, Ridout DA, Hoskote A, Verhulst L, Ricci M, Bull C (2006) Delayed diagnosis of congenital heart disease worsens preoperative condition and outcome of surgery in neonates. Heart 92(9):1298–1302
58. Eckersley L, Sadler L, Parry E, Finucane K, Gentles TL (2015) Timing of diagnosis affects mortality in critical congenital heart disease. Arch Dis Child. doi:10.1136/archdischild-2014-307691 [Epub ahead of print]
59. Bonnet D, Coltri A, Butera G, Fermont L, Le Bidois J, Kachaner J et al (1999) Detection of transposition of the great arteries in fetuses reduces neonatal morbidity and mortality. Circulation 99(7):916–918
60. Copel JA, Tan AS, Kleinman CS (1997) Does a prenatal diagnosis of congenital heart disease alter short-term outcome? Ultrasound Obstet Gynecol 10(4):237–241
61. Franklin O, Burch M, Manning N, Sleeman K, Gould S, Archer N (2002) Prenatal diagnosis of coarctation of the aorta improves survival and reduces morbidity. Heart 87(1):67–69
62. AIUM (2003) AIUM practice guideline for the performance of an antepartum obstetric ultrasound examination. J Ultrasound Med 22(10):1116–1125
63. ISUOG (2006) Cardiac screening examination of the fetus: guidelines for performing the 'basic' and 'extended basic' cardiac scan. Ultrasound Obstet Gynecol Off J Int Soc Ultrasound Obstet Gynecol 27(1):107–113
64. RCOG (2011) Ultrasound screening: supplement to ultrasound screening for fetal abnormalities. http://www.rcog.org.uk/womens-health/clinical-guidance/ultrasound-screening. 2000. Accessed 9 Mar 2014
65. Antenatal Care (n.d.) Routine care for the healthy pregnant woman. http://www.nice.org.uk/CG062
66. Carvalho JS, Allan LD, Chaoui R, Copel JA, DeVore GR, Hecher K et al (2013) ISUOG Practice Guidelines (updated): sonographic screening examination of the fetal heart. Ultrasound Obstet Gynecol 41(3):348–359
67. Yagel S, Cohen SM, Achiron R (2001) Examination of the fetal heart by five short-axis views: a proposed screening method for comprehensive cardiac evaluation. Ultrasound Obstet Gynecol 17(5):367–369
68. Fetal Anomaly Screening Programme (2015) Programme handbook, June 2015. https://www.gov.uk/government/publications/fetal-anomaly-screening-programme-handbook. Accessed 5 Jan 2016
69. Carvalho JS, Doya E, Freeman J, Clough A (1997) Identification of fetal laterality and visceral situs should be part of routine fetal anomaly scans. In: Momma K, Imai Y (eds) World congress of pediatric cardiology and cardiac surgery, May 11–15 1997, Honolulu. Futura Pub. Co, Armonk, p 117
70. Sharland GK, Allan LD (1992) Screening for congenital heart disease prenatally. Results of a 2 1/2-year study in the South East Thames Region. Br J Obstet Gynaecol 99(3):220–225
71. Hunter S, Heads A, Wyllie J, Robson S (2000) Prenatal diagnosis of congenital heart disease in the northern region of England: benefits of a training programme for obstetric ultrasonographers. Heart 84(3):294–298
72. Carvalho JS, Mavrides E, Shinebourne EA, Campbell S, Thilaganathan B (2002) Improving the effectiveness of routine prenatal screening for major congenital heart defects. Heart 88(4):387–391

73. NICOR (2015) The trend towards improvement in antenatal diagnosis. https://nicor4.nicor.org.uk/CHD/an_paeds.nsf/vwContent/Antenatal%20Diagnosis?Opendocument. Accessed 2 Jan 2016
74. Jowett V, Carvalho JS (in press) Antenatal diagnosis of congenital heart disease. In: Gatzoulis MA, Steer P (eds) Heart disease in pregnancy. Cambridge University Press
75. Shinebourne EA, Macartney FJ, Anderson RH (1976) Sequential chamber localization – logical approach to diagnosis in congenital heart disease. Br Heart J 38(4):327–340
76. Anderson RH, Becker AE, Freedom RM, Macartney FJ, Quero-Jimenez M, Shinebourne EA et al (1984) Sequential segmental analysis of congenital heart disease. Pediatr Cardiol 5(4):281–287
77. Carvalho JS, Ho SY, Shinebourne EA (2005) Sequential segmental analysis in complex fetal cardiac abnormalities: a logical approach to diagnosis. Ultrasound Obstet Gynecol 26(2):105–111
78. Hornberger LK, Sanders SP, Rein AJ, Spevak PJ, Parness IA, Colan SD (1995) Left heart obstructive lesions and left ventricular growth in the midtrimester fetus. A longitudinal study. Circulation 92(6):1531–1538
79. Hornberger LK, Sanders SP, Sahn DJ, Rice MJ, Spevak PJ, Benacerraf BR et al (1995) In utero pulmonary artery and aortic growth and potential for progression of pulmonary outflow tract obstruction in tetralogy of Fallot. J Am Coll Cardiol 25(3):739–745
80. Yagel S, Weissman A, Rotstein Z, Manor M, Hegesh J, Anteby E et al (1997) Congenital heart defects: natural course and in utero development. Circulation 96(2):550–555
81. Api O, Carvalho JS (2008) Fetal dysrhythmias. Best Pract Res Clin Obstet Gynaecol 22(1):31–48
82. Carvalho JS (2014) Primary bradycardia: keys and pitfalls in diagnosis. Ultrasound Obstet Gynecol 44(2):125–130
83. Carvalho JS (2012) Clinical management of fetal dysrhythmias. In: Kilby MD, Johnston A, Oepkes D (eds) Fetal therapy. Scientific basis & critical appraisal of clinical benefits. Cambridge University Press, Cambridge
84. Strasburger JF, Wakai RT (2010) Fetal cardiac arrhythmia detection and in utero therapy. Nat Rev Cardiol 7(5):277–290
85. FAST (2016) Therapy trial of fetal tachyarrhythmia. https://clinicaltrials.gov/ct2/show/NCT02624765. Accessed 6 Jan 2016
86. ACOG (2009) ACOG practice bulletin no. 106: intrapartum fetal heart rate monitoring: nomenclature, interpretation, and general management principles. Obstet Gynecol 114(1):192–202
87. Mitchell JL, Cuneo BF, Etheridge SP, Horigome H, Weng HY, Benson DW (2012) Fetal heart rate predictors of long QT syndrome. Circulation 126(23):2688–2695
88. Jaeggi ET, Hamilton RM, Silverman ED, Zamora SA, Hornberger LK (2002) Outcome of children with fetal, neonatal or childhood diagnosis of isolated congenital atrioventricular block. A single institution's experience of 30 years. J Am Coll Cardiol 39(1):130–137
89. Pedra SR, Smallhorn JF, Ryan G, Chitayat D, Taylor GP, Khan R et al (2002) Fetal cardiomyopathies: pathogenic mechanisms, hemodynamic findings, and clinical outcome. Circulation 106(5):585–591
90. Gavilan C, Herraiz I, Granados MA, Moral MT, Gomez-Montes E, Galindo A (2011) Prenatal diagnosis of neonatal Marfan syndrome. Prenat Diag 31(6):610–613
91. Bronshtein M, Siegler E, Yoffe N, Zimmer EZ (1990) Prenatal diagnosis of ventricular septal defect and overriding aorta at 14 weeks' gestation, using transvaginal sonography. Prenat Diag 10(11):697–702
92. Gembruch U, Knopfle G, Chatterjee M, Bald R, Hansmann M (1990) First-trimester diagnosis of fetal congenital heart disease by transvaginal two-dimensional and Doppler echocardiography. Obstet Gynecol 75(3 Pt 2):496–498
93. Carvalho JS, Moscoso G, Ville Y (1998) First-trimester transabdominal fetal echocardiography. Lancet 351(9108):1023–1027

94. Carvalho JS, Moscoso G, Tekay A, Campbell S, Thilaganathan B, Shinebourne EA (2004) Clinical impact of first and early second trimester fetal echocardiography on high risk pregnancies. Heart 90(8):921–926
95. Simpsom JM, Jones A, Callaghan N, Sharland GK (2000) Accuracy and limitations of transabdominal fetal echocardiography at 12–15 weeks of gestation in a population at high risk for congenital heart disease. BJOG 107(12):1492–1497
96. Zidere V, Bellsham-Revell H, Persico N, Allan LD (2013) Comparison of echocardiographic findings in fetuses at less than 15 weeks' gestation with later cardiac evaluation. Ultrasound Obstet Gynecol 42(6):679–686
97. Haak MC, Twisk JW, Van Vugt JM (2002) How successful is fetal echocardiographic examination in the first trimester of pregnancy? Ultrasound Obstet Gynecol 20(1):9–13
98. Khalil A, Suff N, Thilaganathan B, Hurrell A, Cooper D, Carvalho JS (2014) Brain abnormalities and neurodevelopmental delay in congenital heart disease: systematic review and meta-analysis. Ultrasound Obstet Gynecol 43(1):14–24
99. Khalil A, Suff N, Thilaganathan B, Hurrell A, Cooper D, Carvalho JS (2014) Reply. Ultrasound Obstet Gynecol 44(1):119–120
100. Khalil A, Bennet S, Thilaganathan B, Paladini D, Griffiths P, Carvalho JS (2016) Prevalence of prenatal brain abnormalities in fetuses with congenital heart disease: systematic review. Ultrasound Obstet Gynecol. doi 10.1002/uog.15932 [Epub ahead of print]
101. Paladini D, Alfirevic Z, Carvalho JS, Khalil A, Malinger G, Rychik J, Gardiner H. Prenatal counselling for neurodevelopmental delay in congenital heart disease: results of a worldwide survey of experts' attitudes advise caution. Ultrasound Obstet Gynecol 2016;47:667–671
102. Bennett TD, Klein MB, Sorensen MD, De Roos AJ, Rivara FP (2010) Influence of birth hospital on outcomes of ductal-dependent cardiac lesions. Pediatrics 126(6):1156–1164
103. Bartsota M, Judd N, Carvalho JS (2014) When, how and where to deliver the fetus with major congenital heart disease. Fetal Mater Med Rev 25(2):79–94
104. Donofrio MT, Levy RJ, Schuette JJ, Skurow-Todd K, Sten MB, Stallings C et al (2013) Specialized delivery room planning for fetuses with critical congenital heart disease. Am J Cardiol 111(5):737–747
105. Carvalho JS (2016) Antenatal diagnosis of critical congenital heart disease. Optimal place of delivery is where appropriate care can be delivered. Arch Dis Child 101:505–507
106. D'Antonio F, Khalil A, Zidere V, Carvalho JS (2015) Fetuses with right aortic arch multicentre cohort study and meta-analysis. Ultrasound Obstet Gynecol Ultrasound Obstet Gynecol. doi:10.1002/uog.15805

Contraception and Cardiovascular Disease

2

Jan S. Erkamp and Jérôme Cornette

Abbreviations

COC	Combined oral contraceptives
DMPA	Depot-medroxyprogesterone acetate
IUDs	Intrauterine devices
LARC	Long-acting reversible contraceptives
LNG-IUS	Levonorgestrel-releasing intrauterine system
PCOS	Polycystic ovary syndrome
PID	Pelvic inflammatory disease
WHO-MEC	WHO medical eligibility criteria

2.1 Introduction

With improvements in medical and surgical management, most women with congenital or acquired heart disease will reach reproductive age and become sexually active [1, 2]. As for healthy women, contraception is important for women with heart disease for various reasons. Besides preventing unintended pregnancies, it can be used for cycle control, treatment of hyperandrogenism and prevention of

---

J.S. Erkamp, MD
Department of Obstetrics and Gynaecology, Franciscus Gasthuis,
Rotterdam, The Netherlands

J. Cornette, MD, PhD (✉)
Department of Obstetrics and Gynaecology, Erasmus Medical Center,
Rotterdam, The Netherlands
e-mail: j.cornette@erasmusmc.nl

© Springer International Publishing Switzerland 2017
J.W. Roos-Hesselink, M.R. Johnson (eds.), *Pregnancy and Congenital Heart Disease*, Congenital Heart Disease in Adolescents and Adults,
DOI 10.1007/978-3-319-38913-4_2

sexually transmittable diseases [3–5]. However, some issues, like drug interactions with cardiac medication and effects on haemodynamics, are very specific to women with cardiac disease and deserve particular attention.

Women with simple cardiac lesions often have similar pregnancy and contraceptive-related risks as healthy women, but these risks are substantially higher in women with complex heart disease [1, 2, 6]. Adequate contraception prevents unintended pregnancies and thereby the pregnancy associated risk of that particular cardiac condition. If pregnancy is undesired, contraception prevents termination of pregnancy, which, beside the emotional burden, also carries added medical risks in this population.

Contraception can also help to carefully plan and prepare women for pregnancy, which helps achieving better pregnancy outcomes. Some cardiac conditions imply an absolute contraindication for pregnancy, making effective contraception an essential part of disease management [2].

Most women with heart disease are not or, perhaps even worse, inappropriately advised on the use of contraceptives [7]. Oestrogen-containing formulations with their inherent increased risk of thromboembolic disease are still widely prescribed, while safer alternatives with better contraceptive efficacy are available [8, 9]. Each woman deserves personalised contraceptive advice, which takes her specific medical problems and personal preference into account. A team, consisting of general practitioners, cardiologists and gynaecologists, each with their particular area of expertise on the subject, is best paced to provide contraceptive advice to women with cardiac disease. In young girls with heart disease, it is important to address contraception from the menarche, which often starts around the age of 12–13; while this might seem early, up to 30% will have sexual intercourse before the age of 15 and up to 50% by the age of 17 [7, 8]. Usually, this event is not planned and without prior discussion with their parents or healthcare providers.

Most contraceptive advice is based on data from women without heart disease. The first consideration is the efficacy of the contraceptive method. Large studies have determined efficacy of each method, expressing efficacy as the incidence of unplanned pregnancy over a year of theoretical contraceptive use (correct use) or typical use (use in real live) as the main outcome measure [10]. The efficacy of a contraceptive method is based on its mechanism of action and is dependent on correct use. The discrepancy between theoretical and typical use is more pronounced when the method requires a substantial amount of compliance or in case of a smaller safety window (time frame in which contraceptive efficacy persists). Equally, the chances of the patient continuing to use a given contraceptive method are higher if she feels well while using that particular method [6]. Creating realistic expectations during counselling leads to higher satisfaction and helps accepting side effects that may be undesirable, as is the case with abnormal bleeding patterns [11–13]. These factors are important when striving for optimal patient adherence and long-term results.

The modified WHO classification of maternal cardiovascular risk assesses risks and consequences of pregnancy, and WHO medical eligibility criteria (WHO-MEC) for contraceptive use can be used as a guideline in women with specific conditions [14, 15]. Recommendations are made using four categories for each contraceptive

Table 2.1 MEC categories for contraceptive eligibility [15]

1	A condition for which there is no restriction for the use of the contraceptive method
2	A condition where the advantages of using the method generally outweigh the theoretical or proven risks
3	A condition where the theoretical or proven risks usually outweigh the advantages of using the method
4	A condition which represents an unacceptable health risk if the contraceptive method is used

method and medical condition including heart disease. Categories range from 1, where there is no restriction on the use of the contraceptive method, to category 4 where the condition represents an unacceptable health risk if the contraceptive method is used (Table 2.1) [15, 16]. These guidelines are regularly updated based on available evidence or on expert opinion if the evidence is lacking.

2.2 Short-Acting Contraceptives

Barrier contraceptives (male condoms, female condoms, diaphragms), coitus interruptus and fertility awareness-based methods (calendar methods, temperature curves) are considered insufficient as failure rates are substantial [10]. While 1 year of typical use of male condom as a sole form of contraception is associated with pregnancy rates up to 18 %, this method still has its value in protection against sexually transmitted diseases (STDs) or as an additional method of contraception when necessary.

Combined oestrogen and progesterone contraceptives are successful in preventing pregnancies, but their efficacy is highly dependent on correct use [10, 17].

They consist of different combinations and doses of either ethinylestradiol or estradiol along with a progestogen. The progestogen component varies and is classified by generation (1–4), each with specific characteristics. They are usually delivered in the form of a daily oral tablet but can also be administered transdermally (weekly patch) or through the vaginal mucosa (3-week vaginal ring), thereby avoiding the hepatic first-pass effect. This method acts on three different levels. Ovulation is inhibited; cervical mucus is thickened, preventing sperm penetration; and endometrial receptivity is altered, preventing implantation.

An advantage of the combined oral contraceptives (COC) is improved cycle control, with lighter, less painful and more regular periods. Traditionally, they are used for 3 weeks, after which a withdrawal bleed is induced, mimicking the natural cycle. However, the frequency of withdrawal bleeds can easily be reduced if desired by prolonged or continuous use [3, 4, 18]. Combined oral contraceptives can help in managing ovarian cysts, PCOS (polycystic ovary syndrome), or relieve symptoms of hyperandrogenism [5].

Of concern is the two- to sevenfold increased risk of venous thrombosis associated with any type of COC. This is mainly induced by the oestrogen component which elevates the level of circulating vitamin K-depending clotting factors, plasminogen and platelet adhesion and reduces the anti-thrombin levels [16]. While this increase in risk is substantial and consequences are important, one should bear in mind that the absolute risk remains low in the range of 8–10/10,000 women-years exposure.

COC also increase the risk of arterial thrombosis and dyslipidaemia and may induce hypertension through an increase in the circulating blood volume [16, 19, 20].

Therefore, COC are not recommended or are contraindicated when the cardiac condition increases the risk of hypertensive, ischaemic or thrombogenic complications or when the consequences of such complications are more severe [9, 15]. As such, COC are not suitable in women with (a history of) ischaemic heart disease, hypertension and additional thrombogenic factors or women with atrial flutter or fibrillation [9, 21–23]. In women with potential right to left shunts (cyanotic heart disease, unoperated ASD), venous thrombosis might result in paradoxical embolism and stroke.

In women with complicated valvular disease or Fontan circulation, the risks and consequences of thrombogenic complications (mechanical valve thrombosis, pulmonary embolus) are such that this form of contraception is also contraindicated.

While some controversy exists on whether the increased thrombogenic risk of COC persists when anticoagulant drugs are used, most guidelines still recommend against the use of COC in these cases. An exception might be made in women on oral anticoagulants in whom ovulation bleeding leads to a massive life-threatening haemoperitoneum. In these rare cases, COC is the method of contraception that most effectively suppresses ovulation.

Also one should be aware of the potential influence of both progestogens and oestrogens on the metabolism of warfarin, requiring more frequent INR monitoring when COC are initiated in women on established oral anticoagulation therapy [24]. Alternatively, some drugs used in certain cardiac conditions may reduce the efficacy of combined oral contraceptives. Bosentan, which is used in management of pulmonary hypertension, accelerates the metabolism of contraceptive steroids, requiring additional contraceptive measures like a condom [9, 16, 25].

COC may induce some fluid retention, but there is no evidence that contraceptive steroid hormones affect cardiac function directly. Still, combined oral contraceptives are contraindicated in women with a reduced ejection fraction after a myocardial infarction, especially in the presence of other risk factors, like smoking and hypertension.

There is no formal contraindication for COC use in women with isolated arrhythmias (isolated supraventricular or ventricular extra beats, AVNT or VT in long QT syndrome).

Contraceptive pills, containing *progesterone only*, prevent sperm penetration by cervical mucus thickening and prevent implantation by reducing endometrial receptivity. If used in a higher dose, ovulation may be inhibited [17, 26]. No increased risk of thrombosis in women using progesterone-only pills is reported [27]. These pills can contain different types of progestogens with varying efficacy and safety window and are commonly used as additional contraception in lactating women.

Desogestrel (Cerazette)-containing tablets are effective in inhibiting ovulation with a safety window of 12 h and have similar efficacy as the combined oral contraceptive pill [9, 16, 25, 26, 28]. They are therefore the only pills of this type recommended in women with (severe) cardiac disease.

2.3 Long-Acting Reversible Contraceptives (LARC)

Long-acting reversible contraceptives consist of intrauterine devices (IUDs), subdermal implants and intramuscular injections of DMPA (depot-medroxyprogesterone acetate). By eliminating patient adherence, the efficacy of LARC is excellent, even exceeding sterilisation [10, 29]. Two models of IUDs exist: levonorgestrel-releasing intrauterine system (LNG-IUS) and copper-bearing IUDs. LNG-IUS induces endometrial atrophy and causes formation of a cervical mucus plug, impeding sperm penetration and implantation over a 5-year period. Copper is toxic to the ova and sperm and induces endometrial inflammation which prevents implantation, offering contraception for 10 years [30]. IUDs can be used in both nulliparous and multiparous women. IUDs can be inserted at any point of the cycle or directly postpartum [31, 32]. Insertion during menstruation offers immediate contraception and is facilitated by the physiological opening of the cervical ostium.

Fertility rapidly returns upon removal [29]. Uterine perforation and spontaneous expulsion are rare but are recognised complications. Importantly, IUDs are devoid of increased thrombotic risk. LNG-IUSs increase the levels of high-density lipoprotein, making it a good option for women with ischaemic heart disease and hyperlipidaemia [16, 20]. They often reduce menstrual blood loss, sometimes resulting in complete amenorrhea, but the bleeding pattern may become irregular in some women. It can help to control menstrual bleeding problems which occur more often in women using anticoagulants [33–35]. While the natural menstrual cycle is maintained with copper IUDs, an increase in blood loss and discomfort are often observed with menstruation.

The risk of pelvic infection is increased during the first 3 months after insertion, and transient bacteraemia has been documented at replacement but is rare in uncomplicated insertion or removal [36, 37]. Recent studies and guidelines do not recommend the standard use of prophylactic antibiotics to prevent either PID (pelvic inflammatory disease) or endocarditis at insertion [38–43]. Nevertheless, since the introduction of this guideline which limited the indications for antibiotic prophylaxis, an increase in prevalence of endocarditis has been observed in women with cardiac disease in general [44].

As such, the administration of prophylactic antibiotics (ampicillin 2 g and gentamicin 80 mg given intravenously 1 h before IUD insertion) may be considered in women at high risk of endocarditis [45]. Insertion of an IUD requires extra caution in women with pulmonary hypertension or Fontan repair. Vasovagal reactions may occur upon insertion due to pain and cervical manipulation, which is potentially dangerous in these women [9, 16, 21, 25, 46–48]. Insertion is therefore best performed with pain relief (e.g. IV opioids), cardiovascular monitoring and anaesthetic support on standby, to prevent or adequately anticipate the consequences of a vagal reaction [48].

Subdermal implants, containing etonogestrel (Implanon) or levonorgestrel (Norplant), gradually release their progesterone over the course of 3 years, inhibiting ovulation and altering cervical mucus and endometrial receptivity. Subcutaneous insertion just below the medial groove between the biceps and triceps after local anaesthetic infiltration makes it a simple procedure, leading to contraception with an efficacy exceeding that of sterilisation [10]. Failure rates are low due to the elimination of the "patient adherence" factor. The newer easy-to-use insertion devices and incorporation of radioactive filaments prevent failure due to unnoticed loss and facilitate retrieval in the rare occasion of spontaneous migration of the device [29, 49]. The simplicity of insertion (no vasovagal reaction accompanying cervical manipulation), high efficacy and absence of increased thrombogenic risk make that subdermal implants are an excellent option for women with mechanical valves, pulmonary hypertension or Fontan repair [9, 11, 16, 21, 25, 29, 50, 51]. Women often experience a reduction in vaginal blood loss in terms of amount, frequency and duration of bleeding. Endometrial atrophy, which may occur after prolonged exposure to progesterone, may cause vascular fragility, occasionally leading to irregular and unpredictable bleeding or spotting [29, 52–55]. As previously mentioned, additional contraceptive measures should be taken in women using Bosentan.

Depot-medroxyprogesterone acetate offers reliable contraception if used every 13 weeks, with a grace period of 4 weeks, but effects usually last much longer. DMPA injections can induce intramuscular haematoma, but even in women on anticoagulants, this rarely seems to be of clinical significance [9, 16, 21, 25]. Uncertainty regarding a potential thrombogenic effect remains, as evidence is conflicting [27, 51, 56, 57].

2.4 Sterilisation

Sterilisation is a good option for patients with a contraindication for pregnancy or for couples with a completed family [9, 21, 25]. The role of sterilisation has decreased as other highly reliable and reversible contraceptive methods have emerged. Sterilisation does not offer non-contraceptive benefits like reduction of blood loss or cycle control.

Although sterilisation is considered a definitive method of contraception, reversal surgery may restore fertility in some cases. Laparoscopic tubal ligation and hysteroscopic insertion of intratubal stents are all considered good options, but these procedures carry risks. Laparoscopic *tubal ligation* is performed under general anaesthesia and requires a pneumoperitoneum with elevated intra-abdominal pressures and is therefore contraindicated in the presence of pulmonary hypertension or Fontan repair. Alternatively, an open or laparoscopic procedure with minimal inflation can be considered. Perioperative cessation of anticoagulation increases risk of thrombosis, and anaesthesia and the procedure itself create an inherent risk of haemorrhage and infection [9, 21, 25, 58]. Sterilisation at the time of Caesarean section is associated with a slightly higher regret and failure rate as compared to a laparoscopic procedure [59, 60]. The psychological impact of definitive contraception, even in the case of severe heart disease with an absolute contraindication for pregnancy, should be taken into consideration. *Vasectomy* imposes no risk for the woman, but in case of a cardiac condition with a high chance of early demise, vasectomy may lead to male fertility problems in a future relationship.

Hysteroscopic tubal occlusion can also be achieved using various techniques. It does not require a skin incision or abdominal entry. Technical developments mean that hysteroscopes are now very thin and insertion devices allow these procedures to be performed with limited discomfort in an outpatient setting. However, pain relief (e.g. IV opioids), cardiovascular monitoring and anaesthetic support on standby remain necessary in women with pulmonary hypertension or Fontan repair, to prevent or adequately anticipate the consequences of a vagal reaction [48]. Currently, the most commonly used method consists of coils (Essure), which are inserted in the proximal part of the fallopian tube and induce fibrosis and occlusion. This method was approved in Europe and by the FDA and seems to have a low complication and low failure rate after tubal patency is assessed by ultrasound or hysterosalpingography after 3 months [61]. Nevertheless, recently some controversy on its safety emerged after the reports of numerous adverse events by women. This resulted in serious concerns about the risk of chronic pain, device migration and contraceptive efficacy [21, 25, 62–65]. Until these concerns are resolved, it is prudent to avoid this method.

2.5 Emergency Contraception

Emergency or postcoital contraception is essential in women not using any method or in whom a contraceptive method was not used appropriately (e.g. irregular pill intake, condom failure). The method with the highest contraceptive efficacy (failure rate of 0.09%) is the insertion of a *copper IUD* within 120 h after intercourse.

A single dose of 1.5 mg *levonorgestrel* inhibits follicular growth or rupture and is therefore only effective before ovulation. It has a failure rate of 1.1% if taken within 72 h after unprotected coitus. Obesity (BMI >30 kg/m^2) increases the failure rate, and a copper IUD should therefore be preferred in obese women requiring emergency contraception. Drug interactions with warfarin are reported, requiring close control of the INR [24].

Mifepristone 25 mg or *ulipristal acetate* 30 mg can be taken up to 120 h after unprotected intercourse. The superior efficacy of mifepristone and ulipristal over levonorgestrel may arise from ovulation inhibition and its additional postovulatory mechanism of action in inhibiting endometrial receptivity and tubal contractility. Proper counselling on reliable ongoing contraception should be offered at the time of provision of emergency contraception.

Conclusion

Contraceptive counselling in women with cardiovascular disease should begin early, preferably soon after menarche. Choices should be made by a multidisciplinary team, based on impact of pregnancy, safety of use, associated benefits of the contraceptive and the individual's preferences. Efficacy and ease of use are important factors for adequate contraception. Continuation rates are highest when the patient feels well using a particular method. Progestogen-only long-acting reversible contraceptive methods are a good option for patients with cardiovascular disease.

References

1. Baumgartner H, Bonhoeffer P, De Groot NM, de Haan F, Deanfield JE, Galie N et al (2010) ESC Guidelines for the management of grown-up congenital heart disease (new version 2010). Eur Heart J 31(23):2915–2957
2. Roos-Hesselink JW, Ruys TP, Stein JI, Thilen U, Webb GD, Niwa K et al (2013) Outcome of pregnancy in patients with structural or ischaemic heart disease: results of a registry of the European Society of Cardiology. Eur Heart J 34(9):657–665
3. Kaunitz AM (1999) Oral contraceptive health benefits: perception versus reality. Contraception 59(1 Suppl):29s–33s
4. Sulak PJ, Scow RD, Preece C, Riggs MW, Kuehl TJ (2000) Hormone withdrawal symptoms in oral contraceptive users. Obstet Gynecol 95(2):261–266
5. Dragoman MV (2014) The combined oral contraceptive pill – recent developments, risks and benefits. Best Pract Res Clin Obstet Gynaecol 28(6):825–834
6. Wellings K, Brima N, Sadler K, Copas AJ, McDaid L, Mercer CH et al (2015) Stopping and switching contraceptive methods: findings from Contessa, a prospective longitudinal study of women of reproductive age in England. Contraception 91(1):57–66
7. Rogers P, Mansour D, Mattinson A, O'Sullivan JJ (2007) A collaborative clinic between contraception and sexual health services and an adult congenital heart disease clinic. J Family Plan Reprod Health Care Fac Family Plan Reprod Health Care R Coll Obstet Gynaecol 33(1):17–21
8. Pijuan-Domenech A, Baro-Marine F, Rojas-Torrijos M, Dos-Subira L, Pedrosa-Del Moral V, Subirana-Domenech MT et al (2013) Usefulness of progesterone-only components for contraception in patients with congenital heart disease. Am J Cardiol 112(4):590–593
9. Thorne S, Nelson-Piercy C, MacGregor A, Gibbs S, Crowhurst J, Panay N et al (2006) Pregnancy and contraception in heart disease and pulmonary arterial hypertension. J Family Plan Reprod Health Care Fac Family Plan Reprod Health Care, R Coll Obstet Gynaecol 32(2):75–81
10. Trussell J (2011) Contraceptive failure in the United States. Contraception 83(5):397–404
11. Mansour D, Bahamondes L, Critchley H, Darney P, Fraser IS (2011) The management of unacceptable bleeding patterns in etonogestrel-releasing contraceptive implant users. Contraception 83(3):202–210
12. Mansour D, Korver T, Marintcheva-Petrova M, Fraser IS (2008) The effects of Implanon on menstrual bleeding patterns. Eur J Contracept Reprod Health Care Off J Eur Soc Contracept 13(Suppl 1):13–28
13. Modesto W, Bahamondes MV, Bahamondes L (2014) A randomized clinical trial of the effect of intensive versus non-intensive counselling on discontinuation rates due to bleeding disturbances of three long-acting reversible contraceptives. Hum Reprod 29(7):1393–1399
14. Regitz-Zagrosek V, Blomstrom Lundqvist C, Borghi C, Cifkova R, Ferreira R, Foidart JM et al (2011) ESC Guidelines on the management of cardiovascular diseases during pregnancy: the

Task Force on the Management of Cardiovascular Diseases during Pregnancy of the European Society of Cardiology (ESC). Eur Heart J 32(24):3147–3197
15. WHO Guidelines Approved by the Guidelines Review Committee. Medical eligibility criteria for contraceptive use (2015) World Health Organization, Geneva. Copyright (c) World Health Organization 2015
16. Mohan AR, Nelson-Piercy C (2014) Drugs and therapeutics, including contraception, for women with heart disease. Best Pract Res Clin Obstet Gynaecol 28(4):471–482
17. Milsom I, Korver T (2008) Ovulation incidence with oral contraceptives: a literature review. J Family Plan Reprod Health Care Fac Family Plan Reprod Health Care R Coll Obstet Gynaecol 34(4):237–246
18. Anderson FD (2006) Safety and efficacy of an extended-regimen oral contraception utilizing low-dose ethinyl estradiol. Contraception 74(4):355
19. Dong W, Colhoun HM, Poulter NR (1997) Blood pressure in women using oral contraceptives: results from the Health Survey for England 1994. J Hypertens 15(10):1063–1068
20. Lidegaard O, Lokkegaard E, Jensen A, Skovlund CW, Keiding N (2012) Thrombotic stroke and myocardial infarction with hormonal contraception. N Engl J Med 366(24): 2257–2266
21. Silversides CK, Sermer M, Siu SC (2009) Choosing the best contraceptive method for the adult with congenital heart disease. Curr Cardiol Rep 11(4):298–305
22. Camm AJ, Kirchhof P, Lip GY, Schotten U, Savelieva I, Ernst S et al (2010) Guidelines for the management of atrial fibrillation: the Task Force for the Management of Atrial Fibrillation of the European Society of Cardiology (ESC). Eur Heart J 31(19):2369–2429
23. Camm AJ, Lip GY, De Caterina R, Savelieva I, Atar D, Hohnloser SH et al (2012) 2012 focused update of the ESC Guidelines for the management of atrial fibrillation: an update of the 2010 ESC Guidelines for the management of atrial fibrillation. Developed with the special contribution of the European Heart Rhythm Association. Eur Heart J 33(21):2719–2747
24. Ellison J, Thomson AJ, Greer IA, Walker ID (2000) Drug points: apparent interaction between warfarin and levonorgestrel used for emergency contraception. BMJ (Clin Res Ed) 321(7273):1382
25. Thorne S, MacGregor A, Nelson-Piercy C (2006) Risks of contraception and pregnancy in heart disease. Heart 92(10):1520–1525
26. Korver T, Klipping C, Heger-Mahn D, Duijkers I, van Osta G, Dieben T (2005) Maintenance of ovulation inhibition with the 75-microg desogestrel-only contraceptive pill (Cerazette) after scheduled 12-h delays in tablet intake. Contraception 71(1):8–13
27. Mantha S, Karp R, Raghavan V, Terrin N, Bauer KA, Zwicker JI (2012) Assessing the risk of venous thromboembolic events in women taking progestin-only contraception: a meta-analysis. BMJ (Clin Res Ed) 345:e4944
28. Wald RM, Sermer M, Colman JM (2011) Pregnancy and contraception in young women with congenital heart disease: general considerations. Paediatr Child Health 16(4):e25–e29
29. Espey E, Ogburn T (2011) Long-acting reversible contraceptives: intrauterine devices and the contraceptive implant. Obstet Gynecol 117(3):705–719
30. Stephen Searle E (2014) The intrauterine device and the intrauterine system. Best Pract Res Clin Obstet Gynaecol 28(6):807–824
31. Bahamondes MV, Hidalgo MM, Bahamondes L, Monteiro I (2011) Ease of insertion and clinical performance of the levonorgestrel-releasing intrauterine system in nulligravidas. Contraception 84(5):e11–e16
32. Kapp N, Curtis KM (2009) Intrauterine device insertion during the postpartum period: a systematic review. Contraception 80(4):327–336
33. Vigl M, Kaemmerer M, Niggemeyer E, Nagdyman N, Seifert-Klauss V, Trigas V et al (2010) Sexuality and reproductive health in women with congenital heart disease. Am J Cardiol 105(4):538–541
34. Huq FY, Tvarkova K, Arafa A, Kadir RA (2011) Menstrual problems and contraception in women of reproductive age receiving oral anticoagulation. Contraception 84(2):128–132

35. Zingone MM, Guirguis AB, Airee A, Cobb D (2009) Probable drug interaction between warfarin and hormonal contraceptives. Ann Pharmacother 43(12):2096–2102
36. Murray S, Hickey JB, Houang E (1987) Significant bacteremia associated with replacement of intrauterine contraceptive device. Am J Obstet Gynecol 156(3):698–700
37. Everett ED, Reller LB, Droegemueller W, Greer BE (1976) Absence of bacteremia after insertion or removal of intrauterine devices. Obstet Gynecol 47(2):207–209
38. Nishimura RA, Carabello BA, Faxon DP, Freed MD, Lytle BW, O'Gara PT et al (2008) ACC/AHA 2008 Guideline update on valvular heart disease: focused update on infective endocarditis: a report of the American College of Cardiology/American Heart Association Task Force on Practice Guidelines endorsed by the Society of Cardiovascular Anesthesiologists, Society for Cardiovascular Angiography and Interventions, and Society of Thoracic Surgeons. J Am Coll Cardiol 52(8):676–685
39. Centre for Clinical Practice at N. National Institute for Health and Clinical Excellence: Guidance Prophylaxis against infective endocarditis: antimicrobial prophylaxis against infective endocarditis in adults and children undergoing interventional procedures (2008) National Institute for Health and Clinical Excellence (UK) National Institute for Health and Clinical Excellence, London
40. Grimes DA, Schulz KF (2001) Antibiotic prophylaxis for intrauterine contraceptive device insertion. Cochrane Database Syst Rev (2):Cd001327
41. Ladipo OA, Farr G, Otolorin E, Konje JC, Sturgen K, Cox P et al (1991) Prevention of IUD-related pelvic infection: the efficacy of prophylactic doxycycline at IUD insertion. Adv Contracept Off J Soc Adv Contracept 7(1):43–54
42. Sinei SK, Schulz KF, Lamptey PR, Grimes DA, Mati JK, Rosenthal SM et al (1990) Preventing IUCD-related pelvic infection: the efficacy of prophylactic doxycycline at insertion. Br J Obstet Gynaecol 97(5):412–419
43. Walsh TL, Bernstein GS, Grimes DA, Frezieres R, Bernstein L, Coulson AH (1994) Effect of prophylactic antibiotics on morbidity associated with IUD insertion: results of a pilot randomized controlled trial, IUD Study Group. Contraception 50(4):319–327
44. Dayer MJ, Jones S, Prendergast B, Baddour LM, Lockhart PB, Thornhill MH (2015) Incidence of infective endocarditis in England, 2000–13: a secular trend, interrupted time-series analysis. Lancet (Lond, Engl) 385(9974):1219–1228
45. Suri V, Aggarwal N, Kaur R, Chaudhary N, Ray P, Grover A (2008) Safety of intrauterine contraceptive device (copper T 200 B) in women with cardiac disease. Contraception 78(4): 315–318
46. Gemzell-Danielsson K, Mansour D, Fiala C, Kaunitz AM, Bahamondes L (2013) Management of pain associated with the insertion of intrauterine contraceptives. Hum Reprod Update 19(4):419–427
47. Ott J, Promberger R, Kaufmann U, Huber JC, Frigo P (2009) Venous thrombembolism, thrombophilic defects, combined oral contraception and anticoagulation. Arch Gynecol Obstet 280(5):811–814
48. Roos-Hesselink JW, Cornette J, Sliwa K, Pieper PG, Veldtman GR, Johnson MR (2015) Contraception and cardiovascular disease. Eur Heart J 36(27):1728–1734, 34a-34b
49. Jacobstein R, Polis CB (2014) Progestin-only contraception: injectables and implants. Best Pract Res Clin Obstet Gynaecol 28(6):795–806
50. Aznar R, Reynoso L, Ley E, Gamez R, De Leon MD (1976) Electrocardiographic changes induced by insertion of an intrauterine device and other uterine manipulations. Fertil Steril 27(1):92–96
51. Lidegaard O, Nielsen LH, Skovlund CW, Skjeldestad FE, Lokkegaard E (2011) Risk of venous thromboembolism from use of oral contraceptives containing different progestogens and oestrogen doses: Danish cohort study, 2001–9. BMJ (Clin Res Ed) 343:d6423
52. Culwell KR, Curtis KM (2009) Use of contraceptive methods by women with current venous thrombosis on anticoagulant therapy: a systematic review. Contraception 80(4):337–345
53. Kadir RA, Chi C (2007) Levonorgestrel intrauterine system: bleeding disorders and anticoagulant therapy. Contraception 75(6 Suppl):S123–S129

54. Pisoni CN, Cuadrado MJ, Khamashta MA, Hunt BJ (2006) Treatment of menorrhagia associated with oral anticoagulation: efficacy and safety of the levonorgestrel releasing intrauterine device (Mirena coil). Lupus 15(12):877–880
55. Sordal T, Inki P, Draeby J, O'Flynn M, Schmelter T (2013) Management of initial bleeding or spotting after levonorgestrel-releasing intrauterine system placement: a randomized controlled trial. Obstet Gynecol 121(5):934–941
56. Lidegaard O, Nielsen LH, Skovlund CW, Lokkegaard E (2012) Venous thrombosis in users of non-oral hormonal contraception: follow-up study, Denmark 2001–10. BMJ (Clin Res Ed) 344:e2990
57. Goldstein J, Cushman M, Badger GJ, Johnson JV (2007) Effect of depomedroxyprogesterone acetate on coagulation parameter: a pilot study. Fertil Steril 87(6):1267–1270
58. Snabes MC, Poindexter AN 3rd (1991) Laparoscopic tubal sterilization under local anesthesia in women with cyanotic heart disease. Obstet Gynecol 78(3 Pt 1):437–440
59. Hillis SD, Marchbanks PA, Tylor LR, Peterson HB (1999) Poststerilization regret: findings from the United States Collaborative Review of Sterilization. Obstet Gynecol 93(6):889–895
60. Peterson HB, Xia Z, Hughes JM, Wilcox LS, Tylor LR, Trussell J (1996) The risk of pregnancy after tubal sterilization: findings from the U.S. Collaborative Review of Sterilization. Am J Obstet Gynecol 174(4):1161–1168; discussion 8–70
61. Adelman MR, Dassel MW, Sharp HT (2014) Management of complications encountered with Essure hysteroscopic sterilization: a systematic review. J Minim Invasive Gynecol 21(5): 733–743
62. Famuyide AO, Hopkins MR, El-Nashar SA, Creedon DJ, Vasdev GM, Driscoll DJ et al (2008) Hysteroscopic sterilization in women with severe cardiac disease: experience at a tertiary center. Mayo Clin Proc 83(4):431–438
63. Duffy S, Marsh F, Rogerson L, Hudson H, Cooper K, Jack S et al (2005) Female sterilisation: a cohort controlled comparative study of ESSURE versus laparoscopic sterilisation. BJOG 112(11):1522–1528
64. Kerin JF, Cooper JM, Price T, Herendael BJ, Cayuela-Font E, Cher D et al (2003) Hysteroscopic sterilization using a micro-insert device: results of a multicentre phase II study. Hum Reprod 18(6):1223–1230
65. Dhruva SS, Ross JS, Gariepy AM (2015) Revisiting essure – toward safe and effective sterilization. N Engl J Med 373(15), e17

Preconception Counseling 3

M.A.M. Kampman and P.G. Pieper

Abbreviations

ACC	American College of Cardiology
ACE	Angiotensin-converting enzyme
AHA	American Heart Association
ARBs	Angiotensin receptor blockers
AVA	Aortic valve area
CHD	Congenital heart defect
CT	Computed tomography
ESC	European Society of Cardiology
FDA	Food and Drug Administration
ICD	Implantable cardioverter defibrillator
LMWH	Low-molecular-weight heparin
LVOT	Left ventricular outflow tract
MRI	Magnetic resonance imaging
MVA	Mitral valve area
NYHA	New York Heart Association
ROPAC	Registry of Pregnancy and Cardiac Disease
TPVR	Total peripheral vascular resistance
WHO	World Health Organization

M.A.M. Kampman, MD, PhD • P.G. Pieper, MD, PhD (✉)
Department of Cardiology, University Medical Center Groningen,
Groningen, The Netherlands
e-mail: p.g.pieper@umcg.nl

3.1 Introduction

Congenital heart defects (CHDs) are the most common congenital defects in newborns, affecting 9/1000 live-born children worldwide [14, 54]. Due to improved surgical techniques and medical management, the majority of these children survive until adulthood. Nowadays, adults represent two thirds of the total CHD population, and the prevalence of severe CHD in adults is rapidly increasing [30]. It is important to realize that these patients are not cured, and because pregnancy requires major hemodynamic adaptations, these women are at risk of cardiovascular complications and worsening cardiac function.

3.2 Physiological Changes During Pregnancy

Knowledge of the normal physiological changes during pregnancy, labor, and postpartum period is essential for doctors caring for pregnant women with (congenital) heart disease. The most important changes are described here. The initial step is probably a fall in total peripheral vascular resistance (TPVR), as response to the circulating gestational hormones, and later in pregnancy to the low vascular resistance in the uterus and placenta [21]. The fall in TPVR creates a relatively underfilled state, leading to an expansion of the plasma volume, and results in a rise of the cardiac output of 30–50 % above prepregnancy values. This is achieved by increases in stroke volume and heart rate. The changes start early in pregnancy and cardiac output continues to increase until 24 weeks of gestation. The augmented cardiac output is then maintained until term [41]. The hemodynamic changes described result in progressive left ventricular remodeling. Left ventricular end-diastolic and end-systolic dimensions increase during pregnancy, while ejection fraction remains unchanged [12, 45]. Left ventricular mass increases as a result of eccentric hypertrophy of the myocardium.

During labor, cardiac output increases further by approximately 12 % toward the end of labor compared with the end of pregnancy (gestational week 38–39). Pain, anxiety, and autotransfusion because of uterine contraction play an important role in this additional increase in cardiac output [39–41]. The puerperium is characterized by a physiological state of overfilling, due to decompression of the vena cava inferior and autotransfusion from the involution of the uterus [40].

Pregnancy constitutes a hypercoagulable state owing to the increase in coagulation factors and fibrinogen. These changes protect against massive blood loss but also result in increased risk of thromboembolic complications. Venous stasis due to inferior vena cava compression by the growing uterus also contributes to the increased thromboembolic risk.

3.3 Pregnancy in Women with Congenital Heart Disease

The hemodynamic changes of pregnancy can be challenging for women with (congenital) heart disease. Extensive research in the past decades has shown that pregnancy in women with CHD is associated with increased incidence rates of maternal cardiovascular complications and mortality, but obstetric and neonatal complications are also more common [8, 9, 42, 46, 47].

Arrhythmia and heart failure are the most frequently observed cardiac complications. Other important complications are thromboembolic events (especially in women with mechanical heart valves) [8, 9, 42, 47]. Most of the arrhythmias occurring are supraventricular in nature and not life threatening, though they can cause hemodynamic compromise for both mother and child [50].

Data from the European Registry on Pregnancy and Cardiac Disease (ROPAC) showed that the timing of heart failure was dependent on the nature of the underlying heart disease, with heart failure in the second trimester occurring in patients with shunt lesions or valvular heart disease. By contrast, patients with cardiomyopathy or ischemic heart disease developed heart failure shortly after delivery [44].

Common obstetric complications are hypertensive disorders of pregnancy and premature labor. The risk of these complications appears to be associated with the underlying congenital heart disease [9]. Preeclampsia during pregnancy appears an important risk factor for development of heart failure in women with structural CHD [44].

Neonatal mortality, premature birth, and small for gestational age are frequently observed complications in the offspring of women with cardiac disease. Offspring outcome is worse when women experienced heart failure during pregnancy or the peripartum period [44]. There is also a chance of recurrence of congenital heart disease, which is addressed in Chap. 4.

In addition to pregnancy complications, late cardiovascular events also occur more frequently. These occur more frequently in women who have experienced cardiac complications during pregnancy [2, 23]. Deterioration in cardiac function after pregnancy has been described in women with systemic right ventricles and tetralogy of Fallot [6, 10, 17, 53]. Women with congenital aortic valve stenosis, who have been pregnant, have a higher frequency of valvular interventions compared to nulliparous women [52].

Preconception counseling is important in the care for women with congenital heart disease and should be performed before conception or, when this was not possible, as early as possible during pregnancy. It enables women and their partners to make a well-informed choice whether to pursue (or continue) pregnancy or not. Preconception counseling should be multidisciplinary with both cardiac and obstetric input, and it should address at least the cardiovascular risk of pregnancy for the mother and wherever possible fetal risk. Additionally, medication should be reviewed [13].

3.4 Risk Assessment

3.4.1 Maternal Risk

The risk of pregnancy depends on the specific type of congenital heart disease and on the clinical condition of the patient. In general, the risk of pregnancy increases with increasing complexity of the underlying disease, though complexity of disease alone is insufficient for risk prediction [9, 51]. Current European Society of Cardiology (ESC) guidelines on the management of cardiovascular disease during pregnancy

Table 3.1 Modified World Health Organization (WHO) risk classification

WHO I (no increased risk of maternal mortality, mild increased risk of maternal morbidity)
Uncomplicated, small, or mild
Pulmonary valve stenosis
Patent ductus arteriosus
Mitral valve prolapse
Successfully repaired simple lesions
Atrial septal defect
Ventricular septal defect
Patent ductus arteriosus
Anomalous pulmonary venous drainage
WHO II (small increased risk of maternal mortality, moderate increased risk of maternal morbidity)
Unoperated atrial or ventricular septal defect
Repaired tetralogy of Fallot
WHO II-III (depending on individual)
Mild left ventricular impairment
Native or tissue valvular heart disease not considered WHO I or IV
Marfan syndrome without aortic dilatation
Aorta <45 mm in aortic disease associated with bicuspid aortic valve
Repaired coarctation
WHO III (significantly increased risk of maternal mortality or severe morbidity)
Mechanical valve
Systemic right ventricle
Fontan circulation
Cyanotic heart disease (unrepaired)
Other complex congenital heart disease
Aortic dilatation 40–45 mm in Marfan syndrome
Aortic dilatation 45–50 mm in aortic disease associated with bicuspid aortic valve
WHO IV (extremely high risk of maternal mortality or severe morbidity, pregnancy contraindicated)
Pulmonary arterial hypertension of any cause
Severe systemic ventricular dysfunction (LVEF <30%, New York Heart Association functional (NYHA) III–IV)
Previous peripartum cardiomyopathy with any residual impairment of left ventricular function
Severe mitral stenosis, severe symptomatic aortic stenosis
Marfan syndrome with aorta dilated >45 mm
Aortic dilatation >50 mm in aortic disease associated with bicuspid aortic valve
Native severe coarctation

recommend the use of the modified World Health Organization (WHO) risk class to identify maternal cardiovascular risk during pregnancy (Table 3.1) [13]. Since this risk classification integrates all identified maternal cardiovascular risk predictors, including underlying heart disease, residual lesions, and any other comorbidity, this classification is the preferred manner of identifying the cardiovascular risk during pregnancy. For women in modified WHO risk class IV, termination of pregnancy should always be discussed, since maternal mortality and morbidity risk are high.

In the past decade, various predictors of adverse maternal cardiac outcome have been identified, and two widely used prediction models, CARPREG and ZAHARA, have been developed (Table 3.2) [8, 24, 25, 47–49]. These risk scores assign points

Table 3.2 Risk predictors for adverse maternal and neonatal outcome

Maternal outcome	Risk points
CARPREG[a]	
Prior cardiac event (heart failure, stroke/transient ischemic attack) or arrhythmia	1.0
Baseline NYHA functional class >II or cyanosis	1.0
Left heart obstruction (mitral valve area (MVA) <2 cm^2, aortic valve area (AVA) <1.5 cm^2, or peak left ventricular outflow tract gradient (LVOT) >30 mmHg)	1.0
Reduced systemic ventricular systolic function (ejection fraction <40%)	1.0
ZAHARA[b]	
History of arrhythmias	1.5
Use of cardiac medication before pregnancy	1.5
Baseline NYHA functional class ≥2	0.75
Left heart obstruction (peak aortic gradient >50 mmHg or AVA <1.5 cm^2 or mitral valve area <2.0 cm^2)	2.5
Moderate/severe systemic atrioventricular valve regurgitation	0.75
Moderate/severe pulmonary atrioventricular valve regurgitation	0.75
Mechanical valve prosthesis	4.25
Repaired or unrepaired cyanotic heart disease	1.0
Other studies	
Smoking history	
Severe pulmonary valve regurgitation/depressed subpulmonary ventricular ejection fraction	
Mechanical valve prosthesis	
Subpulmonary ventricular dysfunction (TAPSE <16 mm)	
Use of cardiac medication	
Use of anticoagulation	
Pulmonary hypertension	
Dilatation subpulmonary ventricle	
Neonatal outcome	
CARPREG	
NYHA functional class <II or cyanosis	
Heparin/warfarin during pregnancy	
Smoking	
Multiple gestation	
Left heart obstruction (mitral valve area <2 cm^2, aortic valve area <1.5 cm^2 or peak left ventricular outflow tract gradient >30 mmHg)	
ZAHARA	
Multiple gestation	
Smoking	
Repaired or unrepaired cyanotic heart disease	
Mechanical valve prosthesis	
Use of cardiac medication before pregnancy	

AVA aortic valve area, *MVA* mitral valve area, *LVOT* left ventricular outflow tract, *NYHA* New York Heart Association functional class

[a]For each CARPREG predictor present, 1 point is assigned. The risk of maternal cardiovascular complications is 5% with 0 points, 27% with 1 points, and 75% with ≥2 points

[b]For each ZAHARA predictor present, a predictor-specific number of points is assigned. The risk of maternal cardiovascular complications is 2.9% with <0.5 points, 7.5% with 0.5–1.5 points, 17% with 1.51–2.50 points, 43.1% with 2.51–3.5 points, and 70% >3.5 points

when specific risk predictors are present, and the total of points gathered gives an indication of maternal cardiovascular risk during pregnancy. The CARPREG and ZAHARA risk scores have been validated in several studies and appear helpful in predicting maternal cardiac risk [1, 8, 22, 28, 38]. However, in both risk scores, several high-risk populations were underrepresented and because of that several important risk factors were not identified (i.e., dilated aorta and pulmonary arterial hypertension). Recent studies comparing the CARPREG, ZAHARA, and modified WHO risk class indicate that the latter is superior to the CARPREG and ZAHARA risk scores in identifying patients at high risk of cardiovascular complications [1, 28, 38]. Therefore, it should be advised to use the modified WHO risk classification in preconception counseling of women with CHD.

Table 3.2 displays an overview of various identified predictors prior to pregnancy. The use of cardiac medication prior to pregnancy is most likely a surrogate marker for severity of heart disease. This may also be the case for the predictor cyanotic heart disease (corrected and uncorrected), which probably reflects the greater complexity of the underlying lesion.

Two studies thus far investigated the role of increased natriuretic peptide levels in the prediction of cardiovascular complications during pregnancy [24, 49]. Women with cardiovascular complications during pregnancy had higher natriuretic peptide levels compared to women without. More research is required in this field, but natriuretic peptides might provide a valuable tool to identify patients at highest risk of complications when they are already pregnant, as well as to identify women with the lowest risk.

3.4.2 Neonatal Risk

The CARPREG and ZAHARA studies identified predictors of adverse neonatal outcome [8, 47], and data from the European Registry on Pregnancy and Cardiac Disease (ROPAC) indicate that high-modified WHO risk class is associated with adverse offspring outcome, such as low birth weight and premature birth (Fig. 3.1). However, recent validation showed that all three risk assessment strategies failed to accurately identify the risk to the offspring [1].

3.5 Preconception Investigations

Several investigations should be done in order to gather the required information for a full risk assessment (Fig. 3.1). Ideally, these investigations should be performed before pregnancy, otherwise as early as possible during the first trimester. Risk assessment begins with exploring the medical history of the patient. History and clinical assessment are essential in the evaluation of women with CHD who desire to become pregnant, in order to evaluate if the patient is symptomatic (dyspnea or palpitations) or cyanotic or had previous cardiovascular events. Taking a good history and performing an accurate clinical assessment provide instant information about patient well-being and the presence of long-term complications, such as

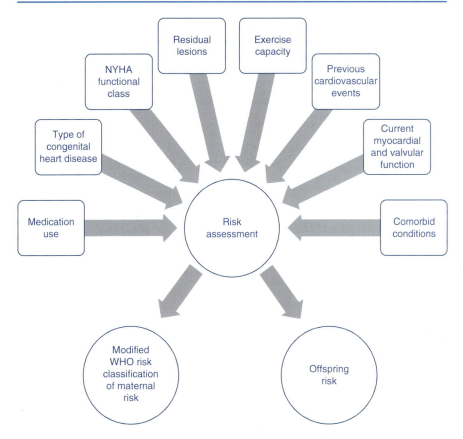

Fig. 3.1 Information required for cardiovascular risk assessment during pregnancy in women with congenital heart disease

hypertension. It also provides an important reference point, in case deterioration occurs during pregnancy.

Echocardiography is an essential tool in the evaluation of cardiac performance. In particular ventricular and valvular function should be assessed, and lesion-specific investigations should be performed (i.e., aortic diameters, signs of re-coarctation, baffle leakage, etc.). These all give important insights in cardiac function and are important to make a good risk assessment. Stress echocardiography using bicycle ergometry may add in the evaluation of patients with valve dysfunction and in patients with reduced systemic ventricular function.

Exercise capacity testing is recommended before pregnancy to assess the functional capacity, chronotropic, and blood pressure response and to identify exercise-induced arrhythmias [13]. Liu et al. found in a population with mainly complex congenital heart disease that abnormal chronotropic response correlated with adverse maternal and neonatal pregnancy outcome [29]. Comparable results were reported by Ohuchi et al. In this study not only peak heart rate but also peak oxygen uptake during exercise testing was associated with maternal and neonatal outcome [37].

Electrocardiography provides valuable information concerning the presence of conduction disorders, which are common in certain types of, mainly complex, congenital heart disease. In patients known with previous arrhythmia or those reporting symptoms of palpitations, Holter monitoring should be performed.

Other imaging modalities, such as magnetic resonance imaging (MRI) or computed tomography (CT), can be useful in situations where echocardiography is not sufficient and are particularly useful for evaluation of aortic disease. There is no place for routine cardiac catheterization as preconception investigation. However, catheterization can be helpful when interventions are necessary before pregnancy and should be done before pregnancy when pulmonary arterial hypertension is suspected, since pulmonary arterial hypertension is a contraindication for pregnancy. All imaging modalities using radiation are relatively contraindicated during early pregnancy [13].

Preconception investigations might reveal that an intervention (i.e., valve interventions, aortic root replacement, and stent placement for re-coarctation) is indicated. It is advised to perform such interventions before pregnancy is actively pursued, since this may reduce cardiovascular risk during pregnancy [13].

3.6   Medication and Devices

The ROPAC registry indicated that cardiac medication is used during one third of the pregnancies in women with cardiac disease [43]. A careful review of all medication used should be performed, since several cardiovascular medications are contraindicated during pregnancy. Whenever possible, these medications should be discontinued or should be switched to an alternative which is safe during pregnancy. When medication is indicated, taking the lowest effective dose can be of benefit for both mother and fetus.

It should be noticed that, although some medications are not recommended by the pharmaceutical industry during pregnancy, the benefit to the mother (especially in case of emergency) may outweigh the potential harmful effects for the fetus, and the drug should then not be withheld from the mother [13].

Until December 2014, the US Food and Drug Administration (FDA) classification was widely used to describe the fetal risks of drugs during pregnancy and breastfeeding:

- Category A: Adequate and well-controlled studies have failed to demonstrate a risk to the fetus in the first trimester of pregnancy (and there is no evidence of risk in later trimesters).
- Category B: Animal reproduction studies have failed to demonstrate a risk to the fetus, but there are no adequate and well-controlled studies in pregnant women, or animal reproduction studies have shown an adverse effect that was not confirmed in controlled studies in women.
- Category C: Either animal reproduction studies have shown an adverse effect on the fetus and there are no adequate and well-controlled studies in humans or

studies in women or animals are not available. Potential benefits may warrant the use of the drug in pregnant women despite potential risks.
- Category D: There is positive evidence of human fetal risk based on adverse reaction data from investigational or marketing experience or studies in humans, but potential benefits may warrant the use of the drug in pregnant women despite potential risks.
- Category X: Studies in animals or humans have demonstrated fetal abnormalities and/or there is positive evidence of human fetal risk based on adverse reaction data from investigational or marketing experience, and the risks involved in the use of the drug in pregnant women clearly outweigh potential benefits.

Because there were major concerns with this classification, it has been replaced by a narrative summary on the risk of each drug during pregnancy and lactation, together with a discussion of the available data. However, in the literature and in the current guidelines, the FDA classification is still widely used. Large databases are available on the Internet, where recommendations for a specific drug can be found (www.embryotox.de; www.safefetus.com; www.lareb.nl).

3.6.1 Beta-Blockers

Beta-blockers are important drugs to modify pregnancy-associated risk of cardiovascular complications (i.e., risk of arrhythmia, prevention of aortic dissection in patients with Marfan syndrome) [13]. They constitute two thirds of the cardiac medication used during pregnancy [43]. A large meta-analysis concluded that there is no increased risk of major congenital anomalies associated with beta-blocker use during the first trimester [57]. However, organ-specific analyses showed a possible small increased risk of cardiovascular defects, cleft lip/palate, and neural tube defects. Various studies indicated an association between the usage of beta-blockers and fetal growth restriction though causality is uncertain [11, 33, 35, 43]. However, beta-blockers should only be discontinued if fetal risk outweighs maternal benefit. Given the wide experience with labetalol and metoprolol during pregnancy, these are preferred, and changing to these medications should be considered before pregnancy. It should be noted that beta-blockers have been associated with hypoglycemia, bradycardia, and hypotension in the neonate; therefore, close observation of neonates exposed to beta-blockers is necessary postpartum.

3.6.2 Angiotensin-Converting Enzyme (ACE) Inhibitors/ Angiotensin Receptor Blockers (ARBs)

ACE inhibitors and ARBs are teratogenic and therefore contraindicated during pregnancy [13]. In women using these drugs, it is wise to introduce an evaluation period before pregnancy without the drugs, in order to see the effect on cardiac function when the patient is not pregnant. If cardiac function remains stable after cessation of the drug (and left ventricular ejection fraction >30%), pregnancy can be pursued, but close follow-up of cardiac function is warranted.

3.6.3 Antiarrhythmic Agents

ESC guidelines state that beta-blockers and digoxin are the preferred choice for the treatment of arrhythmias [13]. Women who use digoxin can continue this during pregnancy since it is safe for the fetus, though it is less effective during strenuous exercise (as pregnancy is considered to be), and dosing can be difficult because of altered pharmacokinetics during pregnancy. Procainamide is safe during pregnancy and no teratogenic effects were reported for flecainide. However, switching to beta-blockers should be considered for women using these drugs. Sotalol has similar concerns for the fetus as other beta-blockers but can be used during pregnancy when necessary.

Amiodarone can cause neonatal hypothyroidism and should be discontinued before pregnancy or switched to one of the drugs considered safe during pregnancy. New antiarrhythmic drugs, such as dronedarone, should not be used in women who pursue pregnancy.

3.6.4 Calcium Channel Blockers

Diltiazem has been demonstrated to be teratogenic in animals; therefore, its use during pregnancy is not recommended [13]. Verapamil does not seem to be associated with congenital anomalies and can be used during pregnancy and is recommended as second-line drug (after beta-blockers) for rate control in atrial fibrillation [13]. Nifedipine can be used during pregnancy.

3.6.5 Diuretics and Aldosterone Antagonists

Furosemide and hydrochlorothiazide are not associated with congenital anomalies but can cause oligohydramnios and underperfusion of the placenta. Therefore, they should not be used during pregnancy unless used to treat acute heart failure in the pregnant patient [13]. Spironolactone has been associated with feminization of male rats and should be discontinued before pregnancy. Data for eplerenone are lacking.

3.6.6 Platelet Aggregation Inhibitors

For low-dose acetylsalicylic acid (<100 mg daily), no teratogenic effects have been reported, and it is considered safe during pregnancy. Clopidogrel did not show any teratogenic effects in animal studies, but data in humans are lacking. Clopidogrel should only be used when strictly indicated (i.e., after stent implantation) and for a shortest period as possible [13]. The use of other platelet aggregation inhibitors is not recommended [13].

3.6.7 Statins

Statins should be discontinued before pregnancy, although the risk appears low [4, 15]. Their safety has not been proven, and maternal negative effects due to its cessation are unlikely during the short period of interruption of therapy for pregnancy [13, 19].

3.6.8 Pulmonary Hypertension Agents

Pulmonary hypertension constitutes a contraindication for pregnancy; therefore, for all drugs used for pulmonary arterial hypertension, only limited data are available. Because of teratogenic effects that have been shown in animal studies, endothelin receptor antagonists (i.e., bosentan, ambrisentan) are contraindicated during pregnancy and are usually discontinued. For the use of epoprostenol, sildenafil, and treprostinil during pregnancy, only limited data are available, but they are preferred over endothelin receptor antagonists [13]. Recent evidence suggests that the use of these medications contributes to reduced mortality in the mother, and their use is advisable in women who choose to continue their pregnancy, after careful counseling of these patients about advantages and disadvantages.

3.6.9 Anticoagulation and Mechanical Valve Prosthesis

Women with mechanical valves on oral anticoagulation medication are of special concern. Because of the hypercoagulable state of pregnancy, the risk of "potentially life-threatening" valve thrombosis is increased. Further, the risk of adverse obstetric outcomes (such as hemorrhage and preterm labor) is increased, as well as adverse offspring events, including miscarriage, neonatal death, and fetal growth restriction [27, 55]. Therefore, preconception counseling about the importance of precise anticoagulation is essential.

In general, three regimens have been widely used:

- Vitamin K antagonist throughout pregnancy
- Unfractionated heparin/low-molecular-weight heparin (LMWH) during the first 12 weeks of gestation and, for 13–36 weeks, vitamin K antagonist
- Unfractionated heparin/LMWH throughout pregnancy

There is no ideal anticoagulation regimen, as every approach has inherent risks and benefits for both mother and fetus [31, 55]. Warfarin and other vitamin K antagonists cross the placental barrier and are associated with embryopathy, late pregnancy loss, and stillbirth [18]. However, several of these effects appear dose dependent, where daily dosage <5 mg warfarin was associated with lower risk of some of the fetal complications [18, 20, 56]. Heparins, on the other hand, do not cross the placenta and therefore do not put the fetus at risk of embryopathy/fetopathy. However, unfractionated and low-molecular-weight heparins are both associated with increased risk of valve thrombosis when compared to treatment with warfarin [3, 7, 32]. Because of this, dosage regimens with unfractionated heparin or LMWH require close monitoring of activated partial thromboplastin time or peak and possibly also through antifactor Xa levels, respectively, to assure an adequate level of anticoagulation [16].

The choice of the regimen depends on patient's preference, expected therapeutic adherence, doctors' experience, and the availability of monitoring facilities and can only be made by the mother-to-be after careful counseling by an experienced cardiologist.

Both ESC and American Heart Association/American College of Cardiology (AHA/ACC) guidelines state that continuation of oral anticoagulation throughout pregnancy should be considered in women taking a daily dose of warfarin <5 mg (phenprocoumon <3 mg or acenocoumarol <2 mg) [13]. In patients taking higher daily doses or not willing to continue oral anticoagulation during the first trimester, a switch to unfractionated heparin or LMWH between the 6th and 12th weeks of pregnancy (under strict dose control) should be considered [13, 36].

Both guidelines explicitly do not recommend usage of any kind of heparin (unfractionated or LMWH) throughout pregnancy, because of the increased risk of valve thrombosis with these regimens in combination with the relatively low fetal risk of vitamin K antagonist in the second and third trimester of pregnancy [13, 36]. The new anticoagulants, such as dabigatran and rivaroxaban, should be avoided during pregnancy since they have shown to be teratogenic in animal studies [26].

3.6.10 Devices

Some women with congenital heart disease wear an implantable cardioverter defibrillator (ICD). Several studies, however, with small populations, indicate that pregnancy had no effect on ICD operation, and no evidence was found to link the presence of an ICD with adverse pregnancy outcome [5, 34]. Women with an ICD and on beta-blocker therapy should continue the drug, as the benefits outweigh the fetal risk. Additional caution might be required during the postpartum period, since one study showed that ICD therapy was mainly necessary in the postpartum period [34].

References

1. Balci A, Sollie-Szarynska KM, van der Bijl AG et al (2014) Prospective validation and assessment of cardiovascular and offspring risk models for pregnant women with congenital heart disease. Heart 100(17):1373–1381. doi:10.1136/heartjnl-2014-305597
2. Balint OH, Siu SC, Mason J et al (2010) Cardiac outcomes after pregnancy in women with congenital heart disease. Heart 96(20):1656–1661. doi:10.1136/hrt.2010.202838
3. Basude S, Hein C, Curtis SL et al (2012) Low-molecular-weight heparin or warfarin for anticoagulation in pregnant women with mechanical heart valves: what are the risks? A retrospective observational study. BJOG 119(8):1008–1013. doi:10.1111/j.1471-0528.2012.03359.x; discussion 1012–1013
4. Bateman BT, Hernandez-Diaz S, Fischer MA et al (2015) Statins and congenital malformations: cohort study. BMJ 350:h1035. doi:10.1136/bmj.h1035
5. Boule S, Ovart L, Marquie C et al (2014) Pregnancy in women with an implantable cardioverter-defibrillator: is it safe? Europace 16(11):1587–1594. doi:10.1093/europace/euu036
6. Bowater SE, Selman TJ, Hudsmith LE et al (2013) Long-term outcome following pregnancy in women with a systemic right ventricle: is the deterioration due to pregnancy or a consequence of time? Congenit Heart Dis 8(4):302–307. doi:10.1111/chd.12001
7. Chan WS, Anand S, Ginsberg JS (2000) Anticoagulation of pregnant women with mechanical heart valves: a systematic review of the literature. Arch Intern Med 160(2):191–196
8. Drenthen W, Boersma E, Balci A et al (2010) Predictors of pregnancy complications in women with congenital heart disease. Eur Heart J 31(17):2124–2132. doi:10.1093/eurheartj/ehq200
9. Drenthen W, Pieper PG, Roos-Hesselink JW et al (2007) Outcome of pregnancy in women with congenital heart disease: a literature review. J Am Coll Cardiol 49(24):2303–2311. doi:10.1016/j.jacc.2007.03.027
10. Egidy Assenza G, Cassater D, Landzberg M et al (2013) The effects of pregnancy on right ventricular remodeling in women with repaired tetralogy of Fallot. Int J Cardiol 168(3):1847–1852. doi:10.1016/j.ijcard.2012.12.071
11. Ersboll AS, Hedegaard M, Sondergaard L et al (2014) Treatment with oral beta-blockers during pregnancy complicated by maternal heart disease increases the risk of fetal growth restriction. BJOG 121(5):618–626. doi:10.1111/1471-0528.12522
12. Estensen ME, Beitnes JO, Grindheim G et al (2013) Altered maternal left ventricular contractility and function during normal pregnancy. Ultrasound Obstet Gynecol 41(6):659–666. doi:10.1002/uog.12296
13. European Society of Gynecology, Association for European Paediatric Cardiology, German Society for Gender Medicine et al (2011) ESC Guidelines on the management of cardiovascular diseases during pregnancy: the Task Force on the Management of Cardiovascular Diseases during Pregnancy of the European Society of Cardiology (ESC). Eur Heart J 32(24):3147–3197. doi:10.1093/eurheartj/ehr218
14. European Surveillance of Congenital Anomalies (EUROCAT) Working Group (2011). http://www.eurocat-network.eu/accessprevalencedata/prevalencetables. Accessed 14 Mar 2012.
15. Godfrey LM, Erramouspe J, Cleveland KW (2012) Teratogenic risk of statins in pregnancy. Ann Pharmacother 46(10):1419–1424. doi:10.1345/aph.1R202
16. Goland S, Schwartzenberg S, Fan J et al (2014) Monitoring of anti-Xa in pregnant patients with mechanical prosthetic valves receiving low-molecular-weight heparin: peak or trough levels? J Cardiovasc Pharmacol Ther 19(5):451–456. doi:10.1177/1074248414524302
17. Guedes A, Mercier LA, Leduc L et al (2004) Impact of pregnancy on the systemic right ventricle after a Mustard operation for transposition of the great arteries. J Am Coll Cardiol 44(2):433–437. doi:10.1016/j.jacc.2004.04.037
18. Hall JG, Pauli RM, Wilson KM (1980) Maternal and fetal sequelae of anticoagulation during pregnancy. Am J Med 68(1):122–140. doi:0002-9343(80)90181-3 [pii]

19. Haramburu F, Daveluy A, Miremont-Salame G (2015) Statins in pregnancy: new safety data are reassuring, but suspension of treatment is still advisable. BMJ 350:h1484. doi:10.1136/bmj.h1484
20. Hassouna A, Allam H (2014) Limited dose warfarin throughout pregnancy in patients with mechanical heart valve prosthesis: a meta-analysis. Interact Cardiovasc Thorac Surg 18(6):797–806. doi:10.1093/icvts/ivu009
21. Hunter S, Robson SC (1992) Adaptation of the maternal heart in pregnancy. Br Heart J 68(6):540–543
22. Jastrow N, Meyer P, Khairy P et al (2011) Prediction of complications in pregnant women with cardiac diseases referred to a tertiary center. Int J Cardiol 151(2):209–213. doi:10.1016/j.ijcard.2010.05.045
23. Kampman MA, Balci A, Groen H et al (2015) Cardiac function and cardiac events 1-year postpartum in women with congenital heart disease. Am Heart J 169(2):298–304. doi:10.1016/j.ahj.2014.11.010
24. Kampman MA, Balci A, van Veldhuisen DJ et al (2014) N-terminal pro-B-type natriuretic peptide predicts cardiovascular complications in pregnant women with congenital heart disease. Eur Heart J 35(11):708–715. doi:10.1093/eurheartj/eht526
25. Khairy P, Ouyang DW, Fernandes SM et al (2006) Pregnancy outcomes in women with congenital heart disease. Circulation 113(4):517–524. doi:10.1161/CIRCULATIONAHA.105.589655
26. Konigsbrugge O, Langer M, Hayde M et al (2014) Oral anticoagulation with rivaroxaban during pregnancy: a case report. Thromb Haemost 112(6):1323–1324. doi:10.1160/TH14-04-0393
27. Lawley CM, Lain SJ, Algert CS et al (2015) Prosthetic heart valves in pregnancy, outcomes for women and their babies: a systematic review and meta-analysis. BJOG. doi:10.1111/1471-0528.13491
28. Lu CW, Shih JC, Chen SY et al (2015) Comparison of 3 risk estimation methods for predicting cardiac outcomes in pregnant women with congenital heart disease. Circ J 79(7):1609–1617. doi:10.1253/circj.CJ-14-1368
29. Lui GK, Silversides CK, Khairy P et al (2011) Heart rate response during exercise and pregnancy outcome in women with congenital heart disease. Circulation 123(3):242–248. doi:10.1161/CIRCULATIONAHA.110.953380
30. Marelli AJ, Ionescu-Ittu R, Mackie AS et al (2014) Lifetime prevalence of congenital heart disease in the general population from 2000 to 2010. Circulation 130(9):749–756. doi:10.1161/CIRCULATIONAHA.113.008396
31. McLintock C (2013) Anticoagulant choices in pregnant women with mechanical heart valves: balancing maternal and fetal risks – the difference the dose makes. Thromb Res 131(Suppl 1):S8–S10. doi:10.1016/S0049-3848(13)70010-0
32. McLintock C, McCowan LM, North RA (2009) Maternal complications and pregnancy outcome in women with mechanical prosthetic heart valves treated with enoxaparin. BJOG 116(12):1585–1592. doi:10.1111/j.1471-0528.2009.02299.x
33. Meidahl Petersen K, Jimenez-Solem E, Andersen JT et al (2012) beta-Blocker treatment during pregnancy and adverse pregnancy outcomes: a nationwide population-based cohort study. BMJ Open 2(4):10.1136/bmjopen-2012-001185. Print 2012. doi:10.1136/bmjopen-2012-001185 [doi]
34. Miyoshi T, Kamiya CA, Katsuragi S et al (2013) Safety and efficacy of implantable cardioverter-defibrillator during pregnancy and after delivery. Circ J 77(5):1166–1170. doi:DN/JST.JSTAGE/circj/CJ-12-1275 [pii]
35. Nakhai-Pour HR, Rey E, Berard A (2010) Antihypertensive medication use during pregnancy and the risk of major congenital malformations or small-for-gestational-age newborns. Birth Defects Res B Dev Reprod Toxicol 89(2):147–154. doi:10.1002/bdrb.20238
36. Nishimura RA, Otto CM, Bonow RO et al (2014) 2014 AHA/ACC guideline for the management of patients with valvular heart disease: a report of the American College of Cardiology/American Heart Association Task Force on Practice Guidelines. Circulation 129(23):e521–e643. doi:10.1161/CIR.0000000000000031
37. Ohuchi H, Tanabe Y, Kamiya C et al (2013) Cardiopulmonary variables during exercise predict pregnancy outcome in women with congenital heart disease. Circ J 77(2):470–476, doi:DN/JST.JSTAGE/circj/CJ-12-0485

38. Pijuan-Domenech A, Galian L, Goya M et al (2015) Cardiac complications during pregnancy are better predicted with the modified WHO risk score. Int J Cardiol 195:149–154. doi:10.1016/j.ijcard.2015.05.076
39. Robson SC, Dunlop W, Boys RJ et al (1987) Cardiac output during labour. Br Med J (Clin Res Ed) 295(6607):1169–1172
40. Robson SC, Dunlop W, Hunter S (1987) Haemodynamic changes during the early puerperium. Br Med J (Clin Res Ed) 294(6579):1065
41. Robson SC, Hunter S, Boys RJ et al (1989) Serial study of factors influencing changes in cardiac output during human pregnancy. Am J Physiol 256(4 Pt 2):H1060–H1065
42. Roos-Hesselink JW, Ruys TP, Stein JI et al (2013) Outcome of pregnancy in patients with structural or ischaemic heart disease: results of a registry of the European Society of Cardiology. Eur Heart J 34(9):657–665. doi:10.1093/eurheartj/ehs270
43. Ruys TP, Maggioni A, Johnson MR et al (2014) Cardiac medication during pregnancy, data from the ROPAC. Int J Cardiol 177(1):124–128. doi:10.1016/j.ijcard.2014.09.013
44. Ruys TP, Roos-Hesselink JW, Hall R et al (2014) Heart failure in pregnant women with cardiac disease: data from the ROPAC. Heart 100(3):231–238. doi:10.1136/heartjnl-2013-304888
45. Savu O, Jurcut R, Giusca S et al (2012) Morphological and functional adaptation of the maternal heart during pregnancy. Circ Cardiovasc Imaging 5(3):289–297. doi:10.1161/CIRCIMAGING.111.970012
46. Siu SC, Colman JM, Sorensen S et al (2002) Adverse neonatal and cardiac outcomes are more common in pregnant women with cardiac disease. Circulation 105(18):2179–2184
47. Siu SC, Sermer M, Colman JM et al (2001) Prospective multicenter study of pregnancy outcomes in women with heart disease. Circulation 104(5):515–521
48. Song YB, Park SW, Kim JH et al (2008) Outcomes of pregnancy in women with congenital heart disease: a single center experience in Korea. J Korean Med Sci 23(5):808–813. doi:10.3346/jkms.2008.23.5.808
49. Tanous D, Siu SC, Mason J et al (2010) B-type natriuretic peptide in pregnant women with heart disease. J Am Coll Cardiol 56(15):1247–1253. doi:10.1016/j.jacc.2010.02.076
50. Tateno S, Niwa K, Nakazawa M et al (2003) Arrhythmia and conduction disturbances in patients with congenital heart disease during pregnancy: multicenter study. Circ J 67(12):992–997
51. Thorne S, MacGregor A, Nelson-Piercy C (2006) Risks of contraception and pregnancy in heart disease. Heart 92(10):1520–1525. doi:10.1136/hrt.2006.095240
52. Tzemos N, Silversides CK, Colman JM et al (2009) Late cardiac outcomes after pregnancy in women with congenital aortic stenosis. Am Heart J 157(3):474–480. doi:10.1016/j.ahj.2008.10.020
53. Uebing A, Arvanitis P, Li W et al (2010) Effect of pregnancy on clinical status and ventricular function in women with heart disease. Int J Cardiol 139(1):50–59. doi:10.1016/j.ijcard.2008.09.001
54. van der Linde D, Konings EE, Slager MA et al (2011) Birth prevalence of congenital heart disease worldwide: a systematic review and meta-analysis. J Am Coll Cardiol 58(21):2241–2247. doi:10.1016/j.jacc.2011.08.025
55. van Hagen IM, Roos-Hesselink JW, Ruys TP et al (2015) Pregnancy in women with a mechanical heart valve: data of the European Society of Cardiology Registry of Pregnancy and Cardiac Disease (ROPAC). Circulation 132(2):132–142. doi:10.1161/CIRCULATIONAHA.115.015242
56. Vitale N, De Feo M, De Santo LS et al (1999) Dose-dependent fetal complications of warfarin in pregnant women with mechanical heart valves. J Am Coll Cardiol 33(6):1637–1641. doi:S0735-1097(99)00044-3 [pii]
57. Yakoob MY, Bateman BT, Ho E et al (2013) The risk of congenital malformations associated with exposure to beta-blockers early in pregnancy: a meta-analysis. Hypertension 62(2):375–381. doi:10.1161/HYPERTENSIONAHA.111.00833

Inheritance of Congenital Heart Disease

Ingrid van de Laar and Marja Wessels

Abbreviations

AS	Aortic valve stenosis
ASD	Atrial septal defect
AVSD	Atrioventricular septal defects
BAV	Bicuspid aortic valve
CGH	Comparative genomic hybridization
CHD	Congenital heart disease
CNVs	Copy number variations
DORV	Double outlet right ventricle
HLHS	Hypoplastic left heart syndrome
LVOTO	Left ventricular outflow tract obstruction
NGS	Next-generation sequencing
PDA	Patent ductus arteriosus
PTA	Persistent truncus arteriosus
SNP	Single-nucleotide polymorphism
TGA	Transposition of great arteries
TOF	Tetralogy of Fallot
VSD	Ventricular septal defects
VUS	Variants of unknown significance
WES	Whole exome sequencing

I. van de Laar, MD, PhD (✉) • M. Wessels, MD, PhD
Department of Clinical Genetics, Erasmus MC, University Medical Center,
's-Gravendijkwal 230, Rotterdam 301 CE, The Netherlands
e-mail: i.vandelaar@erasmusmc.nl

4.1 Introduction

For adult patients with congenital heart disease (CHD), knowledge about the origin and inheritance of their disease and the recurrence risk in (future) offspring is important for several reasons. First, knowledge about the recurrence risk is essential to make informed choices regarding family planning and prenatal screening. While the background risk for CHD in offspring is 0.8 %, the overall risk for babies born to mothers with CHD is in general higher, at about 5–6 %, and disease-specific inheritance risks are available [1, 2]. If CHD is part of a syndrome, the recurrence risks can be as high as 25–50 %. Secondly, in syndromic cases the patient and his or her offspring may be at risk for extracardiac manifestations that may require additional screening and treatment. Third of all, there may be other relatives for whom genetic or cardiologic examination may be appropriate [3]. Therefore, clinical genetic counseling should be part of the multidisciplinary preconception counseling of all women with a CHD who are in the reproductive age. The added value of clinical genetic consultation has been shown by van Engelen et al. who revealed that less than half of the adults with CHD estimated the recurrence risk in a correct range of magnitude [4]. Genetic consultation improves diagnostics by establishing an etiological diagnosis and associated recurrence risk in a substantial proportion of patients and leads to more informed reproductive decisions [5].

In this chapter, we will summarize the genetic and nongenetic causes of CHD and focus on the recurrence risk for a live-born offspring of adults with CHD. In general, both males and females with CHD have a significantly reduced reproductive fitness, e.g., fewer total offspring and more childlessness, as compared to adults without CHD. Not surprisingly, this is even more true for CHD patients with extracardiac manifestations. There is also an increased risk of miscarriage as compared to the normal population [2, 6]. Some of these miscarriages could be due to cardiac disease in the fetus, but this usually remains unclear since generally no pathological examinations are performed of these aborted fetuses.

4.2 Classification and Genetics

Most commonly, CHD occurs as an isolated finding in an otherwise healthy person. Additional noncardiac malformations are present in about a quarter of patients with CHD [7]. CHD can occur as part of many (submicroscopic) chromosomal abnormalities or copy number variations (CNVs) and specific syndromes or as a consequence of teratogenic exposure. The majority of CHD is thought to be due to complex inheritance, involving a multitude of mutations in susceptibility genes superposed on unfavorable environmental and lifestyle factors. In the past decade, tremendous progress has been made in the elucidation of the molecular mechanisms involved in CHD by new technologies that have become available and new insight by alternative inheritance paradigms. Several CHDs have recently been shown to result from de novo genetic aberrations [8]. Epigenetic factors, including imprinting and chromatin remodeling, also play a role in the heart development [8, 9]. Despite of all this progress, many genetic factors contributing to CHD and their interaction with environmental factors are still to be discovered. Also, the relative importance of many DNA alterations (common variants, rare variants, copy number variations (CNVs), de novo mutations) in various known genetic factors remains to be defined.

To establish a recurrence risk for the affected parent, it is essential to determine whether the CHD is:

(a) Non-syndromic (or isolated)
(b) Non-syndromic, but with a family history of CHD
(c) Syndromic
(d) Chromosomal
(e) Due to teratogenic exposure or maternal illnesses

Clinical history, family history, and assessment of dysmorphic features suggestive of a chromosomal or syndromic CHD are essential to discriminate between these different subgroups.

4.2.1 Non-syndromic CHD

Most cases of non-syndromic CHD occur sporadically, and families with clear monogenic inheritance of non-syndromic CHD are scarce. Over the past years, genetic studies in both human patients and animal models have led to the identification of a significant number of genes that are implicated in non-syndromic CHD [10, 11]. The first monogenetic causes of CHD were found by linkage studies in families with clear autosomal dominant inheritance of CHD [12, 13].

By using new DNA techniques such as whole exome sequencing, it was found that damaging de novo gene mutations in genes mainly involved in chromatin remodeling may contribute to approximately 10% of severe non-syndromic CHDs. These de novo mutations occur during the formation of egg or sperm cells or early in embryonic development. As these de novo mutations were found in patients with severe and lethal CHD, it is not yet known what proportion of CHD in patients that reach adulthood or childbearing age are due to de novo mutations. It is thought that the majority of non-syndromic, nonfamilial CHD cannot be explained by a single-gene defect, and interacting genetic and nongenetic (environmental) factors may contribute in these cases. This is also referred to as multifactorial inheritance. Whereas recurrence risks can be given with confidence for CHD caused by single-gene mutations (see below), establishing recurrence risk in multifactorial diseases is more complicated. This is because the number of genes contributing to the disease is usually not known and the extent of environmental effects can vary substantially.

For this large group of non-syndromic CHD, empiric recurrence risk is still used to predict the individual risk of CHD in offspring. In Table 4.1, empiric recurrence risks for different types of CHD in offspring of both males and females are summarized. It is of note that the studies used to establish these risks have limitations: First, most studies have focused on the recurrence risk of CHD in siblings, and data

Table 4.1 Recurrence risks for offspring of a father or mother with different types of CHD

Type of CHD	Father with CHD		Mother with CHD	
	Recurrence risk for offspring (%)	Affected births/ live births among offspring	Recurrence risk for offspring (%)	Affected births/ live births among offspring
TOF				
Chin-Yee et al. [14]	3.4	6/179	6.3	11/174
Burn et al. [15]	1.6	2/124	4.5	6/132
Nora [16]	1.5		2.5	
Drenthen et al. [2]			3	6/202
APVC				
Burn et al. [15]	0	0/10	5.9	1/17
Abnl connection				
Burn et al. [15]	4.5	1/22	5.9	1/17
TGA				
Burn et al. [15]	0	0/14	0	0/6
Drenthen et al. [2]			0.6	1/176
ccTGA (l-TGA)				
Therrien et al. [17]			3.7	1/27
Drenthen et al. [2]			3.6	1/28
AVSD				
Burn et al. [15]	7.7	1/13	7.9	3/38
Nora [16]	1		14	
Drenthen et al. [2]			8	7/88
AS				
Nora [16]	5		18	
Driscoll et al. [18]	1.2	3/251	1.4	1/72
Drenthen et al. [2]			4.1	5/121
PS				
Nora [16]	2		6	
Driscoll et al. [18]	1.7	3/176	3.9	8/205
Drenthen et al. [2]			2.8	3/164
ASD II				
Nora [16]	1.5		6	
Drenthen et al. [2]			2.1	6/291
VSD				
Nora [16]	2.5		9.5	
Driscoll et al. [18]			2.7	2/74
Drenthen et al. [2]	3	10/334	2.9	11/384
CoA				
Nora [16]	2.5		4	
Drenthen et al. [2]			4	10/251
Ebstein				
Drenthen et al. [2]			4	5/126

Data from Refs. [2, 14–18]

on recurrence risk in offspring of affected parents are scarce. Secondly, most papers on this topic originate from the previous century, before many monogenic causes and copy number variants were discovered, and little recent studies are available [19]. Third of all, there are marked limitations of these studies since they are generally based on small numbers of probands and their offspring, and there is a considerable selection bias due to variations in survival patterns of different types of CHD and selective referral of more severely affected patients to tertiary care centers. The last reason that makes the recurrence risk number difficult to interpret is that miscarriage and abortion pregnancies are usually excluded which may result in an underestimation of the recurrence rate.

In general, it is stated that mothers with a CHD have a greater risk of CHD in the offspring than fathers (Table 4.1). The ratio for affected offspring born to affected mothers versus those born to affected fathers is about 2:5. In a national cohort study based on a Swedish population registry, it was even stated that men with both complex and simple CHD did not have an increased risk of having children with a CHD [20]. However, this was not supported by other studies [16, 18]. The excess of malformations in the offspring of affected women might be explained by the recognition that some of the key genes in cardiac development are imprinted. A maternal copy of the gene is necessary for normal heart formation, and therefore a deleterious allele of maternal origin would have a greater effect than those of paternal origin.

4.2.1.1 Diagnostics in Non-syndromic CHD

Traditional genetic testing involved Sanger sequencing of a number of genes in a stepwise manner to try to identify the causal mutation. Currently, many genetic laboratories have introduced next-generation sequencing (NGS) into service, which changed the whole field of genetics. With NGS, or massive parallel sequencing, millions of small DNA fragments can be sequenced at the same time, creating a massive pool of data. Bioinformatic analyses are used to piece together these fragments by mapping the individual reads to the human reference genome providing accurate data on DNA variation. NGS can be used to sequence all 22,000 coding genes (whole exome) or targeted to small numbers of individual genes (panels).

The contribution of the known CHD genes in adults with non-syndromic CHD without a family history of CHD is small. In some countries, target NGS of a panel of genes involved in CHD or whole exome sequencing (WES) is available. However, its usefulness is a matter of debate since many variants of unknown significance (VUS) will be found, and, in the absence of other affected family members, it is challenging to assign causality with certainty to the found variants. The use of a targeted NGS panel for genes involved in CHD might, at this point, be most useful when a monogenetic cause is suspected, for instance, in the case of parental consanguinity or familial CHD [21, 22]. Parental consanguinity is associated with a two- to threefold increased offspring risk of CHD. This is most likely due to the shared genetic variants among parents fitting autosomal recessive inheritance [23, 24].

Traditional G-banding karyotyping has been widely used to look for large (3–5 Mb) deletions or duplications of the genome (copy number variations, CNV) in CHD patients. This technique is gradually being replaced by techniques with higher-resolution, chromosomal microarray testing. Several chromosomal microarray platforms can be used for genome-wide CNV detection, including comparative genomic hybridization (CGH) arrays and single-nucleotide polymorphism (SNP) arrays. The resolution of these platforms has increased tremendously in the past year to up to 5–10 Kb. With these new techniques, smaller deletions and duplications can be found that may be pathogenic, also in isolated CHD cases.

Although the yield of chromosomal microarray testing is higher in patients with CHD and extracardiac anomalies, detection of CNVs by microarray testing can be considered in all adults with non-syndromic CHD. The diagnostic yield for non-syndromic CHD is around 4 % [25, 26]. Some chromosomal microarray platforms can also reveal regions of homozygosity, which might lead to the causal recessive gene underlying the heart defect.

In order to estimate the recurrence risk in offspring of a CHD patient, it might be useful to perform cardiac screening in family members. This is particularly true for left ventricular outflow tract obstructions (LVOTOs), ranging from bicuspid aortic valve to hypoplastic left heart syndrome. LVOTOs have been recognized as a group of CHDs with "high heritability" [27, 28]. Therefore, it is advised to perform cardiac screening of first-degree relatives (parents, siblings, and children) of patients with LVOTO in order to better estimate the recurrence risk in offspring [29].

4.2.2 Non-syndromic CHD with a Significant Family History of CHD

In familial non-syndromic CHD, the inheritance pattern can be autosomal dominant, autosomal recessive, or X-linked recessive. A person affected by an autosomal dominant condition has a 50 % chance of passing the mutated gene to each child. The chance that a child will not inherit the mutated gene is also 50 %. In families with autosomal dominant inheritance of CHD, reduced penetrance and variable expression of CHD are observed. Reduced (or incomplete) penetrance refers to the proportion of persons who are carrier of a mutation in a specific gene that do not exhibit signs and symptoms of the genetic disorder. Variable expressivity refers to the range of signs and symptoms that can occur in different patients with the same genetic condition. In autosomal recessive inheritance, a mutation in both copies of a gene must be present in order for the disease to develop. Someone who has a mutation in one copy of the gene (but no symptoms) is called a carrier. X-linked recessive diseases usually occur in males and are caused by a mutation in a single-recessive gene on the X chromosome. Mothers can be carriers of the disease and may be mildly affected.

In the following paragraphs, we will summarize a subset of genes involved in non-syndromic familial CHD, categorized in different subgroups of CHD. This list is incomplete since new CHD genes are identified in a rapid pace. A nice recent review of all non-syndromic and syndromic genes involved in CHD is given by Lalani et al. [11].

Septal Defects

The first single-gene mutation causing non-syndromic CHD was described in the transcription factor gene *NKX2.5* in families with inherited atrial septal defect (ASD) and atrioventricular block [12]. Subsequently, mutations in *GATA4* were found in two kindreds with apparent non-syndromic septal defects [13]. Mutations in the T-box gene *TBX20* have been implicated in cardiomyopathy and septal defects [30]. Recently, deleterious variants in *MESP1* were identified in patients with ventricular septal defects (VSD) or tetralogy of Fallot (TOF) [31]. Missense mutations in CRELD1 are found in nearly 6% of isolated atrioventricular septal defects (AVSD) and AVSD associated with heterotaxy syndrome [32]. Septal defects are also caused by mutations in several genes encoding for sarcomeric proteins like *ACTC1*, *MYH6*, *MYH7*, and *MYBPC3* [33].

Left Ventricular Outflow Tract Obstruction (LVOTO)

In familial left ventricular outflow tract obstruction (LVOTO), including aortic valve stenosis (AS), bicuspid aortic valve (BAV), coarctation of the aorta (CoA), and hypoplastic left heart syndrome (HLHS), Garg et al. initially described the first pathogenic mutations in the *NOTCH1* gene [34]. In the past years, a limited number of NOTCH1 mutations were published in several small cohorts of LVOTO patients. Recently, a large cohort of 428 LVOTO patients was screened for *NOTCH1*. Pathogenic mutations in *NOTCH1* occur in 1% of sporadic LVOTO and in 7% of familial LVOTO patients [35]. Reduced penetrance occurs in many non-syndromic CHD families, as is exemplified by families with *NOTCH1* gene mutations; cardiovascular malformations are found in 75% of *NOTCH1* mutation carriers. Also marked variable expressivity is seen in the *NOTCH1* families described by Kerstjens et al. as the spectrum of disease does not only involve left-sided heart defects but also right-sided heart defects affecting the pulmonary valve, conotruncal disease including pulmonary atresia, Fallot's tetralogy and truncus arteriosus, thoracic aortic aneurysm, and other CHDs, such as anomalous pulmonary venous return, ASD, and VSD [35].

Other genes involved in non-syndromic LVOTO are *GJA1*, *NKX2.5*, *GATA5*, *SMAD6*, *MYH6*, *GATA4*, *GATA6*, and *MEF2C*, but the number of patients with mutations in these genes is low indicating that many genes need to be discovered [36].

Conotruncal Defects

Homozygous deleterious mutations in the *NKX2.6* gene have been associated with persistent truncus arteriosus (PTA) and might be accompanied by an absent thymus [37]. Also, mutations in *GATA6* have been reported in PTA and TOF and can be associated with pancreatic agenesis [38]. A minority of patients with TOF have a mutation in the *FOG2* gene [39]. Also, rare mutations in *FOXH1*, *TDGF1*, *GDF1*, and *THRAP2* cause isolated conotruncal defects.

Laterality Defects

Laterality disorders refer to a broad group of disorders caused by the embryonic disruption of normal left-right patterning, including situs inversus totalis and heterotaxy (or situs ambiguus). Situs inversus totalis is the mirror image reversal of all visceral organs including the lungs, spleen, liver, and stomach, whereas heterotaxy is the abnormal orientation of one or more organs along the LR axis. The CHDs common in laterality disorders include atrioventricular septal defects (AVSD), transposition of great arteries (TGA), double outlet right ventricle (DORV), abnormal systemic and/or pulmonary venous connection, abnormal position of the heart (dextrocardia), and isomerism of the atrial appendages. A marked proportion of patients with laterality disorders are born to consanguineous parents. Therefore, it is suggested that laterality disorders are more often than other CHDs characterized by autosomal recessive inheritance [40]. Also, X-linked recessive inheritance is more prevalent in patients with laterality disorders [41]. Recently, recessive mutations in MMP21 were identified in 5.9% of non-syndromic heterotaxy cases [40]. Other recessive genes involved in heterotaxy are CCDC11, WDR16, and GDF1 [42–44].

X-linked recessive inheritance of heterotaxy was first described by Gebbia et al. who detected ZIC3 mutations in familial and sporadic heterotaxy patients [41]. ZIC3 mutations typically result in a variable phenotype ranging from situs abnormalities and heart defects to more syndromic heart defects involving additional midline, gastrointestinal, urogenital, and/or central nervous system anomalies. ZIC3 mutations have also been found in both males (5.2%) and females (1.8%) with isolated non-syndromic heterotaxy spectrum CHD such as TGA [45].

Heterozygous mutations in genes of the NODAL pathway, including *NODAL*, *LEFTY2*, *CFC1*, *TDGF1*, *ACVR2B*, *SESN1*, and *FOXH1* and other cilia-related genes like *NPHP4*, are also involved in cardiac laterality defects [46, 47].

4.2.2.1 Diagnostics in Non-syndromic CHD with a Significant Family History of CHD

In familial non-syndromic CHD, it was shown that massive parallel sequencing of a panel of known cardiac genes increased the diagnostic value. In a cohort of families with non-syndromic CHD, targeted NGS of 57 genes known to be involved in CHD identified likely pathogenic mutations in 31% of the families [21]. Jia et al. found potential causative variants in less than half of the families (46%) by using the same technique [22]. However, even in familial non-syndromic CHD, it remains challenging to interpret the large number of identified variants. A chromosomal microarray is also advised in familial non-syndromic CHD patients since small microdeletions or duplications encompassing CHD genes can be the underlying cause [48].

4.2.3 Syndromic

CHD can occur in many genetic syndromes and have been found to be associated with mutations in a variety of single genes associated with syndromic disease. These monogenic syndromes with CHD are present in about 5% of newborn

Table 4.2 Syndromes to consider in different types of CHD

TOF	22q11 microdeletion syndrome, Alagille syndrome, CHARGE syndrome
Interrupted aortic arch	22q11 microdeletion syndrome
Truncus arteriosus	22q11 microdeletion syndrome
LVOTO	Jacobsen syndrome, Turner syndrome, Kabuki syndrome, Potocki-Lupski syndrome
PS	Noonan syndrome, Mowat-Wilson syndrome
PPS	Alagille syndrome, Williams syndrome
SVAS	Williams syndrome
AVSD	Down syndrome, CHARGE syndrome
VSD	Holt-Oram syndrome
ASD	Holt-Oram syndrome, Noonan syndrome, Wolf-Hirschhorn syndrome
PDA	Char syndrome, Mowat-Wilson syndrome

babies with CHD. For the carer who advises adults with CHD in the preconceptional counseling setting, it is important to be aware of monogenic syndromic conditions that might have very subtle characteristics, as these conditions often have a high recurrence risk in the offspring of the patient. Some recognizable syndromes with CHD as a major feature of the condition are discussed below. In Table 4.2, different types of CHD and associated chromosomal causes and monogenic syndromes are listed.

Noonan syndrome, which is the most frequently observed syndrome in CHD patients, is an autosomal dominant condition caused by mutations in the *PTPN11* gene in approximately 40–60% of patients. Also, other genes in the RAS-MAPK signaling pathway, including *SOS1*, *RAF1*, *KRAS*, *NRAS*, *MEK1/2*, *BRAF*, *CBL*, *SHOC2*, and *RIT1*, can cause Noonan syndrome and Noonan-like phenotypes [49]. CHD is present in about 70–80% of Noonan patients, and the most frequently reported CHDs are pulmonary stenosis with dysplastic leaflets, hypertrophic cardiomyopathy, and secundum atrial septal defects. Some genotype-phenotype correlations have been suggested, especially for cardiac anomalies [50]. Other clinical features include dysmorphic features, short stature, pectus, and cryptorchism. In most affected individuals, intelligence is within the normal range, with intelligence quotient generally varying between 70 and 120.

Mutations in the *TBX5* gene cause Holt-Oram syndrome. Individuals with Holt-Oram syndrome display great phenotypic variability with mild to severe limb defects and various types of CHD, including atrial septal defects, ventricular septal defects (especially muscular), and atrioventricular conduction defects. Congenital heart defects are present in about 75% of Holt-Oram patients. Individuals with Holt-Oram syndrome have a normal intelligence.

Alagille syndrome is a disorder characterized by normal intelligence, liver disease, vertebral anomalies, dysmorphic features, and various types of CHD, including peripheral pulmonary artery stenosis, pulmonary valve stenosis, and tetralogy of Fallot [51]. In approximately 90% of patients, a mutation in the *JAG1* gene is found. *NOTCH2* mutations have been found in a minority of patients with Alagille syndrome.

Char syndrome is characterized by the triad of typical facial features (prominent lips), patent ductus arteriosus (PDA), and aplasia or hypoplasia of the middle phalanges of the fifth fingers. It is caused by mutations in the *TFAP2B* gene. No intellectual disability has been described in Char syndrome.

CHARGE syndrome is an autosomal dominant disorder caused by mutations in the CHD7 gene. CHARGE is an acronym for a set of congenital anomalies commonly encountered in this syndrome. The letters stand for coloboma of the eye, heart defects, atresia of the choanae, retardation of growth and/or development, genital and/or urinary abnormalities, and ear abnormalities and deafness. Those features are no longer used in making a diagnosis of CHARGE syndrome, but the name of the syndrome is not changed. CHD occur in approximately 75 % of patients with molecularly diagnosed CHARGE syndrome, and conotruncal defects and atrioventricular septal defects are overrepresented [52].

Another rare syndrome involved in CHD patients is Kabuki syndrome which is characterized by intellectual disability, peculiar facial gestalt, short stature, skeletal and visceral abnormalities, cardiac anomalies, and immunological defects. It is caused mainly by de novo mutations in the *KMT2D* and rarely by mutations in the X-linked *KDM6A* gene. Approximately 40–50 % of individuals with Kabuki syndrome have CHD. Left-sided heart defects, especially coarctation of the aorta, are strongly associated with Kabuki syndrome. Interestingly, de novo mutations in *KMT2D* genes have also been associated with CHD, as previously mentioned [8].

Mowat-Wilson syndrome is characterized by intellectual disability and distinctive facial features in association with variable structural congenital anomalies including CHD, Hirschsprung disease, hypospadias, agenesis of the corpus callosum, short stature, epilepsy, and microcephaly. Mowat-Wilson syndrome is caused by mutation in the transcription factor ZEB2 [53]. In more than half of the patients, cardiac defects are present which frequently involve the pulmonary arteries and/or valves.

Almost all abovementioned syndromes have an autosomal dominant inheritance pattern with a 50 % risk for offspring. Some syndromes generally occur de novo such as CHARGE, Mowat-Wilson, and Kabuki syndrome, and these patients rarely reproduce. Other syndromes display marked variability and can be encountered more frequently in adults with CHD such as Noonan syndrome.

4.2.4 Chromosomal Defects and Copy Number Variations (CNVs)

4.2.4.1 Numeric Chromosomal Defects

Numeric chromosomal defects are known to be the underlying cause in about 10–12 % of newborn babies with CHD. At adult age, this percentage is lower because many children with chromosomal defects die at a young age. Examples of patients with a numeric chromosomal defect who reach adult age are patients with trisomy 21 (Down syndrome) and monosomy X (Turner syndrome). In Down syndrome, the prevalence of CHD is about 50 %, and the most common defect is a complete atrioventricular septal defect although other lesions like ASD, VSD, PDA, and TOF are also seen [54, 55]. Left-sided CHD is most frequently (about 30%) seen in Turner syndrome (45, X) [56, 57] including bicuspid aortic valve, aortic valve stenosis, and coarctation of the aorta. Several studies of Turner patients have shown aortopathy, including dilatation of the ascending aorta, aortic aneurysms, and aortic dissection, supporting stringent cardiac follow-up for all individuals with Turner syndrome [58, 59].

Most patients with Down or Turner syndrome are not reproductive; however, when a mosaic pattern is present, they might be able to have children. The specific karyotype should be considered when counseling adults with Down or Turner syndrome regarding reproduction and potential risks for offspring [60].

4.2.4.2 Copy Number Variants

With the introduction of chromosomal microarray testing, it became clear that CNVs are overrepresented in patients with both syndromic and non-syndromic CHD [61, 62]. These CNVs vary in size and might contain genes involved in the heart development. They account for approximately 15–20% of all newborn babies with syndromic CHD, but the diagnostic yield varies significantly between syndromic (18%) and non-syndromic CHD patients (4.3%) [26, 63, 64]. Many large CNVs are unique to a single CHD patient, but several are recurrent in CHD cohorts. To date, there are over 40 clinically delineated deletion and duplication syndromes associated with CHD. These CNVs can be classified in three groups: (I) CNVs associated with well-described microdeletion syndromes, (II) CNVs that include genes known to be involved in CHD, and (III) CNVs associated with a wide variety of other phenotypes such as autism or intellectual disability, which may include CHD. This group of CNVs often shows reduced penetrance and might be present in a healthy parent. These CNVs are also called susceptibility loci.

Group I CNVs Associated with Well-Described Microdeletion Syndromes

The most frequent microdeletion syndrome associated with CHD is the 22q11.2 deletion syndrome which is due to a deletion of chromosome band 22q11.2 and leads to haploinsufficiency of more than 30 genes including the transcription factor *TBX1* and *CRKL* gene, both implicated as the cause of CHD in this deletion syndrome [65]. About 75% of individuals with 22q11.2 deletion have a CHD, typically a conotruncal defects such as an interrupted aortic arch, truncus arteriosus, or tetralogy of Fallot. It is advised to perform (targeted) microarray testing for 22q11.2 deletion in all newborns with a conotruncal defect.

Williams syndrome is caused by a deletion of chromosome band 7q11.2 including the elastin gene. Haploinsufficiency of the elastin gene causes CHD in Williams syndrome; most typically, patients have supravalvular aortic stenosis. About half of the affected individuals with Wolf-Hirschhorn syndrome (4p16.3 deletion) have a CHD including ASD, PS, VSD, and PDA. Jacobsen syndrome is a condition that is caused by the deletion of the terminal end of chromosome 11q and is also known as the 11q terminal deletion syndrome. Half of the patients have CHD including ventricular septal defects and left ventricular outflow tract obstructions, particularly hypoplastic left heart syndrome.

More recently described microdeletion/duplication syndromes include Kleefstra syndrome and Potocki-Lupski syndrome. Kleefstra syndrome, which is caused by microdeletion of 9q34.3, leads to EHMT1 disruption. CHD is reported in about 50 % of individuals with this syndrome including ASD, VSD, TOF, CoA, BAV, and pulmonic stenosis [66, 67]. Duplication of the 17p11.2 region leads to Potocki-Lupski syndrome and this often leads to BAV and dilated aortas [68, 69].

Group II CNVs That Include Genes Known to Be Involved in Congenital Heart Disease

The most frequent CNVs associated with CHD are duplications or deletions at chromosome 1q21.1, encompassing the *GJA5* gene, which occur in at least 1 % of reported CHD cases [61]. Deletions of chromosome 8p23.1 are found in CHD patients, and this microdeletion includes the *GATA4* gene, involved mainly in familial septal defects as mentioned previously. Submicroscopic deletions of chromosome 6q24–25 include the *TAB2* gene, which is involved in a variety of CHD [48, 70]. The *NKX2.5* gene is deleted in patients with a deletion of chromosome 5q35 and causes ASD and AV conduction defect.

Group III CNV Susceptibility Loci

An example of a CNV susceptibility locus is the 16p11.2 deletion that includes the region known as the "16p11.2 autism susceptibility locus." CHD is reported occasionally; however, no specific recurrent CHD is observed [71].

Also in patients with CNVs, there is a reduced reproductive fitness. Offspring of patients with a microdeletion or duplication will have a 50 % chance of inheriting the chromosomal abnormality.

4.2.5 Exposures

Exogenic risk factors for CHD have been grouped in maternal illnesses and maternal exposures. Well-established maternal diseases that are known to be associated with CHD include maternal insulin-dependent diabetes, phenylketonuria, and first-trimester rubella infection. Other risk factors might be maternal obesity and age. Maternal use of retinoic acid in also a well-established risk factor but also the use of alcohol, cigarettes, amphetamines, anticonvulsive drugs, hormones, lithium, and some selective serotonin reuptake inhibitors increases the risk of having a child with CHD. Some of these risk factors are a good target for intervention, and cessation of the risk factor or treatment of the condition will clearly reduce the recurrence risk.

References

1. Firth H, Hurst J (2005) Oxford desk reference – clinical genetics. Oxford University Press, United Kingdom
2. Drenthen W et al (2007) Outcome of pregnancy in women with congenital heart disease: a literature review. J Am Coll Cardiol 49(24):2303–2311

3. Burchill L et al (2011) Genetic counseling in the adult with congenital heart disease: what is the role? Curr Cardiol Rep 13(4):347–355
4. van Engelen K et al (2013) The value of the clinical geneticist caring for adults with congenital heart disease: diagnostic yield and patients' perspective. Am J Med Genet A 161A(7):1628–1637
5. Parrott A, Ware SM (2012) The role of the geneticist and genetic counselor in an ACHD clinic. Program Pediatr Cardiol 34(1):15–20
6. Morissens M et al (2013) Does congenital heart disease severely jeopardise family life and pregnancies? Obstetrical history of women with congenital heart disease in a single tertiary centre. Cardiol Young 23(1):41–46
7. Ferencz C, Boughman JA (1993) Congenital heart disease in adolescents and adults. Teratology, genetics, and recurrence risks. Cardiol Clin 11(4):557–567
8. Zaidi S et al (2013) De novo mutations in histone-modifying genes in congenital heart disease. Nature 498(7453):220–223
9. Lahm H et al (2015) Tetralogy of Fallot and hypoplastic left heart syndrome – complex clinical phenotypes meet complex genetic networks. Curr Genomics 16(3):141–158
10. Wessels MW, Willems PJ (2010) Genetic factors in non-syndromic congenital heart malformations. Clin Genet 78(2):103–123
11. Lalani SR, Belmont JW (2014) Genetic basis of congenital cardiovascular malformations. Eur J Med Genet 57(8):402–413
12. Schott JJ et al (1998) Congenital heart disease caused by mutations in the transcription factor NKX2-5. Science 281(5373):108–111
13. Garg V et al (2003) GATA4 mutations cause human congenital heart defects and reveal an interaction with TBX5. Nature 424(6947):443–447
14. Chin-Yee NJ, Costain G, Swaby JA, Silversides CK, Bassett AS (2014) Reproductive fitness and genetic transmission of tetralogy of Fallot in the molecular age. Circ Cardiovasc Genet 7(2):102–109
15. Burn J, Brennan P, Little J, Holloway S, Coffey R, Somerville J et al (1998) Recurrence risks in offspring of adults with major heart defects: results from first cohort of British collaborative study. Lancet 351(9099):311–316
16. Nora JJ (1993) Causes of congenital heart diseases: old and new modes, mechanisms, and models. Am Heart J 125(5 Pt 1):1409–1419
17. Therrien J, Barnes I, Somerville J (1999) Outcome of pregnancy in patients with congenitally corrected transposition of the great arteries. Am J Cardiol 84(7):820–824
18. Driscoll DJ et al (1993) Occurrence risk for congenital heart defects in relatives of patients with aortic stenosis, pulmonary stenosis, or ventricular septal defect. Circulation 87(2 Suppl):I114–I120
19. Nora JJ, Nora AH (1988) Update on counseling the family with a first-degree relative with a congenital heart defect. Am J Med Genet 29(1):137–142
20. Kernell K et al (2014) Congenital heart disease in men – birth characteristics and reproduction: a national cohort study. BMC Pregnancy Childbirth 14:187
21. Blue GM et al (2014) Targeted next-generation sequencing identifies pathogenic variants in familial congenital heart disease. J Am Coll Cardiol 64(23):2498–2506
22. Jia Y et al (2015) The diagnostic value of next generation sequencing in familial nonsyndromic congenital heart defects. Am J Med Genet A 167A(8):1822–1829
23. Nabulsi MM et al (2003) Parental consanguinity and congenital heart malformations in a developing country. Am J Med Genet A 116A(4):342–347
24. Yunis K et al (2006) Consanguineous marriage and congenital heart defects: a case-control study in the neonatal period. Am J Med Genet A 140(14):1524–1530
25. Breckpot J et al (2011) Challenges of interpreting copy number variation in syndromic and non-syndromic congenital heart defects. Cytogenet Genome Res 135(3-4):251–259
26. Geng J et al (2014) Chromosome microarray testing for patients with congenital heart defects reveals novel disease causing loci and high diagnostic yield. BMC Genomics 15:1127
27. Hinton RB Jr et al (2007) Hypoplastic left heart syndrome is heritable. J Am Coll Cardiol 50(16):1590–1595

28. Cripe L et al (2004) Bicuspid aortic valve is heritable. J Am Coll Cardiol 44(1):138–143
29. Kerstjens-Frederikse WS et al (2011) Left ventricular outflow tract obstruction: should cardiac screening be offered to first-degree relatives? Heart 97(15):1228–1232
30. Kirk EP et al (2007) Mutations in cardiac T-box factor gene TBX20 are associated with diverse cardiac pathologies, including defects of septation and valvulogenesis and cardiomyopathy. Am J Hum Genet 81(2):280–291
31. Werner P et al (2015) MESP1 mutations in patients with congenital heart defects. Hum Mutat 37(3):308–314
32. Robinson SW et al (2003) Missense mutations in CRELD1 are associated with cardiac atrioventricular septal defects. Am J Hum Genet 72(4):1047–1052
33. Wessels MW, Willems PJ (2008) Mutations in sarcomeric protein genes not only lead to cardiomyopathy but also to congenital cardiovascular malformations. Clin Genet 74(1):16–19
34. Garg V et al (2005) Mutations in NOTCH1 cause aortic valve disease. Nature 437(7056): 270–274
35. Kerstjens-Frederikse WS et al (2016) Cardiovascular malformations caused by NOTCH1 mutations do not keep left: data on 428 probands with left-sided CHD and their families. Genet Med [Epub ahead of print]
36. Kodo K et al (2012) Genetic analysis of essential cardiac transcription factors in 256 patients with non-syndromic congenital heart defects. Circ J 76(7):1703–1711
37. Heathcote K et al (2005) Common arterial trunk associated with a homeodomain mutation of NKX2.6. Hum Mol Genet 14(5):585–593
38. Lin X et al (2010) A novel GATA6 mutation in patients with tetralogy of Fallot or atrial septal defect. J Hum Genet 55(10):662–667
39. Pizzuti A et al (2003) Mutations of ZFPM2/FOG2 gene in sporadic cases of tetralogy of Fallot. Hum Mutat 22(5):372–377
40. Guimier A et al (2015) MMP21 is mutated in human heterotaxy and is required for normal left-right asymmetry in vertebrates. Nat Genet 47(11):1260–1263
41. Gebbia M et al (1997) X-linked situs abnormalities result from mutations in ZIC3. Nat Genet 17(3):305–308
42. Perles Z et al (2012) A human laterality disorder associated with recessive CCDC11 mutation. J Med Genet 49(6):386–390
43. Ta-Shma A et al (2015) A human laterality disorder associated with a homozygous WDR16 deletion. Eur J Hum Genet 23(9):1262–1265
44. Kaasinen E et al (2010) Recessively inherited right atrial isomerism caused by mutations in growth/differentiation factor 1 (GDF1). Hum Mol Genet 19(14):2747–2753
45. Cowan J, Tariq M, Ware SM (2014) Genetic and functional analyses of ZIC3 variants in congenital heart disease. Hum Mutat 35(1):66–75
46. French VM et al (2012) NPHP4 variants are associated with pleiotropic heart malformations. Circ Res 110(12):1564–1574
47. Zhu L, Belmont JW, Ware SM (2006) Genetics of human heterotaxias. Eur J Hum Genet 14(1):17–25
48. Weiss K et al (2015) Familial TAB2 microdeletion and congenital heart defects including unusual valve dysplasia and tetralogy of fallot. Am J Med Genet A 167(11):2702–2706
49. Aoki Y et al (2015) Recent advances in RASopathies. J Hum Genet 61(1):33–39
50. Roberts AE et al (2013) Noonan syndrome. Lancet 381(9863):333–342
51. Turnpenny PD, Ellard S (2012) Alagille syndrome: pathogenesis, diagnosis and management. Eur J Hum Genet 20(3):251–257
52. Corsten-Janssen N et al (2013) The cardiac phenotype in patients with a CHD7 mutation. Circ Cardiovasc Genet 6(3):248–254
53. Zweier C et al (2005) Clinical and mutational spectrum of Mowat-Wilson syndrome. Eur J Med Genet 48(2):97–111
54. Jaiyesimi O, Baichoo V (2007) Cardiovascular malformations in Omani Arab children with Down's syndrome. Cardiol Young 17(2):166–171

55. Irving CA, Chaudhari MP (2012) Cardiovascular abnormalities in Down's syndrome: spectrum, management and survival over 22 years. Arch Dis Child 97(4):326–330
56. Korpal-Szczyrska M et al (2005) [Cardiovascular malformations in Turner syndrome] Wady ukladu sercowo-naczyniowego w zespole Turnera. Endokrynol Diabetol Chor Przemiany Materii Wieku Rozw 11(4):211–214
57. Volkl TM et al (2005) Cardiovascular anomalies in children and young adults with Ullrich-Turner syndrome the Erlangen experience. Clin Cardiol 28(2):88–92
58. Bondy CA (2008) Aortic dissection in Turner syndrome. Curr Opin Cardiol 23(6):519–526
59. Carlson M, Silberbach M (2007) Dissection of the aorta in Turner syndrome: two cases and review of 85 cases in the literature. J Med Genet 44(12):745–749
60. Hadnott TN et al (2011) Outcomes of spontaneous and assisted pregnancies in Turner syndrome: the U.S. National Institutes of Health experience. Fertil Steril 95(7):2251–2256
61. Soemedi R et al (2012) Contribution of global rare copy-number variants to the risk of sporadic congenital heart disease. Am J Hum Genet 91(3):489–501
62. Hitz MP et al (2012) Rare copy number variants contribute to congenital left-sided heart disease. PLoS Genet 8(9):e1002903
63. Glessner JT et al (2014) Increased frequency of de novo copy number variants in congenital heart disease by integrative analysis of single nucleotide polymorphism array and exome sequence data. Circ Res 115(10):884–896
64. Thienpont B et al (2007) Submicroscopic chromosomal imbalances detected by array-CGH are a frequent cause of congenital heart defects in selected patients. Eur Heart J 28(22):2778–2784
65. Verhagen JM et al (2012) Phenotypic variability of atypical 22q11.2 deletions not including TBX1. Am J Med Genet A 158A(10):2412–2420
66. Kleefstra T et al (2006) Loss-of-function mutations in euchromatin histone methyl transferase 1 (EHMT1) cause the 9q34 subtelomeric deletion syndrome. Am J Hum Genet 79(2):370–377
67. Stewart DR, Kleefstra T (2007) The chromosome 9q subtelomere deletion syndrome. Am J Med Genet C Semin Med Genet 145C(4):383–392
68. Jefferies JL et al (2012) Cardiovascular findings in duplication 17p11.2 syndrome. Genet Med 14(1):90–94
69. Potocki L et al (2000) Molecular mechanism for duplication 17p11.2- the homologous recombination reciprocal of the Smith-Magenis microdeletion. Nat Genet 24(1):84–87
70. Thienpont B et al (2010) Haploinsufficiency of TAB2 causes congenital heart defects in humans. Am J Hum Genet 86(6):839–849
71. de Souza KR et al (2015) Cytogenomic evaluation of subjects with syndromic and nonsyndromic conotruncal heart defects. Biomed Res Int 2015:401941

Care During Pregnancy

5

Iris M. van Hagen and Jolien W. Roos-Hesselink

Abbreviations

DIC	Disseminated intravascular coagulation
FDA	Food and Drug Administration
LMWH	Low-molecular-weight heparin
WHO	World Health Organization

5.1 Introduction

Close follow-up of pregnant women with congenital heart disease is essential. In the light of the increasing attention to maternal death and morbidity due to cardiovascular disease, several guidelines have paid attention to the topic [1, 2]. In 2011 a very comprehensive statement was produced by the ESC working group [3], also discussing the cardiac evaluation throughout pregnancy. All recommendations are based on level C evidence, and choices may be individualised based on clinical experience. After the risk assessment during preconception counselling, evaluation of clinical parameters during pregnancy provides information on the status of risk to evolve cardiac deterioration.

I.M. van Hagen, MD (✉) • J.W. Roos-Hesselink, MD, PhD
Department of Cardiology, Division of Adult Congenital Heart Disease,
Erasmus MC, University Medical Center,
POBox 2040, Rotterdam, The Netherlands
e-mail: i.vanhagen@erasmusmc.nl; j.roos@erasmusmc.nl

© Springer International Publishing Switzerland 2017
J.W. Roos-Hesselink, M.R. Johnson (eds.), *Pregnancy and Congenital Heart Disease*, Congenital Heart Disease in Adolescents and Adults,
DOI 10.1007/978-3-319-38913-4_5

5.2 Clinical Follow-Up

Frequency of follow-up during pregnancy can be determined after the risk stratification has been established before pregnancy using the modified World Health Organization (WHO) classification. It consists of four classes: the risk of mortality and morbidity is low in WHO class I, and the risk is extremely high in WHO class IV, where pregnancy should be avoided. Women with WHO class I may have their pregnancy care in a community hospital. However, although the risk of a cardiac event in this group has been estimated at 0 % by two studies [4, 5], another has shown an event rate of up to 7 % in women without atrial fibrillation or signs of heart failure before pregnancy [6]. Consequently, it seems wise to evaluate the cardiac status of these women at least once or twice during pregnancy. This can be organised in the local hospital. In the case of deterioration of cardiac function, there should be a low threshold for referral to a tertiary centre. Patients with WHO class II and higher should be regularly seen in a tertiary centre. Their risk of a cardiac event is mildly to moderately increased, and thus they should be seen at 12, 20 and 30 weeks of pregnancy. An echocardiography at 20 weeks is justified in most cases. In some patients, additional follow-up visits are required, such as monitoring of anticoagulation therapy in women with a mechanical valve. A multidisciplinary team, including an obstetrician, cardiologist and anaesthetist, should formulate a delivery plan between 20 and 30 weeks [3]. Table 5.1 shows a summary of follow-up recommendations for each WHO class.

At 20–25 weeks, a multidisciplinary team should evaluate the progress of each patient. The team should consist of at least a cardiologist, an obstetrician and an anaesthesiologist. Echocardiography or other examinations should be discussed. An individualised labour plan should be made, taking into account the WHO classification, as specified during preconception counselling. It should describe the planned method and timing of delivery, whether there is a need for primary caesarean section, induction, primary epidural anaesthesia and assisted vaginal delivery and the need for postpartum prolonged admission. The delivery plan should be documented electronically if possible and made easily available to all involved specialties.

5.3 Diagnostic Modalities

After taking a careful history and physical examination, an electrocardiogram should be performed as a part of standard care. Heart rate increases by approximately 10–20 % during normal pregnancy [7]. Deviation towards a left axis is observed, which can be explained by elevation of the diaphragm and increase in ventricular mass and/or blood volume. Prominent Q waves may evolve in the inferior leads in 50–68 %, and T-wave abnormalities have been described in 70–80 % of pregnant women. These changes are also thought to be related to a physical shift in the position of the heart. Alternatively, the increased workload of the pregnant heart or the hormonal and serum electrolyte changes have been suggested to cause Q- and T-wave deviations [8].

5 Care During Pregnancy

Table 5.1 Follow-up during pregnancy and delivery

	Risk	Diagnosis	Practical implications for pregnancy	Practical implications for delivery
mWHO I	No to mild increased risk in morbidity compared to normal population	Repaired simple lesion ASD or VSD PDA PAPVR Mild valvular disease Uncomplicated PDA	Follow-up by cardiologist in peripheral or tertiary centre: twice (end of first and end of second trimester)	After uncomplicated pregnancy: as usual Otherwise, as class II
mWHO II	Small increased risk of maternal mortality and moderate increased risk in morbidity	Unrepaired uncomplicated ASD or VSD Repaired tetralogy of Fallot	**Follow-up by expert cardiologist and obstetrician:** 12 weeks 20 weeks + echocardiography 30 weeks	**Multidisciplinary team decides on plan:** Timing of delivery Induction of delivery Mode of delivery: Vaginal delivery (preferred) Assisted delivery (vacuum or forceps) Shortened second stage Anaesthetic approach **Postpartum in-hospital monitoring:** 24, 48 or 72 h, in case of moderate increased risk of heart failure or arrhythmia
mWHO II-III		Mild systemic ventricular dysfunction Repaired coarctation Native or tissue valve disease Marfan (<40 mm) BAV (<45 mm)	Aortic disease with diameter >40 mm: Echocardiography every 4–8 weeks (or MRI)	
mWHO III	Significantly increased risk of maternal mortality and severe morbidity	Mechanical valve Systemic right ventricle Fontan circulation Unrepaired cyanotic heart disease Other complex congenital heart disease Marfan (40–45 mm) BAV (45–50 mm)	Regular intensive monitoring up to monthly	
mWHO IV	Extremely high risk of maternal mortality or severe morbidity	Pulmonary arterial hypertension Severe systemic ventricular dysfunction Severe mitral stenosis Severe symptomatic aortic stenosis Marfan (>45 mm) BAV (>50 mm) Native severe coarctation	Pregnancy contraindicated, if pregnancy occurs: care as for class III	

ASD atrial septal defect, *BAV* bicuspid aortic valve, *PAPVR* partial anomalous pulmonary venous return, *PDA* persistent ductus arteriosus, *VSD* ventricular septal defect

Echocardiography is the basis of the evaluation of cardiac status during pregnancy, both routinely and in the event of a clinical deterioration. In any patient with congenital heart disease, echocardiography should be performed at least once during pregnancy. Ventricular and valvular function as well as ascending aorta dimensions can be assessed and compared to pre-pregnancy values. Left ventricular diastolic dimensions are known to increase approximately 7–12 % throughout pregnancy and to return to preconception values 6–12 months after pregnancy in healthy women [9]. Systolic dimensions remain stable, allowing for the increment of stroke volume. Maximum haemodynamic adaptation takes place beyond 20 weeks up to the end of the second trimester [7], and routine echocardiographic follow-up during pregnancy can therefore be planned between 20 and 24 weeks of gestation. Transoesophageal echocardiography is relatively safe during pregnancy. It is in particular helpful in haemodynamically stable women with a mechanical valve prosthesis and suspected valve thrombosis to determine thrombus size and to guide therapy [10].

Exercise testing during pregnancy has been studied and showed no adverse consequences with regard to the fetal well-being measured by umbilical artery Doppler indices and fetal heart rate [11]. Safety of exercise testing in women with established congenital heart disease has not been studied. Therefore it is recommended to not exceed a heart rate of 80 % of predicted maximum heart rate and a respiratory exchange ratio of 1.0 in VO_2max testing [3]. Dobutamine stress exercise should be avoided, because of limited experience during pregnancy.

MRI is the preferred imaging modality in women with aortic disease in whom aortic diameters need to be assessed during pregnancy and cannot be visualised using echocardiography. In these cases, it is recommended to have an MRI performed before pregnancy, for comparability of diameters. Gadolinium is not routinely used. It readily passes the placental border and thus may enter the fetal circulation and is excreted in the amniotic fluid through the fetal kidneys. The impact of the presence of gadolinium in the amniotic fluid on the fetus is unclear but should be considered harmful [12]. In individual cases, gadolinium use may be considered based on the estimated risk-benefit ratio in favour of the benefits for the mother.

A supine position compresses the inferior vena cava, but not the aorta. A left lateral position with a tilt of 30°, rather than 15°, relieves this compression at least partially [13]. Position should be consistent from early pregnancy to delivery, because of the large influence of position on cardiac haemodynamic parameters [14].

While survival of congenital heart disease patients has increased over the past decades, the imaging burden of this population has similarly grown. The number of tests per patients is partly associated with the disease complexity [15]. Also, utilisation rate of CT during pregnancy increased in the general population [16]. Cardiac catheterisation, chest CT or nuclear imaging leads to a fetal exposure to low-dose ionising radiation and should be avoided during pregnancy. But if a strong indication exists and chest CT is performed, the risks of fetal damage are low. Fetal radiation exposure below 50 mSv is associated with a negligible fetal risk. Chest CT leads to a fetal exposure of approximately 0.01–3 mSv, depending on the target diagnosis. Only abdominal CT and myocardial perfusion scans exceed 50 mSv [17]. CT imaging should be performed in left lateral position, and to further decrease the fetal radiation exposure rate, shielding may be considered, but decrease of exposure is limited and clinically hardly relevant [18, 19]. Iodinated contrast agents cross the placenta and are better avoided, although evidence of serious fetal harm is lacking [17].

Cardiac catheterisation may be needed in rare cases. In the case of fluoroscopy by trans-radial approach, shielding causes double exposure to the patient [20]. To avoid the use of fluoroscopy, an electroanatomical mapping system might be used to navigate and perform intracardiac pressure measurements [21]. Fluoroscopy might be considered in cases of suspected mechanical valve thrombosis, with short exposure times. All imaging modalities including clinical indications are summarised in Table 5.2.

5.4 Incidence and Timing of Events

Most simple types of congenital heart disease are associated with a low risk of events during pregnancy, while women with complex lesions are at higher risk. In a comprehensive literature review, complicated pregnancies were most often seen in patients with a cyanotic heart disease, a Fontan circulation or a partial atrioventricular septal defect [22]. About 35–40% of these pregnancies ended in a miscarriage, compared to approximately 10% in the general population. The highest risk of heart failure, arrhythmia or cardiovascular mortality was found in patients with Eisenmenger's syndrome, cyanotic disease, Fontan circulation and partial atrioventricular septal defect and patients with a transposition of the great arteries.

With a physiologic haemodynamic burden being present from the first weeks of gestation and increasing towards the end of the second trimester [7], cardiac events are likely to happen during the entire pregnancy. The contractions during labour are an additional load, and therefore patients are also at risk of events during the peripartum period.

5.4.1 Heart Failure

Indeed, in a prospective study, heart failure occurred throughout pregnancy, but most typically at the end of the second trimester and in the first week after delivery. In women with congenital heart disease, the incidence of heart failure was 8%, which is much lower than the 19% in pregnant women with valvular heart disease and 40% in women with a cardiomyopathy. Women with signs or symptoms of heart failure before pregnancy and those with pulmonary hypertension are at highest risk [23].

5.4.2 Arrhythmia

In the absence of cardiac disease, pregnancy is very rarely complicated by arrhythmias [24]. In patients with congenital heart disease outside pregnancy, mainly those with multiple previous cardiac surgeries and those with a diminished ventricular

Table 5.2 Imaging modalities and their implications during pregnancy in women with congenital heart disease

	Indication	Disadvantages	Considerations
Electrocardiography	Part of standard evaluation		Physiologic changes: left axis deviation, prominent Q waves inferior leads, T wave abnormalities
Echocardiography			Physiologic changes: increase of dimensions
Cardiac MRI	Routine if follow-up of aortic dimensions is warranted and echocardiography is insufficient	Unknown effect of gadolinium to the fetus	Left lateral position, avoid gadolinium
Transoesophageal echocardiography		Potential increase of intra-abdominal pressure	Fetal monitoring in case of sedation
Exercise test		Safety to fetus unknown	Avoid dobutamin, max 80 % of predicted heart rate, VO2max: respiratory exchange ratio max 1.0
Chest CT	Only if it has clear clinical consequences, and potential benefit to the mother	Fetal radiation exposure: 0.01 - 1 mSv[a]	Consider to use shielding, avoid contrast agents, left lateral position
Catheterization (e.g. intracardiac pressure measurement)		Fetal radiation exposure: up to 0.074 mSv[a]	Preferably use electro-anatomic mapping system
Fluoroscopy (e.g. mechanical valve evaluation)		Fetal radiation exposure: up to 0.244 mSv/min[a]	Shielding, duration as short as possible

Source: Colletti et al. [17]

[a]*CT* computed tomography, *MRI* magnetic resonance imaging

function are at risk. During pregnancy, the risk of arrhythmias in women with congenital heart disease is generally low. The incidence of supraventricular arrhythmias is estimated at 0.4–0.7% [25, 26]. Ventricular arrhythmias occur in approximately 0.4–1.6% in the presence of structural congenital heart disease [27, 28]. However, the incidence is much higher in patients with inherited arrhythmic disease, up to 13% in women with previously diagnosed arrhythmogenic right ventricular cardiomyopathy with an ICD, although this is not increased compared to outside pregnancy [29].

5.4.3 Valve Thrombosis

Hormonal changes cause a hypercoagulable state during pregnancy. Therefore, patients with an increased risk of thrombosis, based on their underlying cardiac disease, should receive adequate anticoagulation and be monitored intensively throughout pregnancy. For instance, women with a mechanical valve prosthesis deserve special attention, and close cooperation with a haematologist is advised. Mechanical valve thrombosis is a hazardous complication that may occur in approximately 5% of pregnancies, with a mortality rate as high as 20% [30]. Several anticoagulant strategies for the prevention of valve thrombosis have been proposed, but none have been proved to be superior. Specific time of risk is presumably when a patient is switched to a different anticoagulant agent. Other patients at risk are those with low flow mechanical valves such as a valve in the mitral position or in the case of ventricular dysfunction, although studies are too small to statistically substantiate these theories.

5.4.4 Aortic Dissection

In line with the haemodynamic changes in pregnancy, the vessel wall integrity is both influenced by different loading conditions and hormonal influences on the smooth muscle cells and reticular fibres of the tunica media of the aortic wall. In women with aortic disease such as Marfan syndrome, but presumably also in patients with Loeys-Dietz or vascular-type Ehlers-Danlos, these changes result in an increased risk of aortic dissection during pregnancy [31–34]. In Marfan syndrome, the incidence of aortic dissection is approximately 4.5% during pregnancy. An aortic dissection may occur throughout the entire pregnancy and up to several weeks after delivery. Because of this elevated risk, women with aortic disease and a dilated aorta should be seen every 4–8 weeks with imaging of the aorta (either echocardiography or MRI).

5.5 Medication During Pregnancy

The treatment of symptoms during pregnancy is limited by the potential fetal toxicity of therapeutic agents. The Food and Drug Administration (FDA) controls a database of drugs and their potential harm to the fetus. Table 5.3 shows the FDA

Table 5.3 FDA classification for drugs in pregnancy

FDA class	Human studies	Animal studies	Implication	Cardiac examples
FDA A	No risk		No risk in human controlled studies	
FDA B	No controlled studies	No risk	No evidence of risk in human studies	Sotalol, LMWH, unfractionated heparin, clopidogrel (no evidence in humans), acetylsalicylic acid (low dose), nitrates, hydrochlorothiazide, PDE5 inhibitors, prostanoids
	No risk	Risk		
FDA C	No controlled studies	Risk	Risk not ruled out	Digoxin, other beta-blockers, calcium channel blockers, clopidogrel, furosemide, most NOACs
FDA D	Risk		Positive evidence of risk in human studies	Amiodarone, *vitamin K antagonists*[a] ACE-inhibitors, ARBs, atenolol
FDA X	Risk		Risk of drug outweighs the potential benefit, contraindicated in pregnancy	Statins, endothelin receptor antagonists, *vitamin K antagonists*[a]
FDA N			FDA has not yet classified the drug	Vernakalant

ARBs angiotensin II receptor blocker, *FDA* Food and Drug Administration, *LMWH* low molecular weight heparin, *PDE5 inhibitors* phosphodiesterase 5 inhibitors

[a]Vitamin K antagonists are only classified FDA D in pregnant women with mechanical heart valves, who are at high risk of thromboembolism, and for whom the benefits of COUMADIN may outweigh the risks. Otherwise FDA X

classification and an overview of cardiac medication. In each woman the balance between maternal benefit and fetal risk of these drugs needs to be taken into account. The physiologic haemodynamic changes of pregnancy alter the pharmacokinetics and pharmacodynamics of drugs. The volume of distribution increases warranting a higher dosage in some drugs to reach therapeutic levels, e.g. in the case of digoxin. Many more complex influences of pregnancy on pharmacokinetics exist [35]. Overall, the absorption is reduced, and drug elimination is increased during pregnancy, generally leading to a lower level of plasma concentration. Close monitoring of drug levels may be necessary during pregnancy, in particular for drugs with a low therapeutic index (therapeutic-toxic dose ratio).

5.5.1 Anticoagulation in Patients with a Mechanical Valve

Several guidelines advise on anticoagulation strategies that are based mainly on small cohort studies and expert opinion [3, 36]. None of the anticoagulation regimens used worldwide seem to be superior, with the use of vitamin K antagonists leading to more frequent fetal demise, while a higher rate of valve thrombosis may be encountered in patients switched to (low molecular weight) heparin [30]. Patients should be changed to low molecular weight or unfractionated heparin as soon as they become pregnant and continue at least up to the end of the first trimester [3]. Strict control of either through levels of anti-Xa (LMWH) [37–41] or APTT (unfractionated heparin) is warranted. The guidelines advise treating women with vitamin K antagonists in the second and third trimester. The period of switching to another anticoagulant agent might put the patient at an increased risk of valve thrombosis, although this is not supported by the evidence. It is recommended to use dual anticoagulation until the INR is at least >2.5 during two consecutive measurements. In the case of a planned vaginal delivery, they should be switched to a form of heparin again by 36 or 37 weeks. At 36 h before planned labour, unfractionated heparin is the first choice of treatment as it can be reversed more easily than LMWH. At 4–6 h before planned delivery, heparin should be stopped temporarily and restarted 4–6 h after delivery [3, 36].

5.6 Cardiac Interventions During Pregnancy

5.6.1 Interventions for Arrhythmia

When pharmacological treatment fails or the arrhythmia is associated with haemodynamic instability in women suffering from tachyarrhythmia, direct current cardioversion is the first choice therapy. It can be used safely in pregnancy, with facilities for emergency delivery readily available [42]. It has been suggested that direct current cardioversion might induce uterine contractions [43], although this was described in the era of monophasic shock protocols [44]. Cardioversion should be performed in left lateral position to relieve the inferior cava compression, and fetal monitoring is advised.

In drug-resistant or recurrent tachyarrhythmias with haemodynamic compromise, radio-frequency ablation can be considered. However, evidence on safety during pregnancy is based only on a few case reports. The use of fluoroscopy can be avoided in the presence of an electroanatomical mapping system, with a minimum of radiation exposure [45].

5.6.2 Device Implantation

The indication for ICD implantation is the same as outside pregnancy [46]. Fluoroscopic guidance should be avoided if possible, for instance, using transoesophageal echocardiography or with reconstructed 3D geometry [47, 48]. Also, temporary pacing or pacemaker implantation can be performed safely. Recently, the use of (3D) electroanatomical reconstruction was reported with subsequent successful pacemaker implantation in early pregnancy free of fluoroscopy [49].

5.6.3 Resuscitation

In principle, cardiopulmonary resuscitation is performed following the standard procedures, except for some adjustments [50]. Basic life support should be performed with manual left uterine displacement to relieve caval compression, specifically in the case of an obvious gravid uterus. Fetal monitors are better removed, as the first goal is to resuscitate the mother and monitoring of the fetus is less important. Intravenous access should be achieved quickly, preferably above the diaphragm level during advanced cardiovascular life support. After 4 min of resuscitation without return of spontaneous circulation, immediate emergency caesarean section should be strongly considered and ideally be performed within 5 min of onset. Table 5.4 presents possible contributing factors which are summarised in acronym 'BEAUCHOPS' [51]. Next to a direct cardiac cause, obstetric indirect causes of cardiac deterioration should be considered. Key knowledge in the further treatment of a pregnant woman in shock is the fact that the uterus, and thus the fetal circulation, is considered a nonvital organ during shock.

Table 5.4 Potential causes of cardiac arrest during pregnancy	BEAUCHOPS
	*B*leeding/DIC
	*E*mbolism: coronary, pulmonary, amniotic
	*A*naesthetic complications
	*U*terine atony
	*C*ardiac disease: MI, ischaemia, aortic dissection, cardiomyopathy
	*H*ypertension/preeclampsia/eclampsia
	*O*thers: differential diagnosis of standard ACLS guidelines
	*P*lacenta abruption/praevia
	*S*epsis

DIC disseminated intravascular coagulation

5.6.4 Percutaneous and Surgical Intervention

If a percutaneous procedure cannot be postponed until after delivery, then the procedure should be performed with limited exposure to fluoroscopy or guided by echocardiography and preferably in the second trimester [3].

The potential benefits of any surgical intervention need to be carefully weighed against the obvious fetal risks. Valve surgery or aortic surgery should be postponed until after delivery whenever possible. The placental perfusion during surgery is compromised, which causes an increased risk of fetal morbidity and mortality. Surgery performed before delivery is associated with a fetal mortality of approximately 20–30 % [52–54]. Therefore, in the case of an indicated emergency surgery and a viable fetus, it is recommended to perform emergency caesarean section before cardiac surgery is carried out. Shorter cardiopulmonary bypass time and aortic cross-clamping time are associated with a better fetal outcome and similar maternal outcome [55]. In addition, normothermia, a higher pump flow and perfusion pressure and left lateral position are recommended [3, 56]. The efficacy and safety of the intra-aortic balloon pump during pregnancy need further investigation [57].

> **Key Messages**
> Every hospital providing tertiary care to pregnant women with cardiovascular disease should constitute a multidisciplinary team of cardiologists, obstetricians and anaesthesiologists with expertise in this field. This team should preferably have a meeting on regular basis and be involved in the delivery plan.
>
> Follow-up of women with congenital heart disease can be based on their WHO class, but may be individualised based on clinical parameters.
>
> Echocardiography is the basis of cardiac evaluation during pregnancy. Routine follow-up with MRI is advised to visualise the aorta in women with aortic pathology, when aortic diameters cannot be measured with echocardiography. Other diagnostic modalities are generally preserved for patients with potential deterioration of their cardiac function or should be postponed until after delivery.
>
> The most common complications during pregnancy in women with congenital heart disease are heart failure and arrhythmias. In 5 % of patients with a mechanical valve, pregnancy is complicated by valve thrombosis. Women with aortic pathology, such as Marfan syndrome or Loeys-Dietz syndrome, are at increased risk of aortic dissection.
>
> Medication during pregnancy should carefully be considered for their potential fetotoxicity. Women with a mechanical valve need close and frequent follow-up after the anticoagulant strategy has been determined.
>
> Emergency cardiac surgery in the case of a viable fetus in situ is preferably preceded by a caesarean section.

References

1. Task Force on the Management of Cardiovascular Diseases During Pregnancy of the European Society of C (2003) Expert consensus document on management of cardiovascular diseases during pregnancy. Eur Heart J 24(8):761–781
2. Vahanian A, Alfieri O, Andreotti F, Antunes MJ, Baron-Esquivias G, Baumgartner H, Borger MA, Carrel TP, De Bonis M, Evangelista A, Falk V, Lung B, Lancellotti P, Pierard L, Price S, Schafers HJ, Schuler G, Stepinska J, Swedberg K, Takkenberg J, Von Oppell UO, Windecker S, Zamorano JL, Zembala M, Guidelines ESCCfP, Joint Task Force on the Management of Valvular Heart Disease of the European Society of C, European Association for Cardio-Thoracic S (2012) Guidelines on the management of valvular heart disease (version 2012): the Joint Task Force on the Management of Valvular Heart Disease of the European Society of Cardiology (ESC) and the European Association for Cardio-Thoracic Surgery (EACTS). Eur J Cardiothorac Surg 42(4):S1–S44
3. Regitz-Zagrosek V, Lundqvist CB, Borghi C, Cifkova R, Ferreira R, Foidart JM, Gibbs JSR, Gohlke-Baerwolf C, Gorenek B, Iung B, Kirby M, Maas AHEM, Morais J, Nihoyannopoulos P, Pieper PG, Presbitero P, Roos-Hesselink JW, Schaufelberger M, Seeland U, Torracca L, Bax J, Auricchio A, Baumgartner H, Ceconi C, Dean V, Deaton C, Fagard R, Funck-Brentano C, Hasdai D, Hoes A, Knuuti J, Kolh P, McDonagh T, Moulin C, Poldermans D, Popescu BA, Reiner Z, Sechtem U, Sirnes PA, Torbicki A, Vahanian A, Windecker S, Baumgartner H, Deaton C, Aguiar C, Al-Attar N, Garcia AA, Antoniou A, Coman I, Elkayam U, Gomez-Sanchez MA, Gotcheva N, Hilfiker-Kleiner D, Kiss RG, Kitsiou A, Konings KTS, Lip GYH, Manolis A, Mebaaza A, Mintale I, Morice MC, Mulder BJ, Pasquet A, Price S, Priori SG, Salvador MJ, Shotan A, Silversides CK, Skouby SO, Stein JI, Tornos P, Vejlstrup N, Walker F, Warnes C, Force T, CPG ECPG (2011) ESC Guidelines on the management of cardiovascular diseases during pregnancy The Task Force on the Management of Cardiovascular Diseases during Pregnancy of the European Society of Cardiology (ESC). Eur Heart J 32(24):3147–3197
4. Balci A, Sollie-Szarynska KM, van der Bijl AG, Ruys TP, Mulder BJ, Roos-Hesselink JW, van Dijk AP, Wajon EM, Vliegen HW, Drenthen W, Hillege HL, Aarnoudse JG, van Veldhuisen DJ, Pieper PG, investigators Z-I (2014) Prospective validation and assessment of cardiovascular and offspring risk models for pregnant women with congenital heart disease. Heart 100(17):1373–1381
5. Lu CW, Shih JC, Chen SY, Chiu HH, Wang JK, Chen CA, Chiu SN, Lin MT, Lee CN, Wu MH (2015) Comparison of 3 risk estimation methods for predicting cardiac outcomes in pregnant women with congenital heart disease. Circ J 79(7):1609–1617
6. van Hagen IM, Boersma E, Johnson MR, Thorne SA, Parsonage WA, Escribano Subías P, Leśniak-Sobelga A, Irtyuga O, Sorour KA, Taha N, Maggioni AP, Hall R, Roos-Hesselink JW, on behalf of the ROPAC investigators and EORP team (2016) Global cardiac risk assessment in the Registry of Pregnancy and Cardiac disease: results of a registry from the European Society of Cardiology. Eur J Heart Fail 18:523–533
7. Robson SC, Hunter S, Boys RJ, Dunlop W (1989) Serial study of factors influencing changes in cardiac output during human pregnancy. Am J Physiol 256(4 Pt 2):H1060–H1065
8. Sunitha M, Chandrasekharappa S, Brid SV (2014) Electrocardiographic Qrs axis, Q wave and T-wave changes in 2nd and 3rd trimester of normal pregnancy. J Clin Diagn Res 8(9):BC17–BC21
9. Melchiorre K, Sharma R, Thilaganathan B (2012) Cardiac structure and function in normal pregnancy. Curr Opin Obstet Gynecol 24(6):413–421
10. Dogan V, Basaran O, Altun I, Biteker M (2014) Transesophageal echocardiography guidance is essential in the management of prosthetic valve thrombosis. Int J Cardiol 177(3):1103–1104
11. Szymanski LM, Satin AJ (2012) Strenuous exercise during pregnancy: is there a limit? Am J Obstet Gynecol 207(3):179, e171–176
12. Expert Panel on MRS, Kanal E, Barkovich AJ, Bell C, Borgstede JP, Bradley WG Jr, Froelich JW, Gimbel JR, Gosbee JW, Kuhni-Kaminski E, Larson PA, Lester JW Jr, Nyenhuis J, Schaefer

DJ, Sebek EA, Weinreb J, Wilkoff BL, Woods TO, Lucey L, Hernandez D (2013) ACR guidance document on MR safe practices: 2013. J Magn Reson Imaging 37(3):501–530
13. Higuchi H, Takagi S, Zhang K, Furui I, Ozaki M (2015) Effect of lateral tilt angle on the volume of the abdominal aorta and inferior vena cava in pregnant and nonpregnant women determined by magnetic resonance imaging. Anesthesiology 122(2):286–293
14. Rossi A, Cornette J, Johnson MR, Karamermer Y, Springeling T, Opic P, Moelker A, Krestin GP, Steegers E, Roos-Hesselink J, van Geuns RJ (2011) Quantitative cardiovascular magnetic resonance in pregnant women: cross-sectional analysis of physiological parameters throughout pregnancy and the impact of the supine position. J Cardiovasc Magn Reson 13:31
15. Beausejour Ladouceur V, Lawler PR, Gurvitz M, Pilote L, Eisenberg MJ, Ionescu-Ittu R, Guo L, Marelli AJ (2016) Exposure to low-dose ionizing radiation from cardiac procedures in patients with congenital heart disease: 15-year data from a population-based longitudinal cohort. Circulation 133(1):12–20
16. Lazarus E, Debenedectis C, North D, Spencer PK, Mayo-Smith WW (2009) Utilization of imaging in pregnant patients: 10-year review of 5270 examinations in 3285 patients – 1997–2006. Radiology 251(2):517–524
17. Colletti PM, Lee KH, Elkayam U (2013) Cardiovascular imaging of the pregnant patient. AJR Am J Roentgenol 200(3):515–521
18. Damilakis J, Theocharopoulos N, Perisinakis K, Manios E, Dimitriou P, Vardas P, Gourtsoyiannis N (2001) Conceptus radiation dose and risk from cardiac catheter ablation procedures. Circulation 104(8):893–897
19. Chatterson LC, Leswick DA, Fladeland DA, Hunt MM, Webster S, Lim H (2014) Fetal shielding combined with state of the art CT dose reduction strategies during maternal chest CT. Eur J Radiol 83(7):1199–1204
20. Musallam A, Volis I, Dadaev S, Abergel E, Soni A, Yalonetsky S, Kerner A, Roguin A (2015) A randomized study comparing the use of a pelvic lead shield during trans-radial interventions: threefold decrease in radiation to the operator but double exposure to the patient. Catheter Cardiovasc Interv 85(7):1164–1170
21. Tuzcu V, Gul EE, Erdem A, Kamali H, Saritas T, Karadeniz C, Akdeniz C (2015) Cardiac interventions in pregnant patients without fluoroscopy. Pediatr Cardiol 36(6):1304–1307
22. Drenthen W, Pieper PG, Roos-Hesselink JW, van Lottum WA, Voors AA, Mulder BJ, van Dijk AP, Vliegen HW, Yap SC, Moons P, Ebels T, van Veldhuisen DJ, Investigators Z. (2007) Outcome of pregnancy in women with congenital heart disease: a literature review. J Am Coll Cardiol 49(24):2303–2311
23. Ruys TP, Roos-Hesselink JW, Hall R, Subirana-Domenech MT, Grando-Ting J, Estensen M, Crepaz R, Fesslova V, Gurvitz M, De Backer J, Johnson MR, Pieper PG (2014) Heart failure in pregnant women with cardiac disease: data from the ROPAC. Heart 100(3):231–238
24. Shotan A, Ostrzega E, Mehra A, Johnson JV, Elkayam U (1997) Incidence of arrhythmias in normal pregnancy and relation to palpitations, dizziness, and syncope. Am J Cardiol 79(8):1061–1064
25. Whittemore R, Hobbins JC, Engle MA (1982) Pregnancy and its outcome in women with and without surgical treatment of congenital heart disease. Am J Cardiol 50(3):641–651
26. Salam AM, Ertekin E, van Hagen IM, Al Suwaidi J, Ruys TPE, Johnson MR, Gumbiene L, Frogoudaki AA, Sorour KA, Iserin L, Ladouceur M, van Oppen ACC, Hall R, Roos-Hesselink JW (2015) Atrial fibrillation or flutter during pregnancy in patients with structural heart disease data from the ROPAC (Registry on Pregnancy and Cardiac Disease). JACC Clin Electrophysiol 1(4):284–292
27. Siu SC, Sermer M, Colman JM, Alvarez AN, Mercier LA, Morton BC, Kells CM, Bergin ML, Kiess MC, Marcotte F, Taylor DA, Gordon EP, Spears JC, Tam JW, Amankwah KS, Smallhorn JF, Farine D, Sorensen S, Cardiac Disease in Pregnancy I (2001) Prospective multicenter study of pregnancy outcomes in women with heart disease. Circulation 104(5):515–521
28. Tateno S, Niwa K, Nakazawa M, Akagi T, Shinohara T, Yasuda T, Study Group for Arrhythmia Late after Surgery for Congenital Heart D (2003) Arrhythmia and conduction disturbances in patients with congenital heart disease during pregnancy: multicenter study. Circ J 67(12):992–997

29. Hodes AR, Tichnell C, Te Riele AS, Murray B, Groeneweg JA, Sawant AC, Russell SD, van Spaendonck-Zwarts KY, van den Berg MP, Wilde AA, Tandri H, Judge DP, Hauer RN, Calkins H, van Tintelen JP, James CA (2015) Pregnancy course and outcomes in women with arrhythmogenic right ventricular cardiomyopathy. Heart [Epub ahead of print]
30. van Hagen IM, Roos-Hesselink JW, Ruys TP, Merz WM, Goland S, Gabriel H, Lelonek M, Trojnarska O, Al Mahmeed WA, Balint HO, Ashour Z, Baumgartner H, Boersma E, Johnson MR, Hall R, Investigators R, the ERPT (2015) Pregnancy in women with a mechanical heart valve: data of the European Society of Cardiology Registry of Pregnancy and Cardiac Disease (ROPAC). Circulation 132(2):132–142
31. Rossiter JP, Repke JT, Morales AJ, Murphy EA, Pyeritz RE (1995) A prospective longitudinal evaluation of pregnancy in the Marfan syndrome. Am J Obstet Gynecol 173(5):1599–1606
32. Meijboom LJ, Vos FE, Timmermans J, Boers GH, Zwinderman AH, Mulder BJ (2005) Pregnancy and aortic root growth in the Marfan syndrome: a prospective study. Eur Heart J 26(9):914–920
33. Loeys BL, Schwarze U, Holm T, Callewaert BL, Thomas GH, Pannu H, De Backer JF, Oswald GL, Symoens S, Manouvrier S, Roberts AE, Faravelli F, Greco MA, Pyeritz RE, Milewicz DM, Coucke PJ, Cameron DE, Braverman AC, Byers PH, De Paepe AM, Dietz HC (2006) Aneurysm syndromes caused by mutations in the TGF-beta receptor. N Engl J Med 355(8): 788–798
34. Pepin M, Schwarze U, Superti-Furga A, Byers PH (2000) Clinical and genetic features of Ehlers-Danlos syndrome type IV, the vascular type. N Engl J Med 342(10):673–680
35. Dawes M, Chowienczyk PJ (2001) Drugs in pregnancy. Pharmacokinetics in pregnancy. Best Pract Res Clin Obstet Gynaecol 15(6):819–826
36. Nishimura RA, Otto CM, Bonow RO, Carabello BA, Erwin JP 3rd, Guyton RA, O'Gara PT, Ruiz CE, Skubas NJ, Sorajja P, Sundt TM 3rd, Thomas JD, American College of Cardiology/American Heart Association Task Force on Practice G (2014) 2014 AHA/ACC guideline for the management of patients with valvular heart disease: executive summary: a report of the American College of Cardiology/American Heart Association Task Force on Practice Guidelines. J Am Coll Cardiol 63(22):2438–2488
37. Goland S, Schwartzenberg S, Fan J, Kozak N, Khatri N, Elkayam U (2014) Monitoring of anti-xa in pregnant patients with mechanical prosthetic valves receiving low-molecular-weight heparin: peak or trough levels? J Cardiovasc Pharmacol Ther 19(5):451–456
38. Abildgaard U, Sandset PM, Hammerstrom J, Gjestvang FT, Tveit A (2009) Management of pregnant women with mechanical heart valve prosthesis: thromboprophylaxis with low molecular weight heparin. Thromb Res 124(3):262–267
39. Quinn J, Von Klemperer K, Brooks R, Peebles D, Walker F, Cohen H (2009) Use of high intensity adjusted dose low molecular weight heparin in women with mechanical heart valves during pregnancy: a single-center experience. Haematologica 94(11):1608–1612
40. James AH, Brancazio LR, Gehrig TR, Wang A, Ortel TL (2006) Low-molecular-weight heparin for thromboprophylaxis in pregnant women with mechanical heart valves. J Matern Fetal Neonatal Med 19(9):543–549
41. McLintock C, McCowan LM, North RA (2009) Maternal complications and pregnancy outcome in women with mechanical prosthetic heart valves treated with enoxaparin. BJOG 116(12):1585–1592
42. Tromp CH, Nanne AC, Pernet PJ, Tukkie R, Bolte AC (2011) Electrical cardioversion during pregnancy: safe or not? Neth Heart J 19(3):134–136
43. Barnes EJ, Eben F, Patterson D (2002) Direct current cardioversion during pregnancy should be performed with facilities available for fetal monitoring and emergency caesarean section. BJOG 109(12):1406–1407
44. Brown O (2003) Direct current cardioversion during pregnancy. BJOG 110(7):713–714
45. Szumowski L, Szufladowicz E, Orczykowski M, Bodalski R, Derejko P, Przybylski A, Urbanek P, Kusmierczyk M, Kozluk E, Sacher F, Sanders P, Dangel J, Haissaguerre M, Walczak F (2010) Ablation of severe drug-resistant tachyarrhythmia during pregnancy. J Cardiovasc Electrophysiol 21(8):877–882

46. Authors/Task Force M, Priori SG, Blomstrom-Lundqvist C, Mazzanti A, Blom N, Borggrefe M, Camm J, Elliott PM, Fitzsimons D, Hatala R, Hindricks G, Kirchhof P, Kjeldsen K, Kuck KH, Hernandez-Madrid A, Nikolaou N, Norekval TM, Spaulding C, Van Veldhuisen DJ (2015) 2015 ESC guidelines for the management of patients with ventricular arrhythmias and the prevention of sudden cardiac death: the Task Force for the Management of Patients with Ventricular Arrhythmias and the Prevention of Sudden Cardiac Death of the European Society of Cardiology (ESC) Endorsed by: Association for European Paediatric and Congenital Cardiology (AEPC). Eur Heart J 36(41):2793–2867
47. Abello M, Peinado R, Merino JL, Gnoatto M, Mateos M, Silvestre J, Dominguez JL (2003) Cardioverter defibrillator implantation in a pregnant woman guided with transesophageal echocardiography. Pacing Clin Electrophysiol 26(9):1913–1914
48. Tuzcu V, Kilinc OU (2012) Implantable cardioverter defibrillator implantation without using fluoroscopy in a pregnant patient. Pacing Clin Electrophysiol 35(9):e265–e266
49. Kuhne M, Schaer B, Reichlin T, Sticherling C, Osswald S (2015) X-ray-free implantation of a permanent pacemaker during pregnancy using a 3D electro-anatomic mapping system. Eur Heart J 36(41):2790
50. Jeejeebhoy FM, Zelop CM, Lipman S, Carvalho B, Joglar J, Mhyre JM, Katz VL, Lapinsky SE, Einav S, Warnes CA, Page RL, Griffin RE, Jain A, Dainty KN, Arafeh J, Windrim R, Koren G, Callaway CW, American Heart Association Emergency Cardiovascular Care Committee CoCCCP, Resuscitation CoCDitY, Council on Clinical C (2015) Cardiac arrest in pregnancy: a scientific statement from the American Heart Association. Circulation 132(18): 1747–1773
51. Lipman S, Cohen S, Einav S, Jeejeebhoy F, Mhyre JM, Morrison LJ, Katz V, Tsen LC, Daniels K, Halamek LP, Suresh MS, Arafeh J, Gauthier D, Carvalho JC, Druzin M, Carvalho B, Society for Obstetric A, Perinatology (2014) The Society for Obstetric Anesthesia and Perinatology consensus statement on the management of cardiac arrest in pregnancy. Anesth Analg 118(5):1003–1016
52. Elassy SM, Elmidany AA, Elbawab HY (2014) Urgent cardiac surgery during pregnancy: a continuous challenge. Ann Thorac Surg 97(5):1624–1629
53. John AS, Gurley F, Schaff HV, Warnes CA, Phillips SD, Arendt KW, Abel MD, Rose CH, Connolly HM (2011) Cardiopulmonary bypass during pregnancy. Ann Thorac Surg 91(4):1191–1196
54. Patel A, Asopa S, Tang AT, Ohri SK (2008) Cardiac surgery during pregnancy. Tex Heart Inst J 35(3):307–312
55. Hosseini S, Kashfi F, Samiei N, Khamoushi A, Ghavidel AA, Yazdanian F, Mirmesdagh Y, Mestres CA (2015) Feto-maternal outcomes of urgent open-heart surgery during pregnancy. J Heart Valve Dis 24(2):253–259
56. Pomini F, Mercogliano D, Cavalletti C, Caruso A, Pomini P (1996) Cardiopulmonary bypass in pregnancy. Ann Thorac Surg 61(1):259–268
57. Willcox TW, Stone P, Milsom FP, Connell H (2005) Cardiopulmonary bypass in pregnancy: possible new role for the intra-aortic balloon pump. J Extra Corp Technol 37(2):189–191

The Management of Labour and the Post-partum Period in CHD

6

Matt Cauldwell, Mark Cox, Roisin Monteiro, and Mark R. Johnson

Abbreviations

ARBs	Angiotensin receptor blockers
CFM	Continuous fetal monitoring
CHD	Congenital heart disease
CS	Caesarean section
GA	General anaesthesia
M/P	Milk to plasma
PCC	Preconception care
SVR	Systemic vascular resistance

6.1 Introduction

Maternal mortality in developed countries is in the region of 1 per 10,000 births [1]; in emerging nations, the rate is 25 times higher [2]. These risks are greater in the context of pre-existing heart disease, where the overall risk of dying during pregnancy is 1%, 0.6% in the developed and 3.4% in the developing world [3]. Labour is a critical time, when cardiac work is maximal and major changes in blood

---

M. Cauldwell, MD, PhD • M.R. Johnson, MD, PhD (✉)
Department of Obstetrics and Gynaecology, Institute of Reproductive and Developmental Biology, Imperial College School of Medicine, Chelsea and Westminster Hospital, 369 Fulham Road, London SW10 9NH, UK
e-mail: mark.johnson@imperial.ac.uk

M. Cox, MD, PhD • R. Monteiro, MD, PhD
Anesthetic Department, Chelsea and Westminster Hospital,
369 Fulham Road, London SW10 9NH, UK

© Springer International Publishing Switzerland 2017
J.W. Roos-Hesselink, M.R. Johnson (eds.), *Pregnancy and Congenital Heart Disease*, Congenital Heart Disease in Adolescents and Adults,
DOI 10.1007/978-3-319-38913-4_6

volumes occur [4]. Timely and appropriate management decisions are essential as women with heart disease can deteriorate rapidly [5]. Most problems can be anticipated in the antenatal period, making the formulation of the plan for delivery vitally important. Decisions need to be individualised and based on the risks and benefits of the mode of delivery in a given clinical situation.

6.2 Antenatal Care

The ideal provision of pregnancy care for women with CHD should begin with preconception care (PCC), which should be delivered by both an obstetrician and cardiologist. This then allows the individual with CHD to be fully informed and aware of the impact that pregnancy is likely to have on their clinical status and any potential complications they may encounter. As part of this consultation, it is helpful to advise women on aspects of pregnancy care that may be unique to them because of their CHD and also how their care is likely to be delivered and co-ordinated throughout the 9 months of pregnancy. PCC is also an opportunity to review and organise any outstanding investigations prior to pregnancy so as to provide the team who is delivering pregnancy care with complete and up-to-date clinical data. PCC also permits an assessment of the patient's own individual clinical risk which in turn is likely to dictate how their care is delivered.

6.3 Clinical Management Plan for Delivery

1. Place of birth
2. Mode of delivery
3. Induction of labour
4. First stage of labour monitoring, antibiotics, maternal monitoring, fetal monitoring, ECG, SA02, arterial line, CVP
5. Second-stage time-assisted delivery
6. Third stage
7. Postdelivery

6.3.1 Place of Delivery

Early in the first trimester, women with CHD should meet their obstetrician and cardiologist for a review of their clinical status, to discuss the schedule of antenatal care, and the timing and mode of delivery. Women should be made aware that delivery within a hospital setting is recommended, on a consultant-led delivery suite/labour ward, regardless of their underlying lesion. Although the exact level of care required will be decided later in pregnancy for those individuals who are assessed as having low-risk lesions (such as small left to right shunts or valvular regurgitation with normal ventricular function), it may be appropriate to receive their obstetric care in a local obstetric unit rather than in a specialist centre. Local care can be enhanced by a comprehensive cardiac assessment at PCC or early in the first trimester, so that any pertinent issues can be clarified and further investigations and follow-up arranged. If the local obstetric unit feels unable to care for these patients, then their care should be transferred to specialist centres, which routinely manage women with CHD.

6.3.2 Multidisciplinary Delivery Planning

Every woman with CHD should have a detailed delivery plan completed in the third trimester. This delivery plan should follow from a joint co-ordinated assessment by the obstetricians, cardiologists and anaesthetists. Within this plan there should be clear written information regarding the proposed place of delivery; mode of delivery; the type of monitoring the patient needs to receive, which members of the medical team need to be informed should any problems arise; the recommended pain relief required; and the specific management of the second and third stage of labour and postdelivery monitoring.

6.3.3 Mode of Delivery: Vaginal Delivery or Planned Caesarean Section?

Rates of Caesarean section are much higher in women with CHD [6], reflecting the desire to avoid an emergency Caesarean section in this group of patients. To date, advice regarding the mode of delivery in women with congenital heart disease (CHD) has been based exclusively on expert opinion with little or no data to guide clinicians. The recent paper based on the ROPAC dataset from over 1,200 deliveries showed that a planned Caesarean section did not confer any maternal advantage when compared with attempted vaginal delivery [7]. In fact, comparing planned vaginal delivery with planned Caesarean section showed that babies were delivered earlier and were consequently of a lower birthweight, whilst maternal outcomes were worse with higher maternal mortality and rates of heart failure. This could reflect the fact that planned Caesareans were more common in women with worse heart disease, but even when this was corrected for, the differences remained, with higher rates of heart failure, lower birthweight and shorter gestation, suggesting that elective CS was associated with no maternal benefit and a worse fetal outcome. Most importantly, from a maternal point of view, the outcome of emergency CS performed in labour was no worse than for those having a pre-labour elective CS. These data suggest that vaginal delivery can be attempted in most women, with CS reserved for those with an obstetric indication. The ESC guidelines suggest that women on oral anticoagulation in preterm labour and patients with Marfan syndrome and an aortic diameter of greater than 45 mm should be delivered by CS [8]. The current data suggest that attempted vaginal delivery is safe in all others and that emergency CS carries no greater risk than elective CS. More research, focussed on the outcome of labour in women with severe heart disease, needs to be performed.

6.3.4 Timing of Delivery and Induction of Labour

A spontaneous onset of labour followed by a vaginal delivery is the best option for women with CHD and, in the absence of obstetric factors (preterm ruptured membranes, fetal growth restriction, pre-eclampsia); there are no data to support early induction of labour. However, in the noncardiac population, induction of labour in many groups has been shown to be safe and does not increase the rate of Caesarean section before 40 weeks of gestation and to actually reduce CS rates after 40 weeks [9, 10]. Perhaps more importantly, induction at 40 weeks reduces stillbirth rates by around 50% [11]. Consequently, in women with CHD who experience higher rates of stillbirth, a policy to induce labour at 40 weeks may be beneficial and consistent with improving pregnancy outcomes but currently has no evidence base. Should induction of labour be required, then artificial rupture of membranes and oxytocin infusion are preferred. If prostaglandins are required to promote cervical ripening, caution should be used as there is the risk of uterine hyperstimulation, which may then require emergency delivery. It may be preferable to consider mechanical methods of cervical ripening such as a Foley catheter or cervical laminaria.

6.3.5 First Stage of Labour

During labour in normal (noncardiac patients) women, cardiac output progressively increases to reach a maximum in the second stage [12]. There are no equivalent data in women with heart disease, and the data from Robson et al. are taken from women without epidural anaesthesia and may therefore be a response to pain. Current recommendations are for women with CHD to have an early epidural to minimise pain and so the increase in cardiac output, but there are no data to support this. In the non-pregnant state, adverse cardiac events are infrequently associated with exercise. However, these data are on the background of a normal cardiac workload, which is not the case in pregnancy where the cardiac output is increased by up to 50% from non-pregnant levels.

At the onset of the second stage, passive descent of the fetal head is permitted. For women with an epidural, this increases the chance of a spontaneous vaginal birth, reduces the overall time required for pushing and reduces the likelihood of an assisted delivery [13]. An active second stage is considered to be appropriate for the majority of women with CHD. Prior studies demonstrated a preference to replace the active second stage with an immediate assisted delivery [14]. However, this is currently only routinely recommended for patients with a dilated aorta [8]. More recent data demonstrate that despite an active second stage, women with CHD are still more likely to have an assisted vaginal delivery because of an imposed shortened stage [14]. At present there are no studies examining how the active second stage should be managed in this group and whether a shortened second stage is beneficial. Information regarding the recommended length of an active second stage should be clearly documented in the patient's labour plan.

6.3.6 Third Stage of Labour

Present guidance recommends that women without heart disease may opt for a physiological third stage if the risk of post-partum haemorrhage is deemed to be low [15]. However, women with cardiac disease have a reported greater risk of post-partum haemorrhage, which may complicated up to a quarter of deliveries, and so an "active" third stage of labour is recommended [16]. Obstetric haemorrhage should be avoided in this group because of the large associated fluid shifts at delivery, which may be poorly tolerated in the parturient with cardiac disease. Oxytocin is widely used to counter uterine atony, as first-line uterotonic agent for the active management of the third stage of labour, as it shortens the length of the third stage and reduces blood loss and the rate of post-partum haemorrhage [17]. A UK postal survey of obstetricians and midwives found that Syntometrine was the most commonly used agent for the active management of the third stage of labour [18]. However, the use of ergometrine in women with cardiac disease is not advised because of its marked hypertensive effect [19] and association with coronary artery spam and myocardial ischaemia [20]. Furthermore, oxytocin is not without its own side effects, most notably, vasodilatation of the subcutaneous vessels combined with vasoconstriction in the splanchnic bed and coronary arteries as well as an effect on cardiac receptors to increase heart rate [21], the overall effect being a tachycardia and hypotension. These effects are dose related so the minimum effective dose of oxytocin is suggested. At present no studies have directly evaluated different oxytocin regimens for the management of the third stage with reduced rates of haemorrhage as a primary endpoint. Should second- or third-line agents be required, misoprostol and Hemabate can be utilised for the treatment of post-partum haemorrhage, but the former is associated with pyrexia and the latter with marked gastrointestinal upset.

6.4 Antibiotic Prophylaxis

The overall incidence of infective endocarditis in pregnancy is extremely rare and thought to be about 0.006 % [22]. There exists some variation in international guidance, but the indications for patients to receive prophylaxis have certainly reduced in recent years [23, 24]. In pregnancy, there is no specific guidance to advise which women with CHD if any require antibiotic at the point of delivery. We therefore suggest a pragmatic approach and to discuss this information with the patient in the antenatal period. For women who feel strongly about receiving antibiotics at delivery, especially those with an artificial valve, we would agree that this is a reasonable option. We further refer to the recent ESC guidelines on endocarditis [23]. Furthermore women having a Caesarean section should routinely be offered antibiotic prophylaxis prior to skin incision as this has been shown to reduce the risk of maternal infection [25].

6.4.1 Monitoring in Labour

During labour, women should have both continuous fetal monitoring (CFM) and maternal cardiac monitoring. Basic non-invasive monitoring should include an ECG for the detection of maternal arrhythmia in labour. A 12-lead ECG can be performed in the event of signs or symptoms of ischaemia. There are clear limitations of basic non-invasive monitoring, and so regular medical review by an appropriately experienced doctor monitoring is necessary. For women with high-risk cardiac lesions, invasive cardiovascular may be prudent, usually in the form of an arterial and of uncertain benefit line and occasionally a central venous line. A Swan-Ganz catheter is rarely indicated. The need for these additional forms of monitoring should be included in the antenatal delivery plan.

6.4.2 Obstetric Analgesia and Anaesthesia for Cardiac Patients

Anaesthetic involvement in the antenatal care of women with cardiac disease is essential. Anaesthetists must be part of the team who assess these patients and monitor them through their pregnancy. In more complex cases, anaesthetists will need time to understand the patient's cardiovascular physiology and how labour, anaesthetic and obstetric interventions might affect it. Plans for the timing and mode of delivery, and how best to provide analgesia or anaesthesia for this, should be made by a multidisciplinary team of anaesthetists, obstetricians and cardiologists. Even if vaginal delivery is planned, emergency operative delivery may be indicated for obstetric reasons, so an anaesthetic plan must be made for both the expected mode of delivery and emergency intervention. The vast majority of women with cardiac disease will have an anaesthetic intervention, either in the form of regional analgesia for labour or anaesthesia for operative delivery.

6.4.3 Labour Analgesia

Although women in labour can choose or decline a range of analgesic options, when a woman with cardiac disease is in labour, epidural analgesia is usually recommended. In addition to providing superior pain relief to other modes of analgesia, epidural analgesia can attenuate the cardiovascular stresses of labour [26]. Cardiac output increases by 50% through pregnancy and may increase by a further 25% during the first stage of labour and by 40% during the second stage, with further increases during contractions [12]. This is mediated through increased venous return and pain-related catecholamine release. An established early epidural before labour pain should be recommended to all patients who may not cope with increased cardiac demands; this has been shown to significantly reduce maternal catecholamine levels which may lead to tachycardia, hypertension and ventricular stress [27]. Alternatively, a low-dose combined spinal-epidural can be sited which affords quicker analgesia if labour progression is advanced. Whichever technique is used, regional analgesia should be initiated carefully, allowing titration to effect with close haemodynamic monitoring. An effective epidural can also be used to facilitate a passive second stage if necessary or deliver anaesthesia if a surgical delivery is required.

Alternative options to epidural analgesia are available but do not carry the same cardiovascular benefits for the cardiac patient as they cannot abolish pain and the associated catecholamine release. Nitrous oxide and oxygen in a 50:50 mix (Entonox or "gas and air") provides very variable levels of analgesia [28]. Whilst readily accessible, its use is limited by side effects such as nausea, vomiting and dizziness. Intramuscular diamorphine and pethidine are commonly used parenteral opioids. They are readily available, as they can be prescribed by midwives, but provide only moderate levels of pain relief [29]. Cardiovascular benefits are not seen, and side effects include nausea, sedation and respiratory depression. Hypercarbia associated with respiratory depression may exacerbate arrhythmias, myocardial ischaemia or pulmonary hypertension in women at risk. Remifentanil patient-controlled intravenous analgesia is a more recent technique. Remifentanil is an ultrashort-acting opiate with a half-life of 3 min. Whilst it provides better analgesia than other opiates and Entonox, it is inferior to epidural analgesia in terms of analgesia and therefore cardiovascular benefit [30]. It can result in profound respiratory depression and can lead to reduced FHR variability so is usually offered only when epidural analgesia is contraindicated [31].

6.4.4 Delivery Anaesthesia

Anaesthetic options for delivery include general anaesthesia and regional techniques. Providing anaesthesia by either technique can lead to more dramatic haemodynamic changes than providing analgesia; consideration must be given to whether invasive cardiovascular monitoring is necessary. For either technique, systemic vasoconstrictors such as phenylephrine and ephedrine should be prepared to treat reductions in blood pressure. Greater control may be obtained with a carefully titrated infusion commenced at induction.

Regional techniques include:

- A single-shot spinal anaesthetic
- Catheter techniques, commonly epidural catheters or less commonly intrathecal catheters
- A combination of the two (combined spinal-epidural anaesthesia)

The reduction in systemic vascular resistance (SVR) is a concern with regional techniques in cardiac patients. Catheter techniques are therefore usually recommended to allow a more gradual titration than that which can be achieved with a single-shot technique. Regional anaesthetic techniques with a slower onset reduce cardiovascular instability and have the added advantage that they can be abandoned if not tolerated. The addition of an opiate is beneficial as it reduces the dose of local anaesthetic needed and thus the haemodynamic consequences. Contraindications to neuraxial blockade include concurrent anticoagulation, deranged platelet/clotting parameters, local or generalised sepsis and patient refusal. Further, neuraxial blockade should be used with caution in patients with a fixed cardiac output such as stenotic valvular lesions and hypertrophic cardiomyopathy as cardiac output cannot increase to compensate for the reduction in SVR and reduced venous return is poorly tolerated.

6.4.5 General Anaesthesia

General anaesthesia (GA) carries a higher risk in pregnant compared to non-pregnant women. Concerns relate to:

- Intubation may be more challenging, with a difficult airway experienced in 1/224 obstetric patients and 1/2,000 in non-obstetric patients [32, 33].
- The risk of aspiration is increased due to raised intra-abdominal pressure, reduced lower oesophageal sphincter tone and delayed gastric emptying.
- Oxygen desaturation may occur more quickly due to lower oxygen reserve and a reduced functional residual capacity, coupled with increased oxygen consumption.
- In addition, the fetus may be affected through the placental transfer of drugs.

There are also some concerns specific to cardiac patients. Induction of general anaesthesia results in a drop in SVR, but this is not usually as precipitous as with neuraxial blockade. GA drugs may, however, cause myocardial depression; this includes the usual drugs used for induction and maintenance of anaesthesia in the obstetric population, e.g. thiopental, propofol and volatile inhalational agents. Anaesthetists may choose to deliver a "cardiac" anaesthetic, which tends to involve a slower induction using drugs that are more cardiovascularly stable such as high doses of opioids. This may result in a less responsive baby, so the neonatal team must be informed of drugs used. Laryngoscopy and intubation may result in tachycardia and raised pulmonary artery pressures; this may be attenuated by altering the anaesthetic technique and using a short-acting opiate, beta blocker or intravenous lignocaine prior to induction. Consideration must also be given to how the patient's circulation will cope with positive pressure ventilation and its effects on venous return, which is usually reduced in these circumstances. Nitrous oxide is often used as part of the maintenance of anaesthesia in the obstetric population, but as it can increase pulmonary vascular resistance, it should be avoided in patients with pulmonary hypertension.

For these reasons, GA is usually second choice to RA, reflected in the National Obstetric Anaesthetic Database for 2012, which reported a rate of 7.6% use of GA for CS overall in the UK [34]. However, there has been little research looking into the incidence of CS under GA in the cardiac population. A single-centre study reported a rate of 27% in 2003 [35], and anecdotal experience suggests that rates of GA for CS in this group have decreased since then but remain higher than the non-cardiac population. The higher rates of GA may be because the need for an urgent CS or because of contraindications to RA, such as clotting abnormalities, which are more frequent in this group of women. In some patients with cardiac disease, anaesthetists prefer to avoid the more dramatic drop in SVR seen in regional anaesthesia. For the highest-risk patients, GA allows rapid emergency investigation and intervention, e.g. TOE or CPB if needed.

6.4.6 Postdelivery Care

Vigilant monitoring does not end with delivery; major cardiovascular changes occur over 12–24 h following delivery. Uterine blood flow returns to the systemic circulation, and the low resistance uteroplacental circulation is lost, meaning that this is a high-risk time for patients susceptible to volume overload and heart failure. Cardiovascular monitoring is therefore imperative during this period, especially for women with a high risk of developing heart failure, for up to 48 h, usually in a high-dependency setting on the labour ward or in intensive care if the underlying cardiac disease is more severe. Basic, non-invasive monitoring should be the baseline standard of care of all women with cardiac disease, including intermittent non-invasive BP, continuous ECG monitoring and pulse oximetry. The need for invasive monitoring should be dictated by the patient's clinical status and evolving clinical picture. Furthermore, regular and timely review should be made by the healthcare team to ensure appropriate and timely intervention if needed. Some patients require specific surveillance after delivery, for example, patients with an aortopathy and a history of peripartum cardiomyopathy. Thought should be given to the implications for breastfeeding of any drugs used.

6.4.7 Postdelivery Imaging

In certain cases, it may be wise to consider additional imaging prior to a patient's discharge. This is particularly true of women with aortopathy as they are a concern regarding the risk of dissection. This appears to be greatest in the third trimester and the post-partum period particularly for those with Marfan syndrome [36]. It is postulated that this greater risk of dissection may be due to increased cardiac output, which peaks after delivery, following the uterine autotransfusion, but changes in blood pressure and hormonal changes may also play a role. Aortic dissection can have devastating consequences with high rates of maternal mortality of up to 30% [37]. Re-imaging of the aorta with echocardiography or MRI prior to discharge will identify patients that have undergone an acute change in aortic dimensions and who are therefore at greater risk of dissection in the puerperium.

6.4.8 Thromboprophylaxis

In the postnatal period, women are at greatest risk of venous thromboembolism [38]. CHD alone is not an indication for thromboprophylaxis, but risk stratification should be employed to determine which women require thromboprophylaxis and for how long. Women with heart failure, after Fontan operation, and those with cyanotic heart disease who are polycythaemic should be considered high risk for thromboembolism and so should be treated. The Royal College of Obstetricians and Gynaecologists has recently updated its guidance and provides risk assessment tools [39].

6.4.9 Breastfeeding

Many women with cardiac disease will have been on medications prior to pregnancy some of which may have been stopped because of risks of teratogenicity. The benefits of breastfeeding are well established, but a few drugs are contraindicated in breastfeeding.

Beta Blockers The majority of beta blockers are considered safe with breastfeeding. However, the level of drug that is excreted into breast milk differs and will be influenced by the milk to plasma (M/P) ratio. Nevertheless, the majority of studies of beta blockers in breastfeeding demonstrate that despite the higher M/P levels of agents such as metoprolol and nadolol, the dose delivered to the infant would have no clinical effect; however, it may also be prudent to choose a beta blocker with a lower M/P ratio if there is any suggestion of impaired renal or hepatic function in the mother or infant.

ACE Inhibitors There are limited data, but concern has been raised about severe neonatal hypotension with these agents, particularly in premature infants. Consequently, they should be used with caution and those with low availability in breast milk, such as enalapril, captopril and quinapril chosen [40].

Calcium Channel Blockers All calcium channel blockers pass into breast milk in small amounts [41]; however, their use in breastfeeding is generally considered to be safe.

Furosemide Although excreted into breast milk, no adverse effects have been reported with regard to breastfeeding.

ARBs At present angiotensin receptor blockers are not recommended during pregnancy and breastfeeding because of insufficient data to support their use [42].

Anticoagulants Warfarin is predominantly protein bound so only small amounts are freely available in breast milk. Heparin, neither low molecular weight nor unfractionated heparin, are detectable in breast milk because of their high molecular weight. Currently there are no data published on the use of clopidogrel during breastfeeding.

6.4.10 Postnatal Review

All women with CHD should be offered a postnatal review jointly with their obstetrician and cardiologists between 6 and 12 weeks after delivery. At this visit, women should not only have a basic medical review but future pregnancies also discussed. Women should be made aware that a short pregnancy interval of less than 18 months may be associated with higher rates of preterm delivery. Furthermore, there is some evidence that pregnancy may impair long-term functional status for some women with CHD, and so discussions about future pregnancy need to be considered carefully. In the short term, at least women should be advised about the use of long-acting reversible contraceptive devices such as the Mirena IUD or progesterone implants.

References

1. MBRACE-UK- saving mothers, improving mothers care. https://www.npeu.ox.ac.uk/mbrrace-uk/reports. Last accessed 15 Feb 2016
2. Lawson GW, Keirse MJ (2013) Reflections on the maternal mortality millennium goal. Birth 40(2):96–102
3. Roos-Hesselink JW, Ruys TP, Stein JI, Thilén U, Webb GD, Niwa K, Kaemmerer H, Baumgartner H, Budts W, Maggioni AP, Tavazzi L, Taha N, Johnson MR, Hall R, ROPAC Investigators (2013) Outcome of pregnancy in patients with structural or ischaemic heart disease: results of a registry of the European Society of Cardiology. Eur Heart J 34(9):657–665
4. Meah VL, Cockcroft JR, Backx K, Shave R, Stöhr EJ (2016) Cardiac output and related haemodynamics during pregnancy: a series of meta-analyses. Heart 102:518–526
5. Bhatt AB, DeFaria Yeh D (2015) Pregnancy and adult congenital heart disease. Cardiol Clin 33(4):611–623
6. Siu SC, Colman JM, Sorensen S et al (2002) Adverse neonatal and cardiac outcomes are more common in pregnant women with cardiac disease. Circulation 105:2179–2184
7. Ruys TP, Roos-Hesselink JW, Pijuan-Domènech A, Vasario E, Gaisin IR, Iung B, Freeman LJ, Gordon EP, Pieper PG, Hall R, Boersma E, Johnson MR, ROPAC investigators (2015) Is a planned caesarean section in women with cardiac disease beneficial? Heart 101(7):530–536
8. ESC Committee for Practice Guidelines (2011) ESC guidelines on the management of cardiovascular diseases during pregnancy: the Task Force on the Management of Cardiovascular Diseases during Pregnancy of the European Society of Cardiology (ESC). Eur Heart J 32(24):3147–3197
9. Walker KF, Malin G, Wilson P, Thornton JG (2016) Induction of labour versus expectant management at term by subgroups of maternal age: an individual patient data meta-analysis. Eur J Obstet Gynecol Reprod Biol 197:1–5
10. Gibson KS, Waters TP, Bailit JL (2014) Maternal and neonatal outcomes in electively induced low-risk term pregnancies. Am J Obstet Gynecol 211(3):249.e1–249.e16
11. Mozurkewich E, Chilimigras J, Koepke E, Keeton K, King VJ (2009) Indications for induction of labour: a best-evidence review. BJOG 116(5):626–636
12. Robson SC, Dunlop W, Boys RJ, Hunter S (1987) Cardiac output during labour. Br Med J (Clin Res Ed) 295(6607):1169–1172
13. Brancato RM, Church S, Stone PW (2008) A meta-analysis of passive descent versus immediate pushing in nulliparous women with epidural analgesia in the second stage of labor. J Obstet Gynecol Neonatal Nurs 37(1):4–12

14. Robertson JE, Silversides CK, Mah ML, Kulikowski J, Maxwell C, Wald RM, Colman JM, Siu SC, Sermer M (2012) A contemporary approach to the obstetric management of women with heart disease. J Obstet Gynaecol Can 34(9):812–819
15. National Institute of Clinical Excellence-Intrapartum care for healthy women and babies- https://www.nice.org.uk/guidance/cg190/chapter/1-recommendations
16. Cauldwell M, Von Klemperer K, Uebing A, Swan L, Steer PJ, Gatzoulis M, Johnson MR (2016) Why is post-partum haemorrhage more common in women with congenital heart disease? Int J Cardiol 218:285–290
17. Prendiville WJP, Elbourne D, McDonald SJ (2003) Active versus expectant management in the third stage of management of the third stage of labour to prevent post-partum haemorrhage (joint statement). International Confederation of Midwives and International Federation of Gynaecology and Obstetrics, The Hague
18. Farrar D, Tuffnell D, Airey R, Duley L (2010) Care during the third stage of labour: a postal survey of UK midwives and obstetricians. BMC Pregnancy Childbirth 10:23. doi:10.1186/1471-2393-10-23
19. Begley CM, Gyte GM, Devane D, McGuire W, Weeks A (2015) Active versus expectant management for women in the third stage of labour. Cochrane Database Syst Rev (3):CD007412
20. Yaegashi N, Miura M, Okamura K (1999) Acute myocardial infarction associated with post-partum ergot alkaloid administration. Int J Gynaecol Obstet 64(1):67–68
21. Svanström MC, Biber B, Hanes M, Johansson G, Näslund U, Bålfors EM (2008) Signs of myocardial ischaemia after injection of oxytocin: a randomized double-blind comparison of oxytocin and methylergometrine during caesarean section. Br J Anaesth 100(5):683–689
22. Dajani AS Jr (1997) Prevention of bacterial endocarditis. Recommendations by the American Heart Association. JAMA 277:1794–1801
23. Habib G, Lancellotti P, Antunes MJ, Bongiorni MG, Casalta JP, Del Zotti F et al (2015) ESC guidelines for the management of infective endocarditis: the Task Force for the Management of Infective Endocarditis of the European Society of Cardiology (ESC). Endorsed by: European Association for Cardio-Thoracic Surgery (EACTS), the European Association of Nuclear Medicine (EANM). Eur Heart J 36(44):3075
24. Nishimura RA, Carabello BA, Faxon DP et al (2008) ACC/AHA guideline update on valvular heart disease: focused update on infective endocarditis. Circulation 118:887–896
25. National Institute for Health and Care Excellence (NICE) Guideline CG132 http://www.nice.org.uk/guidance/cg132/chapter/1-Guidance#planned-cs
26. Anim-Somuah M, Smyth RM, Jones L (2011) Epidural versus non-epidural or no analgesia in labour. Cochrane Database Syst Rev (12):CD000331
27. Shnider SM, Abboud TK, Artal R et al (1983) Maternal catecholamines decrease during labor after lumbar epidural anesthesia. Am J Obstet Gynecol 147:13–15
28. Klomp T, van Poppel M, Jones L, Lazet J, Di Nisio M, Lagro-Janssen AL (2012) Inhaled analgesia for pain management in labour. Cochrane Database Syst Rev (9):CD009351
29. Ullman R, Smith LA, Burns E, Mori R, Dowswell T (2010) Parenteral opioids for maternal pain relief in labour. Cochrane Database Syst Rev (9):CD007396
30. Ismail MT, Hassanin MZ (2012) Neuraxial analgesia versus intravenous remifentanil for pain relief in early labor in nulliparous women. Arch Gynecol Obstet 286(6):1375–1381. doi:10.1007/s00404-012-2459-3
31. Tveit TO, Seiler S, Halvorsen A, Rosland JH (2012) Labour analgesia: a randomised, controlled trial comparing intravenous remifentanil and epidural analgesia with ropivacaine and fentanyl. Eur J Anaesthesiol 29(3):129–136
32. Muchatuta NA, Kinsella SM (2013) Remifentanil for labour analgesia: time to draw breath? Anaesthesia 68(3):231–235. doi:10.1111/anae.12153
33. Quinn AC, Milne D, Columb M, Gorton H, Knight M (2013) Failed tracheal intubation in obstetric anaesthesia: 2 yr national case-control study in the UK. Br J Anaesth 110:74–80
34. Obstetric Anaesthetists Association- 2012 Database- http://www.oaa-anaes.ac.uk/home

35. Boyle RK (2003) Anaesthesia in parturients with heart disease: a five year review in an Australian tertiary hospital. IJA 12:173–177
36. Lind J, Wallenburg HC (2001) The Marfan syndrome and pregnancy: a retrospective study in a Dutch population. Eur J Obstet Gynecol Reprod Biol 98(1):28–35
37. Immer FF, Bansi AG, Immer-Bansi AS, McDougall J, Zehr KJ, Schaff HV, Carrel TP (2003) Aortic dissection in pregnancy: analysis of risk factors and outcome. Ann Thorac Surg 76(1):309–314
38. Kourlaba G, Relakis J, Kontodimas S, Holm MV, Maniadakis N (2016) A systematic review and meta-analysis of the epidemiology and burden of venous thromboembolism among pregnant women. Int J Gynaecol Obstet 132(1):4–10
39. Royal College of Obstetricians and Gynaecologists- Green-top Guideline number 37a- https://www.rcog.org.uk/globalassets/documents/guidelines/gtg-37a.pdf
40. Briggs GG, Freeman RK, Yaffe SJ (2011) Drugs in pregnancy and lactation: a reference guide to fetal and neonatal risk. Lippincott, Williams and Wilkins, Philadelphia, pp 408–409
41. Ghanem FA, Movahed A (2008) Use of antihypertensive drugs during pregnancy and lactation. Cardiovasc Ther 26(1):38–49
42. Podymow T, August P (2011) Antihypertensive drugs in pregnancy. Semin Nephrol 31(1):70–85

Part II

Specific Lesions

Pregnancy in Repaired Tetralogy of Fallot

7

Sonya V. Babu-Narayan, Wei Li, and Anselm Uebing

Abbreviations

CMR	Cardiovascular magnetic resonance
ECG	Electrocardiogram
MAPCAs	Major aortopulmonary collateral arteries
PR	Pulmonary regurgitation
RA	Right atrium
RPA	Right pulmonary artery
RV	Right ventricle
RVOT	Right ventricular outflow tract
WHO	World Health Organisation

S.V. Babu-Narayan, MB BS, BSc, PhD, FRCP (✉)
Cardiovascular Biomedical Research Unit and Adult Congenital Heart Programme,
Royal Brompton Hospital, Sydney Street, London SW3 6NP, UK
e-mail: s.babu-narayan@rbht.nhs.uk

W. Li, MD, PhD
Department of Echocardiography and Adult Congenital Heart Programme,
Royal Brompton Hospital, London, UK

National Heart and Lung Institute, Imperial College, London, UK

A. Uebing, MD, PhD
Adult Congenital Heart Programme, Royal Brompton Hospital, London, UK

© Springer International Publishing Switzerland 2017
J.W. Roos-Hesselink, M.R. Johnson (eds.), *Pregnancy and Congenital Heart Disease*, Congenital Heart Disease in Adolescents and Adults,
DOI 10.1007/978-3-319-38913-4_7

> **Key Facts**
>
> *Incidence*: 400 per million live births, the most common, complex cyanotic defect.
> *Inheritance*: 3–5 % inheritance. Fifteen percent have DiGeorge syndrome due to 22q11 deletion, which has 50 % inheritance.
> *Medication*: ACE inhibitors, AT1 antagonists and some antiarrhythmic agents are contraindicated during pregnancy.
> *World Health Organisation class*: II (*if otherwise well and uncomplicated*).
> *Risks of pregnancy*: maternal arrhythmia, heart failure, low birthweight.
> *Life expectancy*: Depends on underlying anatomy and nature and timing of previous interventions, excellent for those with uncomplicated anatomy, early primary repair and good biventricular function.

> **Key Management**
>
> *Preconception*: Clinical assessment, BNP, 12-lead ECG, echocardiography, cardiopulmonary exercise testing, cardiovascular magnetic resonance (CMR) including to assess for residual pulmonary stenosis or consequent pulmonary regurgitation, right and left ventricular function, QRS duration and objective exercise capacity. Genetic testing to assess for DiGeorge syndrome.
> *Pregnancy*: Each trimester with ECG and echo. Complicated patients, those that have functional deterioration or develop symptoms will require closer follow-up.
> *Labour*: Vaginal delivery with early epidural anaesthesia and assisted delivery for aortic root dilatation (>5.0 cm) and symptomatic heart failure. Continuous ECG telemetry may be useful particularly if there is history of arrhythmia.
> *Post-partum*: Observation for 12–24 h.

7.1 The Condition

7.1.1 Tetralogy of Fallot

Tetralogy of Fallot comprises a "tetrad" of an overriding aorta, ventricular septal defect, pulmonary stenosis and right ventricular hypertrophy all explained anatomically by anterocephalad deviation of the outlet ventricular septum. Congenital heart disease is the most common birth defect and has a 0.8 % incidence [1]. Tetralogy of Fallot has an incidence of 421 per million [2] and is the underlying cause of up to 10 % of cyanotic heart disease. Patients born in developed countries reaching childbearing age will have usually undergone surgical repair with closure of the ventricular septal defect and relief of pulmonary stenosis with resection of muscle bundles in the right ventricular outflow tract with or without more extensive right ventricular outflow reconstruction. The anatomical spectrum varies from double outlet right ventricle of Fallot type to Fallot with absent pulmonary valve or pulmonary atresia with major aortopulmonary collateral arteries (MAPCAs). Survival to 20 years and beyond is now excellent [3] since the advent of surgical repair in the 1950s [4]. We can increasingly expect survival rates of 90% and above at 40 years post-repair [5]. For this reason, repaired tetralogy of Fallot constitutes one of the most common conditions seen in adult congenital heart disease outpatient care. At least 40% of these patients are women and the population is ever growing.

7.1.2 Repaired Tetralogy of Fallot

The emphasis of this chapter focuses on the most common patient within the adult congenital heart disease population, namely, the woman with repaired tetralogy of Fallot. Adult patients may have residual lesions such as residual ventricular septal defect or pulmonary stenosis. More common than haemodynamically significant residual native lesions perhaps is postoperative severe pulmonary regurgitation consequent to adequate surgical relief of the native right ventricular obstruction at the time of repair. Although most patients may wish to proceed with pregnancy, the increased risk of maternal and neonatal complications warrants preconception counselling. The risks of pregnancy depend on the status of the surgical repair. Pregnancy is low risk for women who have no significant residual defects or postoperative sequelae [6] and who have good ventricular function following repair of tetralogy of Fallot (Fig. 7.1).

7.1.3 Repaired Tetralogy of Fallot with Significant Pulmonary Regurgitation

Pulmonary regurgitation is a common consequence of repair of tetralogy of Fallot in particular where more extensive right ventricular outflow and pulmonary artery reconstruction were needed to relieve the original obstruction. It is generally well tolerated by patients and may be asymptomatic from the cardiac viewpoint for several decades. However, with time, pulmonary regurgitation results in right ventricular dilatation, right heart dysfunction, arrhythmia, heart failure and death. In the last 15 years, a lot of progress has been made regarding the timing of reoperation or transcatheter intervention to replace the pulmonary valve. This is now more commonly offered at an earlier stage, based on investigations and before patients become symptomatic. The status of the right ventricle is a more important arbiter of pregnancy-related risk than the degree of pulmonary regurgitation

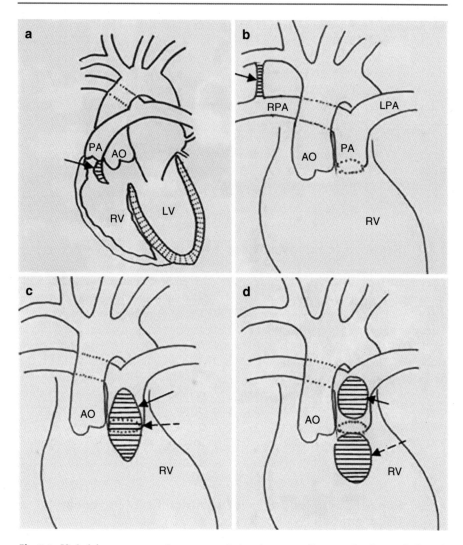

Fig. 7.1 Underlying anatomy and common variations in nature of intervention for surgical repair of tetralogy of Fallot. Image (**a**) depicts the underlying anatomical substrate of tetralogy of Fallot. Anterocephalad deviation of the outlet septum (*arrow*) is the key anatomical feature leading to subpulmonary stenosis, ventricular septal defect, aortic override and right ventricular hypertrophy. Image (**b**) depicts a right-sided modified Blalock-Taussig shunt (*arrow*) from the right subclavian artery to the right pulmonary artery. Image (**c**) depicts the use of a transannular patch (*block arrow*) to augment the right ventricular outflow tract and main pulmonary artery (pulmonary valve annulus level *dotted line*; *dashed arrow*). This is associated with pulmonary regurgitation in follow-up. Image (**d**) depicts the use of a pulmonary artery patch (*solid arrow*) and a right ventricular outflow tract patch (*dashed arrow*) allowing augmentation of the pulmonary artery and right ventricular outflow tract whilst sparing the pulmonary valve (pulmonary valve annulus level marked by *dotted line*). If outflow tract patching is avoidable, the patient can be spared right ventriculotomy (Adapted from Babu-Narayan PhD thesis, University of London, Imperial College, 2010. Pathophysiology and management of adults with repaired tetralogy of Fallot studied using cardiovascular magnetic resonance)

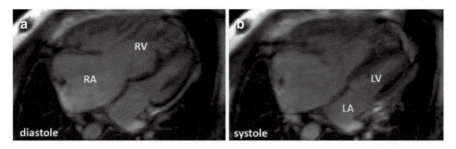

Fig. 7.2 Cardiovascular magnetic resonance still frames in diastole (**a**) and systole (**b**) from a four-chamber steady-state free precession cine showing severe right ventricular dilatation consequent to severe pulmonary regurgitation late after repair of tetralogy of Fallot with functional moderate tricuspid regurgitation and impaired systolic function. There is right atrial dilatation and history of sustained clinical atrial arrhythmia. Using cardiovascular magnetic resonance imaging, accurate assessment of right as well as left ventricular volumes can be made without geometric assumptions which can be particularly misleading in the context of the postoperative right ventricle. In this case, the RV is dramatically dilated with indexed RV volume above 200 mL/m^2 and impaired right ventricular ejection fraction of 41 %

(Fig. 7.2). If both right and left ventricular functions are preserved, pregnancy is likely to be well tolerated despite severe pulmonary regurgitation. However, the risks of pregnancy are increased in the setting of pulmonary regurgitation with right ventricular dilatation and dysfunction and associated clinical symptoms (New York Heart Association class II or higher) [7]. As pregnancy results in an increased circulating volume, this further compounds the right ventricle volume overload. In some cases, irreversible cardiac remodelling can develop especially during the late stage of pregnancy.

When planning pregnancy, a full assessment of the impact of any pulmonary regurgitation should be made. If criteria are met for elective pulmonary valve replacement, this may be preferable prior to embarking on pregnancy. The decision regarding indications for elective pulmonary valve replacement to treat asymptomatic pulmonary regurgitation is individualised as for the patient not planning pregnancy. Echocardiography is the routine test of choice for screening patients with significant pulmonary regurgitation and right heart dilatation and for assessing ventricular function (Figs. 7.3, 7.4). Cardiovascular magnetic resonance imaging is used for accurate right ventricular volume and function assessment and cardiopulmonary exercise testing for objective measure of exercise capacity, and heart assessment also includes 12-lead electrocardiogram and chest x-ray for cardiothoracic ratio. Pregnancy planning may bring forward detailed heart assessment that culminates in recommendation that there are sufficient criteria to warrant haemodynamic intervention prior to pregnancy. In the author's institution, a recovery period of 6 months post-operatively is recommended before then attempting to conceive.

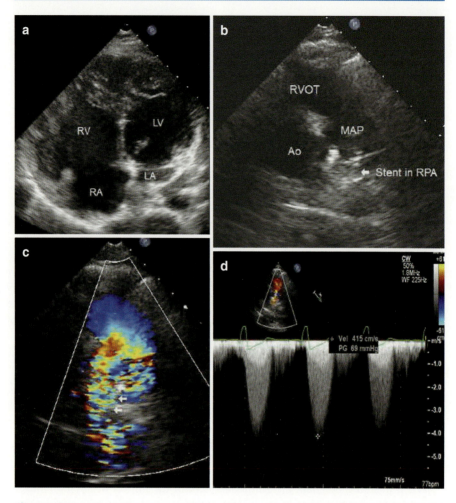

Fig. 7.3 Echocardiography images are from a 28-year-old woman born with tetralogy of Fallot and aortopulmonary window who underwent repair of aortopulmonary window at 8 weeks after birth and repair of tetralogy of Fallot at age 4 years. She also had a history of transcatheter stent insertion to the right pulmonary artery at 19 years old. Echocardiography images at 6 months after delivery are shown. (**a**) Apical four-chamber view showing severely dilated and hypertrophied right ventricle (RV) and dilated right atrium (RA). (**b**) Parasternal short axis view of the right ventricular outflow tract (RVOT). Stent seen in RPA (*arrow*). (**c**) Colour Doppler showing a narrow jet and turbulent flow in the stented right pulmonary artery (RPA). (**d**) Continuous wave Doppler recording of flow across RPA with peak flow velocity 4.2 m/s and calculated peak gradient of 69 mmHg, suggesting severe RPA stenosis

7.1.4 Repaired Tetralogy of Fallot with Significant Residual Pulmonary Stenosis

In general stenotic lesions are less well tolerated than regurgitant lesions. Doppler flow velocity, hence calculated pressure gradient across the stenotic RVOT, will

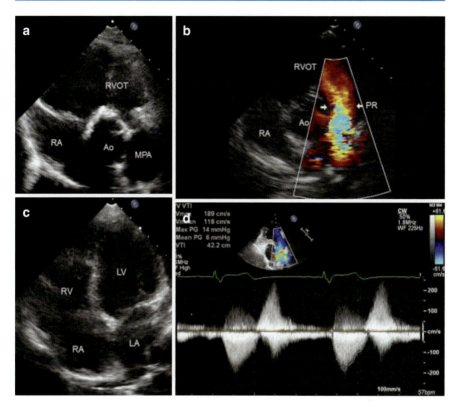

Fig. 7.4 Echo images of a 36-year-old patient at 13 weeks gestation. (**a**) Parasternal short axis view showing aneurysmal dilatation of RVOT with mild infundibular narrowing and thickened pulmonary valve. (**b**) Colour Doppler of RVOT showing a broad jet of regurgitation suggesting severe pulmonary regurgitation (PR). (**c**) Apical four-chamber view showing severely dilated RV and dilated RA. (**d**) Continuous wave Doppler recording of flow in the RVOT. The very short pulmonary regurgitation duration suggests free PR

increase to double, or even triple baseline during pregnancy as the circulating volume increases. Moderate stenosis before pregnancy is very likely to become severe with pregnancy judged by pressure gradient on Doppler. Although patients with mild to moderate right ventricular outflow tract obstruction may go through pregnancy without major cardiovascular or obstetric complications, relief of right ventricular outflow tract obstruction is indicated by a peak-to-peak gradient of more than 50 mmHg or a peak-right ventricular pressure more than 75 mmHg and should be performed prior to pregnancy. If pregnancy is already embarked on and right ventricular function remains preserved, even severe right ventricular outflow tract obstruction may be tolerated [8], but it may also be complicated by right heart failure and the onset of atrial arrhythmia. If early right heart failure is precipitated by pregnancy, balloon valvuloplasty may need to be considered as part of maternal care.

7.1.5 Repaired Tetralogy of Fallot with Aortic Dilatation and Other Risk Factors

Aortic dilatation is prevalent in tetralogy of Fallot [9]. For those patients with Caesarean section or more marked aortic dilatation, for example, with aortic dilatation exceeding 50 mm, early epidural and assisted delivery may be advisable. Current guidelines do not suggest intervention for aortic dilatation in the setting or repaired tetralogy of Fallot below diameters of 55 mm [10]. Though aortopathy could potentially complicate pregnancy management in repaired tetralogy of Fallot, acute aortic dissection in the setting of repaired tetralogy of Fallot is extremely rare. To date aortic dissection has only been described in four men all with significantly dilated aortas greater than or equal to 55 mm.

Left ventricular dysfunction as for all patients considering pregnancy confers additional risk. During pregnancy, mild LV dilatation and reduced ejection fraction is a common finding for repaired congenital heart disease including repaired tetralogy of Fallot. Pulmonary hypertension also confers additional risk. This can be secondary to historic use of Waterston surgical shunt though this will become increasingly rare in women with repaired tetralogy of Fallot of childbearing age; it may rarely occur due to small pulmonary arteries in repaired tetralogy of Fallot. Women with the native diagnosis for pulmonary atresia with ventricular septal defect who had pulmonary blood supply via aortopulmonary collateral arteries are discussed below.

For patients with co-morbidity due to coronary artery disease, obesity or diabetes or for those requiring anticoagulation, specific recommendations for these should be followed.

7.1.6 Tetralogy of Fallot with MAPCAs and Other More Complex Situations

Pulmonary atresia with ventricular septal defect and MAPCAs may be regarded as an extreme variant of tetralogy of Fallot. There is absence of any direct connection between the heart and the pulmonary arterial tree, a large VSD and two ventricles. Blood reaches the pulmonary bed via a patent ductus arteriosus and or major aortopulmonary collateral arteries. Those patients that have successfully undergone a biventricular repair surgical strategy with closure of the ventricular septal defect and right ventricular outflow tract reconstruction with a conduit are acyanotic. However, biventricular dysfunction especially diastolic dysfunction is more prevalent than in patients with simple Fallot variant. Those repaired patients that embark on pregnancy may be regarded similarly to other repaired tetralogy of Fallot patients but with precise risks depending on the status of the repair including the conduit function. However, remaining patients that have more complex anatomy may remain cyanotic. The risks depend on severity of cyanosis and degree of pulmonary hypertension (which can be subsegmental). In general, resting oxygen saturations less than 85 % are unlikely to result in successful pregnancy.

7.1.7 Unrepaired Tetralogy of Fallot

Clinical presentation with pregnancy and unrepaired tetralogy of Fallot is rare but described [11]. Patients may present to specialist adult congenital heart disease services already pregnant with less favourable haemodynamics. Late repair in adulthood of tetralogy of Fallot prior to embarking on pregnancy is preferable.

7.2 Pregnancy Outcome

Most pregnancy outcome studies are small or single centre or retrospective. However, such data as exist suggest that for tetralogy of Fallot patients, most can have successful uneventful pregnancies, but maternal cardiac complications occur in 7–10% [12], most commonly atrial arrhythmia (6–7%) [12] and symptomatic right heart failure (2–5%) [12]. Adverse maternal cardiac events are associated with severe pulmonary regurgitation combined with right ventricular dysfunction, particularly when these occur in combination with left ventricular dysfunction or pulmonary hypertension [10]. In a study of pregnancy in women with repaired tetralogy of Fallot which included 123 completed pregnancies in two centres, the use of cardiac medications prior to pregnancy was the most important predictor of both maternal cardiac events and of small-for-gestational-age babies [13].

Atrial arrhythmia is the most common pregnancy-related cardiac event in patients with repaired tetralogy of Fallot [12, 14]. This is due to the increased circulating volume, which exacerbates the risk of arrhythmia related to scarring caused by atriotomy at previous reparative surgery and by worsening existing chamber dilatation and right ventricular dysfunction. Not surprisingly, a history of arrhythmia increases the chance of recurrence [12, 15, 16].

Ventricular function and cyanosis during pregnancy are the major determinants of outcome for patients with *Fallot and pulmonary atresia* [16], and careful surveillance of both throughout pregnancy is needed. For the mother, cyanosis may progressively worsen in pregnancy with increasing right to left shunting further reducing pulmonary blood flow and oxygenation. Furthermore, maternal complications related to cyanosis include thrombosis, bleeding diathesis, arrhythmia and heart failure [17]. The risks of fetal complications are high and include fetal loss, low birth weight and prematurity. For sicker patients, bed rest, oxygen therapy and low molecular weight heparin may be required to address maternal oxygen consumption and prevent thromboembolic complications.

Vaginal delivery remains desirable given the higher risk of haemorrhage, thromboembolic complications and infections post-Caesarean section. Antibiotic prophylaxis is prudent in labour and delivery.

7.2.1 Obstetric and Fetal Risks

The most common fetal complication is impaired fetal growth, with small for gestational age occurring in 9, 19 and 35% depending on series [12, 16, 19] with pulmonary regurgitation a predisposing factor for low birthweight [18]. The use of cardiac medications prior to pregnancy predicts small-for-gestational-age babies [15]. This may reflect the severity of the condition and its associated negative effects on placental blood flow as well as the direct effects of medication or a combination of both [15]. Prematurity occurs in 6.3 % [13] to 18 % [16].

The risk of vertical transmission of congenital heart disease is 2–3 %, which is two to three times that of the background general population risk of 0.8 %. Patients with unrepaired tetralogy of Fallot and those with hypoplastic, disconnected or ductal origin pulmonary arteries are even more likely to have low birthweight babies [10]. Fetal mortality related to prematurity, intrauterine growth restriction and congenital heart defect recurrence is 2–6 % [16]. The risks of miscarriage, prematurity and having a small-for-gestational-age baby are highest for the unrepaired patient with tetralogy of Fallot or tetralogy of Fallot with pulmonary atresia and MAPCAs and are predicted by resting oxygen saturations.

7.3 Care During Pregnancy and Labour

7.3.1 Management of Pregnancy in Repaired Tetralogy of Fallot

Patients with repaired tetralogy of Fallot are best managed by or with guidance from a *specialist heart disease and pregnancy clinical service*. There, the multidisciplinary team (cardiologist with specific expertise in the care of women with heart disease during pregnancy, an anaesthetist, obstetrician and midwife) will make an *individualised pregnancy and birth plan*. All notes, including antenatal records, results of up-to-date heart investigations and the delivery plan, should be available to all caregivers. The frequency of outpatient review is adjusted according to the individual's cardiac lesion and functional status.

Fetal echocardiography should be offered in all cases at 13–16 weeks and or at 20–22 weeks according to local expertise and resource. If congenital heart disease is identified, support including multidisciplinary case discussion involves fetal cardiologists, paediatric cardiologists and surgeons and the adult congenital heart disease team to facilitate decision-making for the parents.

During pregnancy, *periodic assessments* should focus on clinical and or echocardiographic signs of right or left ventricular dysfunction and the exclusion of clinically significant arrhythmia. All cardiac medications need to be reviewed, although most contemporary female patients of childbearing age with repaired tetralogy of Fallot will not be on cardiac medication. ACE inhibitors should be stopped before pregnancy, but beta blockers may be continued with close surveillance of fetal growth.

Where the volume overload related to pregnancy further complicates pre-pregnancy right ventricular dilatation, diuretics and other heart failure treatment such as beta blockers may be indicated. Standard physical signs such as jugular venous pulsation, mild ankle oedema and right ventricular heave are not necessarily discriminating in later stages of pregnancy, and other investigations including chest x-ray may be needed. Rarely, *residual pulmonary valve and right ventricular outflow tract stenosis* are problematic in pregnancy, and in these cases balloon dilatation and stenting of the right ventricular outflow tract obstruction may warrant discussion.

For the woman with repaired tetralogy of Fallot, the ideal is to await spontaneous onset of labour and *aim for vaginal delivery* with adequate and effective pain relief unless obstetric complications indicate otherwise. Patients at high risk of cardiac complications may need to plan tertiary-centre delivery where combined specialist care for women with heart disease is available. However, this will not be necessary for many women with repaired tetralogy of Fallot, for whom local general hospital antenatal and postnatal care is sufficient. Assisted delivery should be available to avoid a prolonged second stage of labour where necessary. This is especially desirable in the case of associated aortic dilatation to reduce maternal Valsalva efforts. The practice of elective assisted delivery may however be associated with higher rates of post-partum haemorrhage and 3rd-/4th-degree lacerations [19]. Although, for most patients, no specific monitoring is required, continuous ECG is advised for those with a history of arrhythmia. In the case of unrepaired tetralogy of Fallot or cyanotic pulmonary atresia, invasive arterial monitoring may be warranted. The use of Oxytocin should also be limited due to related vasodilatation and arterial hypotension.

In the case of Caesarean section for obstetric reasons, prophylactic antibiotics should be given. In addition, a repaired tetralogy of Fallot patient with a residual ventricular septal defect or previous endocarditis warrants prophylactic antibiotics, independent of mode of delivery as significant bacteraemia is associated with delivery [20]. For those that present with fever, a high index of suspicion of endocarditis should be maintained with repeated blood cultures performed.

For patients with Fallot with *pulmonary atresia*, close surveillance of ventricular function and degree of cyanosis are needed, as these are the main mediators of an adverse pregnancy outcome [12]. Patients with left ventricular diastolic dysfunction may develop pulmonary oedema during labour and around the delivery period. Close monitoring of haemodynamics with prompt treatment can prevent adverse events. Follow-up for these patients needs to be more frequent.

Post-partum follow-up should be individualised; at a minimum low risk women should have a 6-week follow-up. ACE inhibitors, if prescribed previously, are safe to recommence during breastfeeding. From 6 months to 1 year, a new set of cardiac investigations to reassess heart and circulatory status will be useful in particular for those patients with pulmonary regurgitation and right heart dilatation where surveillance needs to be re-established. This assessment will help inform frequency of their on-going adult congenital heart disease follow-up.

7.4 Impact of Physiological Changes

7.4.1 Impact of Pregnancy Adaptation in Repaired Tetralogy of Fallot

Pregnancy-induced cardiac adaptations include initial arterial vasodilatation, followed by a rapid increase in blood volume and cardiac output and a more gradual increase in ventricular mass. These changes reverse over the subsequent 6 months after pregnancy, but a major question is whether pregnancy is associated with a progressive right ventricular dysfunction. A large retrospective data analysis including available echocardiography showed that right ventricular size progressively increased at follow-up in the subgroup of 16 pregnancy patients with repaired tetralogy of Fallot to a degree not present in the 13 controls [21]. The series may have included patients representative of an earlier era of less proactive elective treatment of pulmonary regurgitation, but another retrospective series of 13 pregnancies in women with tetralogy of Fallot investigated the serial changes in indexed right ventricular volumes, documented with cardiovascular magnetic resonance, and demonstrated an apparent accelerated progression of RV dilation. This increased progression compared to matched controls (tetralogy of Fallot without pregnancy) appeared to be driven by those women whose RV dilation was already at the current threshold to merit elective pulmonary valve replacement [22].

Left ventricular diastolic dysfunction is a predictor of adverse outcome in patients with repaired tetralogy of Fallot. In a small prospective data series, progression of diastolic dysfunction related to pregnancy was demonstrated in a cohort of 35 women including six with tetralogy of Fallot (one with severe aortic regurgitation pre-pregnancy) [23]. Progressive aortic dilatation has been raised as a potential concern but there are few data [10].

7.5 Preconception Counselling

For unrepaired patients or those at higher risk of thrombus formation, oestrogen-containing contraceptives should be avoided. If patients are on regular cardiac medications, specific instructions regarding stopping or continuing each drug during planned conception and pregnancy should be given.

In some patients, tetralogy of Fallot is part of the DiGeorge syndrome (15%) for which genetic testing (22Q11 deletion) is available and should be offered to all patients at the time of preconception counselling. The risk of recurrence of DiGeorge syndrome is 50%, but the risk of recurrence in its absence is around 3% [24].

Maternal death is rare. Patients with significant left ventricular dysfunction or severe pulmonary hypertension are those in whom pregnancy-associated risks are high, and pregnancy therefore is inadvisable [10].

Conclusions

Pregnancy outcomes for asymptomatic women with repaired tetralogy of Fallot are good, certainly for those cared for in recognised centres from where the limited data available are derived. Nevertheless, a minority of contemporary childbearing women with repaired tetralogy of Fallot may be at risk, and patient-specific risk stratification is needed in all. Those presenting to antenatal services without recent follow-up of their congenital heart disease, for example, due to migration or loss to follow-up after childhood care, may be most at risk of having entered pregnancy in a suboptimal cardiac condition. The most common maternal complications are arrhythmia and heart failure, both of which usually respond to treatment. Pulmonary regurgitation, the most common adult sequelae of repair of tetralogy of Fallot, does not preclude pregnancy but is less well tolerated if associated with significant right ventricular dilatation or dysfunction prior to pregnancy. Complications in pregnancy are highest in those with associated significant pulmonary hypertension (discussed elsewhere), pulmonary regurgitation with right ventricular dysfunction and or left ventricular dysfunction. Registry data including patient phenotyping using gold standard heart investigation at standard serial intervals remains vital to define which subgroups of women are at risk of deterioration of ventricular function due to pregnancy so that counselling and care can be further individualised.

Acknowledgements Sonya V. Babu-Narayan is supported by an Intermediate Clinical Research Fellowship from the British Heart Foundation (FS/11/38/28864). This project was supported by the NIHR Cardiovascular Biomedical Research Unit of Royal Brompton and Harefield NHS Foundation Trust and Imperial College London. This report is an independent research by the National Institute for Health Research Biomedical Research Unit Funding Scheme. The views expressed in this publication are those of the author(s) and not necessarily those of the NHS, the National Institute for Health Research or the Department of Health.

References

1. Nieminen HP, Jokinen EV, Sairanen HI (2001) Late results of pediatric cardiac surgery in Finland: a population-based study with 96% follow-up. Circulation 104(5):570–575, PMID: 11479255
2. Hoffman JI, Kaplan S (2002) The incidence of congenital heart disease. J Am Coll Cardiol 39(12):1890–1900, PMID: 12084585
3. Nollert G, Fischlein T, Bouterwek S, Böhmer C, Klinner W, Reichart B (1997) Long-term survival in patients with repair of tetralogy of Fallot: 36-year follow-up of 490 survivors of the first year after surgical repair. J Am Coll Cardiol 30(5):1374–1383, PMID: 9350942
4. Lillehei CW, Cohen M, Warden HE, Varco RL (1955) The direct-vision intracardiac correction of congenital anomalies by controlled cross circulation; results in thirty-two patients with ventricular septal defects, tetralogy of Fallot, and atrioventricularis communis defects. Surgery 38(1):11–29, No abstract available. PMID: 14396676
5. Cuypers JA, Menting ME, Konings EE, Opić P, Utens EM, Helbing WA, Witsenburg M, van den Bosch AE, Ouhlous M, van Domburg RT, Rizopoulos D, Meijboom FJ, Boersma E, Bogers AJ, Roos-Hesselink JW (2014) Unnatural history of tetralogy of Fallot: prospective follow-up of 40 years after surgical correction. Circulation 130(22):1944–1953. doi:10.1161/CIRCULATIONAHA.114.009454, Epub 2014 Oct 23.PMID: 25341442
6. Singh H, Bolton PJ, Oakley CM (1982) Pregnancy after surgical correction of tetralogy of Fallot. Br Med J (Clin Res Ed) 285(6336):168–170
7. Khairy P, Ouyang DW, Fernandes SM, Lee-Parritz A, Economy KE, Landzberg MJ (2006) Pregnancy outcomes in women with congenital heart disease. Circulation 113(4):517–524
8. Elkayam U, Bitar F (2005) Valvular heart disease and pregnancy part I: native valves. J Am Coll Cardiol 46(2):223–230, PMID: 16022946, Review
9. Mongeon FP, Gurvitz MZ, Broberg CS, Aboulhosn J, Opotowsky AR, Kay JD, Valente AM, Earing MG, Lui GK, Fernandes SM, Gersony DR, Cook SC, Ting JG, Nickolaus MJ, Landzberg

MJ, Khairy P, Alliance for Adult Research in Congenital Cardiology (AARCC) (2013) Aortic root dilatation in adults with surgically repaired tetralogy of fallot: a multicenter cross-sectional study. Circulation 127(2):172–179. doi:10.1161/CIRCULATIONAHA.112.129585, PMID: 23224208, Epub 2012 Dec 6
10. Baumgartner H, Bonhoeffer P, De Groot NM, de Haan F, Deanfield JE, Galie N, Gatzoulis MA, Gohlke-Baerwolf C, Kaemmerer H, Kilner P, Meijboom F, Mulder BJ, Oechslin E, Oliver JM, Serraf A, Szatmari A, Thaulow E, Vouhe PR, Walma E, Task Force on the Management of Grown-up Congenital Heart Disease of the European Society of Cardiology (ESC), Association for European Paediatric Cardiology (AEPC), ESC Committee for Practice Guidelines (CPG) (2010) ESC Guidelines for the management of grown-up congenital heart disease (new version 2010). Eur Heart J 31(23):2915–2957. doi:10.1093/eurheartj/ehq249, Epub 2010 Aug 27. No abstract available. PMID: 20801927
11. Veldtman GR, Connolly HM, Grogan M, Ammash NM, Warnes CA (2004) Outcomes of pregnancy in women with tetralogy of Fallot. J Am Coll Cardiol 44(1):174–180
12. Drenthen W, Pieper PG, Roos-Hesselink JW, van Lottum WA, Voors AA, Mulder BJ, van Dijk AP, Vliegen HW, Yap SC, Moons P, Ebels T, van Veldhuisen DJ, ZAHARA Investigators (2007) Outcome of pregnancy in women with congenital heart disease: a literature review. J Am Coll Cardiol 49(24):2303–2311, PMID: 17572244, Epub 2007 Jun 4. Review
13. Balci A, Drenthen W, Mulder BJ, Roos-Hesselink JW, Voors AA, Vliegen HW, Moons P, Sollie KM, van Dijk AP, van Veldhuisen DJ, Pieper PG (2011) Pregnancy in women with corrected tetralogy of Fallot: occurrence and predictors of adverse events. Am Heart J 161(2):307–313. doi:10.1016/j.ahj.2010.10.027, PMID: 21315213, Epub 2011 Jan 15
14. Drenthen W, Boersma E, Balci A, Moons P, Roos-Hesselink JW, Mulder BJ, Vliegen HW, van Dijk AP, Voors AA, Yap SC, van Veldhuisen DJ, Pieper PG, ZAHARA Investigators (2010) Predictors of pregnancy complications in women with congenital heart disease. Eur Heart J 31(17):2124–2132. doi:10.1093/eurheartj/ehq200, PMID: 20584777, Epub 2010 Jun 28
15. Silversides CK, Harris L, Haberer K, Sermer M, Colman JM, Siu SC (2006) Recurrence rates of arrhythmias during pregnancy in women with previous tachyarrhythmia and impact on fetal and neonatal outcomes. Am J Cardiol 97(8):1206–1212, Epub 2006 Mar 3.PMID: 16616027
16. Presbitero P, Somerville J, Stone S, Aruta E, Spiegelhalter D, Rabajoli F (1994) Pregnancy in cyanotic congenital heart disease. Outcome of mother and fetus. Circulation 89(6):2673–2676, PMID: 8205680
17. Neumayer U, Somerville J (1997) Outcome of pregnancies in patients with complex pulmonary atresia. Heart 78(1):16–21, PMID: 9290396
18. Gelson E, Gatzoulis M, Steer PJ, Lupton M, Johnson M (2008) Tetralogy of Fallot: maternal and neonatal outcomes. BJOG 115(3):398–402. doi:10.1111/j.14710528.2007.01610.x, PMID: 18190378
19. Ouyang DW, Khairy P, Fernandes SM, Landzberg MJ, Economy KE (2010) Obstetric outcomes in pregnant women with congenital heart disease. Int J Cardiol 144(2):195–199. doi:10.1016/j.ijcard.2009.04.006, PMID: 19411123, Epub 2009 May 2
20. Mitchell SC, Korones SB, Berendes HW (1971) Congenital heart disease in 56,109 births. Incidence and natural history. Circulation 43(3):323–332, PMID: 5102136
21. Uebing A, Arvanitis P, Li W, Diller GP, Babu-Narayan SV, Okonko D, Koltsida E, Papadopoulos M, Johnson MR, Lupton MG, Yentis SM, Steer PJ, Gatzoulis MA (2010) Effect of pregnancy on clinical status and ventricular function in women with heart disease. Int J Cardiol 139(1):50–59
22. Egidy Assenza G, Cassater D, Landzberg M, Geva T, Schreier J, Graham D, Volpe M, Barker N, Economy K, Valente AM (2013) The effects of pregnancy on right ventricular remodeling in women with repaired tetralogy of Fallot. Int J Cardiol 168(3):1847–1852. doi:10.1016/j.ijcard.2012.12.071, PMID: 23369674, Epub 2013 Jan 28
23. Cornette J, Ruys TP, Rossi A, Rizopoulos D, Takkenberg JJ, Karamermer Y, Opić P, Van den Bosch AE, Geleijnse ML, Duvekot JJ, Steegers EA, Roos-Hesselink JW (2013) Hemodynamic adaptation to pregnancy in women with structural heart disease. Int J Cardiol 168(2):825–831. doi:10.1016/j.ijcard.2012.10.005, PMID: 23151412, Epub 2012 Nov 11
24. Nora JJ (1994) From generational studies to a multilevel genetic-environmental interaction. J Am Coll Cardiol 23(6):1468–1471

Transposition of the Great Arteries

8

Daniel Tobler and Matthias Greutmann

Abbreviations

BNP	Brain natriuretic peptide
CHD	Congenital heart disease
d-TGA	D-loop transposition of the great arteries
FAC	Fractional area change
LVOTO	Left ventricular outflow tract obstruction
NR	Not reported
NYHA	New York Heart Association
TGA	Transposition of the great arteries
VSDs	Ventricular septal defects

D. Tobler, MD (✉)
Department of Cardiology, University Hospital Basel,
Petersgraben 4, Basel CH-4031, Switzerland
e-mail: daniel.tobler@hin.ch

M. Greutmann, MD
University Heart Center, Department of Cardiology, University Hospital Zurich,
Raemistrasse 100, Zurich CH-8091, Switzerland
e-mail: Matthias.Greutmann@usz.ch

© Springer International Publishing Switzerland 2017
J.W. Roos-Hesselink, M.R. Johnson (eds.), *Pregnancy and Congenital Heart Disease*, Congenital Heart Disease in Adolescents and Adults,
DOI 10.1007/978-3-319-38913-4_8

Key Facts of Preconception
Incidence: 0.3 per 1000 live births.
Inheritance: Not an elevated risk of congenital heart disease in the offspring.
Medication: ACE inhibitors, AT1 antagonists and some antiarrhythmic agents are contraindicated during pregnancy and should be stopped or replaced.
Typical WHO grade: After atrial repair operation: III (or IV in case of diminished ventricular function or other complications). After uncomplicated arterial switch: II.
Risk of pregnancy: After atrial repair, atrial arrhythmias and heart failure; after arterial switch, aortic dilatation.
Life expectancy: Clearly diminished after atrial repair and slightly diminished after arterial switch.

Key Management
Preconception: Clinical assessment for signs of heart failure, ECG/Holter for arrhythmia. Ventricular and valve function need to be assessed by echocardiography specifically in patients with the atrial repair left-to-right shunt due to baffle leaks and should be actively sought. Screening for systemic and pulmonary venous obstruction and, if relevant, preconception interventions should be discussed. After arterial switch: careful aortic root assessment. Cardiopulmonary exercise testing can be useful for predicting exercise intolerance during pregnancy. It may also detect silent ischaemia in patients after the arterial switch repair. Cardiac MRI should be performed in patients with subaortic RV dysfunction and neo-aortic root dilation as a baseline assessment. Baseline elevated brain natriuretic peptide (BNP) can unmask patients at risk for cardiac complications during pregnancy.

Pregnancy: Atrial repair, at least every trimester with ECG and echo. After arterial switch: at least once at 20 weeks with echo. In patients with functional deterioration, clinical signs of heart failure or arrhythmia or dilated neo-aortic root dimensions, a closer follow-up is required.

Labour: Vaginal delivery is the preferred method. Caesarean section for cardiac reason is reserved for those with aortic root dilatation (>4.5 cm) and those with symptomatic heart failure at the onset of labour. Early epidural anaesthesia or a low-dose combined spinal-epidural is suggested for most women with atrial repair. Continuous telemetric monitoring is advised in women at high risk for arrhythmias.

Postpartum: Atrial repair at least 48 h; arterial switch, at least 6 h.

8.1 The Condition

8.1.1 Anatomy, Surgical Techniques and Cardiac Outcomes of d-TGA

D-loop transposition of the great arteries (d-TGA) is the second most frequent cyanotic congenital heart defect with a prevalence of about 0.3 per 1000 live births [1] and a male preponderance of 2:1. In d-TGA the atrial chambers are connected to their morphologically appropriate ventricles (atrioventricular concordance), whereas the aorta arises from the right ventricle and the pulmonary artery from the left ventricle (ventriculo-arterial discordance). This anatomy leads to separated pulmonary and systemic circulations in parallel: Deoxygenated blood returning to the heart from the systemic circulation is pumped back to the systemic circulation by the right ventricle, while oxygenated pulmonary venous blood is pumped back into the lungs through the left ventricle (Fig. 8.1). Associated congenital cardiac lesions

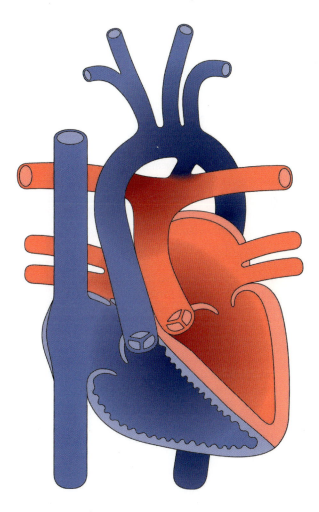

Fig. 8.1 d-Transposition of the great arteries with intact ventricular septum (Copyright © 2014 New Media Center, University of Basel. All Rights Reserved)

in d-TGA include ventricular septal defects (VSDs) in about 40–50% and, less commonly, left ventricular outflow tract obstruction and coarctation of the aorta.

8.1.1.1 Surgical Repair Techniques

Before surgical repair became available, d-TGA was a lethal condition with an average life expectancy at birth of 0.65 years [2]. When open-heart surgery became feasible in the mid-1950s, survival changed dramatically. In the contemporary era, d-TGA has become a well-treatable condition and survival to adulthood is the rule [3, 4].

The first widely used repair technique was the atrial switch operation (Senning or Mustard procedure) with redirection of the venous blood flow at the atrial level [5, 6]. By the late 1980s, the arterial switch operation (Jatene operation) with redirection of blood flow at the level of the great arteries superseded the atrial switch procedure [7]. For the small subset of patients with d-TGA, concomitant ventricular septal defect and pulmonary stenosis, the Rastelli operation was and is an important surgical option [8]. Although the atrial switch operation is no longer performed today, the majority of patients who underwent this operation are still alive and there remains a substantial cohort of women in the childbearing age. As a consequence, all three repair techniques may be encountered in women of childbearing age. Relevant aspects of physiology, long-term complications and pregnancy-specific problems regarding these three types of repair will be discussed below.

(i) *The atrial switch operation* (*the Senning and Mustard procedure*): The principle of the atrial switch operation is illustrated in Fig. 8.2. Although technically slightly different procedures, the physiological result after the Senning and the Mustard operation is the same: redirection of systemic venous blood at the atrial level by surgically created baffles. The atrial switch operation leaves the morphological right ventricle as the systemic (subaortic) ventricle and the tricuspid valve as the systemic atrioventricular valve.

(ii) *The arterial switch operation* (*the Jatene procedure*): The principle of the arterial switch operation is illustrated in Fig. 8.3. The operation anatomically corrects the transposed arteries by transection of the aorta and the pulmonary artery above the valve level, reimplantation of the coronary arteries into the neo-aortic root and forward translocation of the pulmonary artery into its new position anterior to the aorta. The benefit of the Jatene technique is that the anatomic left ventricle is located in the systemic (subaortic) position and surgical manipulation of the atria is avoided. With refinement of the surgical technique, the arterial switch operation has become the standard procedure for patients with d-TGA since the late 1980s/early 1990s. Therefore, the cohort of women after the ASO of childbearing age is younger than the atrial switch cohort, and data regarding pregnancy issues and outcomes in this novel adult patient cohort are less robust.

(iii) *The Rastelli operation*: The Rastelli operation was introduced in 1969 to repair patients with d-TGA with concomitant ventricular septal defect and obstruction to pulmonary outflow. The principle of the Rastelli operation is illustrated

Fig. 8.2 Atrial switch operation (Copyright © 2014 New Media Center, University of Basel. All Rights Reserved)

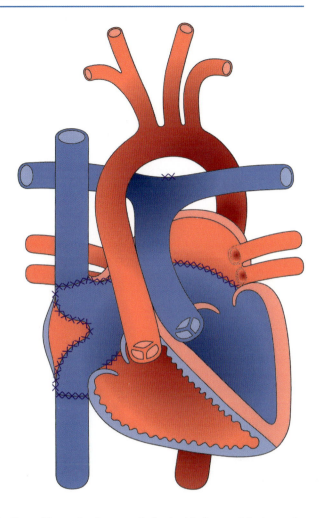

in Fig. 8.4. After the Rastelli repair, the morphological left ventricle is established in subaortic position, and the continuity between the subpulmonic right ventricle and the pulmonary artery is created by implantation of a bioprosthetic valved conduit.

Long-term outcomes of patients with repaired d-TGA are largely determined by the type of repair and type and severity of residual haemodynamic lesions. The most common long-term complications in patients after atrial switch repair are arrhythmias (particularly atypical atrial flutter and sinus node dysfunction) and progressive dysfunction of the subaortic right ventricle with or without progressive systemic tricuspid valve regurgitation. Furthermore, baffle obstruction and baffle leaks as well as pulmonary hypertension can occur. On average, this patient group has substantially reduced exercise capacity compared to the general population [9]. Cardiac complications become more common as patients age. These patients have a reduced life expectancy, which is important for pre-pregnancy counselling. There is however

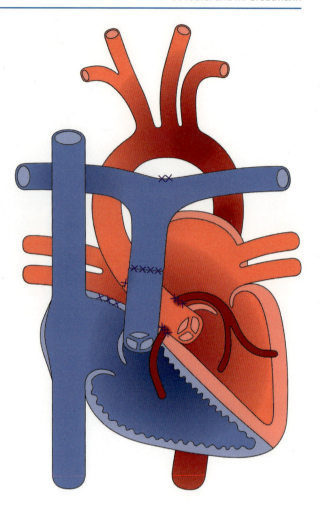

Fig. 8.3 Arterial switch operation (Copyright © 2014 New Media Center, University of Basel. All Rights Reserved)

a wide range in individual variation of disease courses. Long-term follow-up data beyond the fifth decade of life is not yet available.

The majority of adult survivors after the arterial switch operation are still young, and their outcome beyond the third decade of life is not yet known. To date, it seems that subaortic ventricular dysfunction and arrhythmias are less common compared to patients after the atrial switch operation [10–12]. The main reason for re-intervention is obstruction of the branch pulmonary arteries. Potential long-term complications include neo-aortic root dilatation, neo-aortic valve regurgitation or obstruction of the reimplanted coronary arteries [13, 14]. Survival to adulthood is the rule but lifelong specialised follow-up remains mandatory.

In patients after the Rastelli repair, re-intervention due to deterioration of the right ventricular-pulmonary artery conduit is inevitable. Subaortic left ventricular

Fig. 8.4 Rastelli operation (Copyright © 2014 New Media Center, University of Basel. All Rights Reserved)

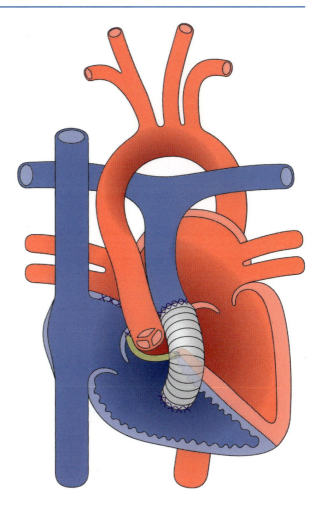

dysfunction and arrhythmias are relatively common. In the largest published series on long-term outcomes after Rastelli repair, overall freedom from death and transplantation was 52 % at 20 years [15]. In contrast, in the Canadian cohort, the estimated survival at 17 years of follow-up was 89 % [16].

8.2 Pregnancy Outcome

Data regarding pregnancy outcomes in women with the atrial switch operation are limited to several medium-sized and smaller retrospective case series [17–23]. Reports of pregnancy outcomes in women after the arterial switch operation and Rastelli repair are sparse [24, 25]. Reported pregnancy outcomes of series of patients with repaired d-TGA are summarised in Table 8.1 [26].

Table 8.1 Summary of pregnancy outcomes of women with repaired d-TGA

Study	Atrial switch							Arterial switch	Rastelli
	Clarkson et al.	Genoni et al.	Drenthen et al.	Canobbio et al.	Metz et al.	Trigas et al.	Cataldo et al.	Tobler et al.	Radford, Stafford
Publication year	1994	1999	2005	2006	2011	2014	2015	2010	2005
Number of women	9	11	28	40	10	34	21	9	6[a]
Number of pregnancies	15	13	69	70	21	60	34	17	12
Cardiac outcomes									
Women with cardiac complications (%)	0	9	61	45	14 (baffle obstruction in 36%)	NR	62	22	50 (LVOTO 100% in d-TGA)
Arrhythmia (%)	0	0	16	36 (no further specification)	7	5	14	6	0
Heart failure (%)	0	9	3		7	6	0	0	0
Deteriorating NYHA class (%)	0	23	25		NR	12	14	0	NR
Obstetric and fetal outcomes									
Hypertension-associated complications (%)	20	NR	13	17	7	2	NR	NR	NR
Miscarriages in first trimester (%)	13	15	25	14	29	18	NR[b]	23	41
Live births (%)	80	77	71	77	67	73	NR[b]	76	50 (25% in d-TGA)
Live births at <35 weeks of gestation (%)	0	0	33	39	50	25	38 (<37 weeks)	0	16 (50% in d-TGA)
Number of infants with CHD	0	0	0	0	0	0	0	1	0

Modified from Roche [26]

CHD congenital heart disease, *LVOTO* left ventricular outflow tract obstruction, *NYHA* New York Heart Association, *NR* not reported, *TGA* transposition of the great arteries

[a]Three women with d-TGA, three women with other types of CHD
[b]Report on completed pregnancies only

8.2.1 Cardiac Risks

Cardiac events during pregnancy and peripartum in women after the Mustard or Senning operation include arrhythmias, heart failure and thromboembolic or cerebrovascular events. In a meta-analysis of peer-reviewed literature, Drenthen et al. reported pregnancy outcomes of 170 pregnancies in women after the atrial switch operations. The most frequently encountered cardiac complication was arrhythmia (15.6%) followed by heart failure (10.8%) [27].

The major concern of pregnancy in women after the atrial switch operation is the fact that in two reported series, the risk of worsening subaortic ventricular function during pregnancy was reported to be as high as 25% of pregnancies, with no recovery in the majority of cases [22, 28]. Although the mortality risk is small, pregnancy-related deaths have been reported [18, 29]. In a recent report from three tertiary care centres, five life-threatening events occurred in 60 pregnancies (8%), two of which were cardiac arrest complicating delivery, with successful resuscitation [22]. In a North American cohort of 14 pregnancies that resulted in live births, symptomatic baffle obstruction was observed in five (36%) pregnancies [21]. In three of these five women, baffle obstruction became symptomatic in their second pregnancy. In all instances, the superior limb of the systemic venous atrial baffle was affected.

There are limited data on the late effects of pregnancy on subaortic right ventricle function. In a recently published series in women with the atrial switch operation, 21 women were followed after pregnancy and were compared with 15 women affected by the same condition who had never had a pregnancy [23]. Follow-up duration was 95 months in the pregnancy group. There were no differences in cardiovascular events (62% versus 53%, P-value 0.7) or worsening systemic ventricular function (29% versus 27%, P-value 0.9), but worsening systemic tricuspid valve regurgitation was significantly more common in the pregnancy group compared to controls (52% versus 0%, P-value 0.001). Additionally, in 14% of women in the pregnancy group, there was worsening of the functional class during pregnancy, which did not improve during follow-up. In contrast, no woman in the control group had worsening of the function class during follow-up.

So far, pregnancy outcomes in women after the arterial switch operation have been described in only one series [24]. The outcomes of 17 pregnancies in nine women managed in two large tertiary care hospitals have been reported. Two women developed cardiac complications during pregnancy; one woman with impaired left ventricular systolic function had non-sustained ventricular tachycardia and one woman with a mechanical systemic atrioventricular valve developed postpartum valve thrombosis. A large proportion of women in this cohort had important residual lesions that confer risk for adverse events in pregnancy, likely related to the fact that these women had the arterial switch operation performed in the early surgical era. With later modifications of the operative technique (i.e. the Lecompte manoeuvre), contemporary cohorts of arterial switch patients may have less residual lesions, which may positively impact their risk of pregnancy complications.

Pregnancy outcomes in women with the Rastelli operation have been reported in one series of six women with a total of 12 pregnancies [25]. Three women had

Rastelli repair for d-TGA and the remaining three women had other types of congenital heart disease. Remarkably, all three women with complex d-TGA developed more severe subaortic obstruction during pregnancy, and further surgery was needed during follow-up.

8.2.2 Obstetric and Fetal Risks

Some series report high rates of preeclampsia and pregnancy-induced hypertension (Table 8.1). Other obstetric complications included premature rupture of membranes and thromboembolic complications [17–20, 22]. In the reported series, induction of labour was commonly utilised (up to 50%). In most women with repaired d-TGA, vaginal delivery with epidural anaesthesia is the preferred mode of delivery. Caesarean section for cardiac reasons should be considered for women with significant neo-aortic root dilatation after the arterial switch operation or women after the atrial switch operation with severe symptomatic heart failure.

Premature deliveries are common in women with repaired d-TGA (25–50% in reported series). In the meta-analysis of Drenthen et al., premature delivery was reported in 34% of pregnancies. The reported reasons for premature delivery were mainly obstetric (preterm premature rupture of membranes, severe preeclampsia, placenta praevia with bleeding) [21]. The number of babies born small for gestational age was 19% in the meta-analysis of Drenthen et al. Fetal risks may differ substantially among cohorts of women with different types of repair, and there are very little data on fetal risks in pregnancies of women after the Rastelli operation and the arterial switch operation. In the only series of pregnancies after the arterial switch, there was no preterm delivery and no fetal or neonatal death. In those with birth weights available, the mean birth weight was 3.3 ± 0.5 kg. One child had a birth weight that was small for its gestational age (2330 g, delivered at 38 weeks of gestation). Perinatal mortality has been reported in two children of women with the atrial switch operation [27]. Congenital heart disease in the offspring is rare (<1%) [27]. In all reported pregnancies of women with repaired d-TGA ($n=311$), only one newborn was described having congenital heart disease (Table 8.1).

8.3 Care During Pregnancy and Labour

All women with repaired d-TGA should have a cardiac assessment early in pregnancy (first trimester) to determine their baseline status. Serial follow-up during pregnancy should include clinical assessment and serial transthoracic echocardiography. In patients after the Mustard or Senning repair, quantitative assessment of systolic right ventricular function is challenging. In our practice, for comparison of serial measurements, we recommend to record the fractional area change (FAC), lateral tricuspid annular plane systolic excursion (TAPSE), lateral RV systolic motion velocities by tissue Doppler and the rate of systolic RV pressure increase (dP/dt). In a small series of ten women who underwent serial echocardiograms, dP/

dt decreased during pregnancy with an average value of 1168 ± 156 mmHg/s before pregnancy, compared with 859 ± 228 mmHg/s at week 28 of gestation, and was not regained completely (dP/dt 1081 ± 109 mmHg/s) postpartum [21]. However, the onset of functional deterioration or overt heart failure is not predictable by echocardiographic measurements, and most pregnancies in repaired TGA are tolerated even in the setting of decreased systolic function of the subaortic RV [21, 22].

Echocardiographic follow-up should be performed at the time of peak haemodynamic stress (28–32 weeks of gestation) as well as postpartum. In patients with functional deterioration, clinical signs of heart failure or arrhythmia or dilated neoaortic root dimensions, close follow-up during pregnancy is required. In symptomatic patients with functional deterioration, measurement of BNP or NT-Pro-BNP might be useful to distinguish cardiac complications from other causes of similar symptoms [35]. Increased BNP levels at 20 weeks of gestational age have been shown to predict adverse cardiac events in pregnant women with CHD [36]. Women with heart failure and arrhythmia during pregnancy should be treated according to current guidelines for non-pregnant patients, respecting contraindications for some drugs in pregnancy [31, 37].

A detailed delivery plan is mandatory in all patients with repaired d-TGA. A multidisciplinary team approach is key for optimal peripartum care with the lowest possible risk for the affected woman. In most women vaginal delivery is the preferred method of delivery [31, 38]. Caesarean section for cardiac reason is reserved for those with marked aortic root dilatation (>4.5 cm) and those with symptomatic heart failure at the onset of labour. Early epidural anaesthesia or a low-dose combined spinal-epidural is suggested for most women with repaired d-TGA. The haemodynamic benefit is reduction of cardiac output peaks during labour which are largely mediated by catecholamine surges due to pain and anxiety. Reduction in catecholamine release may lead to reduction of arrhythmia risk, prothrombotic effects and hypertension, which would be an added stress on the systemic ventricle. In patients with progressive heart failure, progressive deterioration of ventricular function or uncontrolled arrhythmia, early involvement of experienced obstetric anaesthetists is important and, if required, the input of cardiac anaesthetists. If overt heart failure occurs, patients should be admitted to a specialised centre, and precipitating factors, such as infection or arrhythmias, should be actively sought and excluded. Bed rest, supplemental oxygen and careful fluid balance with daily weight measurements should be initiated. Careful administration of diuretics may be used but with great caution to avoid overdiuresis which can reduce uteroplacental blood flow. Caesarean section should be considered in women with overt heart failure and haemodynamic instability. The timing of Caesarean section or induced delivery is complex and needs individual consideration based on a multidisciplinary decision. Patients at high risk for cardiac complications need early and extended in-hospital surveillance ante- and postpartum. Continuous electrocardiographic monitoring can be useful, especially in women at high risk for arrhythmias. Invasive monitoring is not generally advised. In patients with residual shunts (i.e. baffle leaks), air- and particulate-eliminating filters should be used on IV lines to avoid paradoxical embolism, because during the profound haemodynamic shifts of labour and delivery, transient reversal of shunt may occur. However, if the delivery of large volumes or radiopaque contrast is required, administration without bubble filters is required; on these occasions, meticulous de-bubbling of IV lines is important.

8.4 Impact of Physiological Changes

Pregnancy, the time of labour and delivery and the postpartum period are associated with profound haemodynamic changes. Plasma volume, stroke volume, cardiac output and heart rate increase importantly. In women with repaired d-TGA, residual haemodynamic lesions, arrhythmias or ventricular dysfunction may hamper the normal adaptation of the cardiovascular system to the demands of pregnancy and so precipitate cardiovascular complications.

8.5 Preconception Counselling

General aspects of preconception counselling in repaired d-TGA: Ideally, all women with repaired d-TGA should have specialist preconception assessment and counselling. Counselling about effective use of contraception and potential risks of pregnancy should begin in adolescence. Educational strategies should be tailored to strengthen the knowledge and appropriate use of *contraception* to avoid unplanned pregnancies and to identify women at increased risk from oestrogen-containing contraceptives. Education should include the maternal and fetal risks of pregnancy, as well as long-term prognosis and risks of long-term complications of the underlying heart defect and the potential impact of pregnancy on long-term outcomes. It should also include information about risks of delayed pregnancies and the need for family planning, particularly in women after an atrial switch repair. Only open and detailed counselling and discussion of these risks will allow the affected woman with d-TGA to make an informed decision about whether or not to proceed with a high-risk pregnancy.

The method of contraception has to combine the highest efficacy and safety profile. Women with residual intracardiac shunt lesions (e.g. women with baffle leaks after the atrial switch repair) should avoid oestrogen-containing contraceptives [30]. Routine testing for residual intracardiac shunts may be considered in these women.

All women with repaired d-TGA need an up-to-date assessment before conception. Individual risk stratification is performed, and risk estimation is based on residual lesions, ventricular function and functional status. Patients with more than moderate impairment of subaortic ventricular function or severe tricuspid regurgitation in the setting of a subaortic right ventricle should be advised against pregnancy [31]. Pre-pregnancy assessment requires a review of the patient's medication, as some may be contraindicated in pregnancy (i.e. angiotensin-converting enzyme inhibitors, angiotensin or aldosterone antagonists). Ideally, such drugs should be stopped well before conception and, when indicated and possible, should be substituted by drugs compatible with pregnancy.

Women with the atrial switch operation should be informed that pregnancy might have an unfavourable long-term impact on subaortic ventricular function. RV function declines in some women during pregnancy, often without complete return to baseline in the postpartum period [21]. Pregnancy might be potentially harmful in the long term and may have an impact on functional status and cardiac morbidity. A seldom-considered issue is that pregnancy increases the likelihood of HLA sensitization, which may return as an issue later in life in a woman being considered for cardiac transplantation [32].

Apart from detailed discussions about maternal and fetal risks of pregnancy in women with repaired d-TGA, pre-pregnancy counselling includes discussion about timely family planning. Risk of pregnancy complications increases as patients age, particularly in women with the atrial switch operation. While RV function was normal in 69% after 14 years of follow-up, 10 years later only 6% of the patients had normal ventricular function ($P<0.0001$) and 61% of patients have moderate to severe RV dysfunction [33]. As a consequence of progressive RV failure and arrhythmia, the risk of premature death is already increasing in young adulthood [34], irrespective of pregnancy risks. As the prognosis of the woman with a failing systemic ventricle may interfere with the ability to raise children, discussions about the prognosis and potential long-term complications should be offered to women seeking advice for risks of pregnancy. It should also be emphasised that it is important to offer these discussions not only to our female patients but also to our male patients with repaired d-TGA when they contemplate to start a family.

Counselling about the risk of inheritance is another important aspect. Although the risk is elevated in patients with CHD in general compared to parents without CHD, inheritance risk seems to be low in parents with d-TGA. In the meta-analysis of Drenthen et al., the CHD recurrence rate was 0.6%, lower than reported in the general population [27]. Nevertheless, we recommend offering fetal echocardiography between 18 and 20 weeks of gestation for all women with d-TGA.

8.5.1 Specific Pre-pregnancy Testing

A thorough clinical assessment for signs of heart failure or arrhythmia should be carried out. Ventricular and valve function needs to be assessed by comprehensive transthoracic echocardiography in all patients with repaired d-TGA. Specifically, in patients with the atrial switch operation, left-to-right shunt due to baffle leaks should be actively sought by using agitated saline contrast echocardiography. Screening for systemic and pulmonary venous obstruction is important, and if relevant, preconception interventions should be discussed. In patients after the arterial switch repair, there should be careful aortic root assessment as neo-aortic root dilatation is a frequent finding in these patients. Conduit dysfunction (obstruction and regurgitation) needs to be assessed in patients with the Rastelli repair. In patients with severe conduit dysfunction, intervention might be necessary before the woman embarks on pregnancy. Cardiopulmonary exercise testing may be a useful tool for predicting exercise intolerance during pregnancy. It may also detect silent ischaemia in patients after the arterial switch repair. Cardiac MRI should be performed in patients with subaortic RV dysfunction and neo-aortic root dilation as a baseline assessment. Baseline elevated brain natriuretic peptide (BNP) can unmask patients at risk for cardiac complications during pregnancy, and routine measurement should be considered in all patients with repaired d-TGA.

Acknowledgement We wish to thank Prof. Jack M. Colman for the thorough review of the manuscript.

References

1. van der Linde D et al (2011) Birth prevalence of congenital heart disease worldwide: a systematic review and meta-analysis. J Am Coll Cardiol 58(21):2241–2247
2. Liebman J, Cullum L, Belloc NB (1969) Natural history of transposition of the great arteries. Anatomy and birth and death characteristics. Circulation 40(2):237–262
3. Losay J et al (2001) Late outcome after arterial switch operation for transposition of the great arteries. Circulation 104(12 Suppl 1):I121–I126
4. Moons P et al (2010) Temporal trends in survival to adulthood among patients born with congenital heart disease from 1970 to 1992 in Belgium. Circulation 122(22):2264–2272
5. Senning A (1959) Surgical correction of transposition of the great vessels. Surgery 45(6):966–980
6. Mustard WT (1964) Successful two-stage correction of transposition of the great vessels. Surgery 55:469–472
7. Jatene AD et al (1976) Anatomic correction of transposition of the great vessels. J Thorac Cardiovasc Surg 72(3):364–370
8. Rastelli GC, McGoon DC, Wallace RB (1969) Anatomic correction of transposition of the great arteries with ventricular septal defect and subpulmonary stenosis. J Thorac Cardiovasc Surg 58(4):545–552
9. Kempny A et al (2012) Reference values for exercise limitations among adults with congenital heart disease. Relation to activities of daily life – single centre experience and review of published data. Eur Heart J 33(11):1386–1396
10. Tobler D et al (2010) Cardiac outcomes in young adult survivors of the arterial switch operation for transposition of the great arteries. J Am Coll Cardiol 56(1):58–64
11. Kempny A et al (2012) Outcome in adult patients after arterial switch operation for transposition of the great arteries. Int J Cardiol 10;167(6):2588–2593
12. Khairy P et al (2013) Cardiovascular outcomes after the arterial switch operation for d-transposition of the great arteries. Circulation 127(3):331–339
13. Losay J et al (2006) Aortic valve regurgitation after arterial switch operation for transposition of the great arteries: incidence, risk factors, and outcome. J Am Coll Cardiol 47(10):2057–2062
14. Schwartz ML et al (2004) Long-term predictors of aortic root dilation and aortic regurgitation after arterial switch operation. Circulation 110(11 Suppl 1):II128–II132
15. Kreutzer C et al (2000) Twenty-five-year experience with rastelli repair for transposition of the great arteries. J Thorac Cardiovasc Surg 120(2):211–223
16. Williams WG et al (2003) Outcomes of 829 neonates with complete transposition of the great arteries 12–17 years after repair. Eur J Cardiothorac Surg 24(1):1–9; discussion 9–10
17. Clarkson PM et al (1994) Outcome of pregnancy after the Mustard operation for transposition of the great arteries with intact ventricular septum. J Am Coll Cardiol 24(1):190–193
18. Genoni M et al (1999) Pregnancy after atrial repair for transposition of the great arteries. Heart 81(3):276–277

19. Drenthen W et al (2005) Risk of complications during pregnancy after Senning or Mustard (atrial) repair of complete transposition of the great arteries. Eur Heart J 26(23):2588–2595
20. Canobbio MM et al (2006) Pregnancy outcomes after atrial repair for transposition of the great arteries. Am J Cardiol 98(5):668–672
21. Metz TD, Jackson GM, Yetman AT (2011) Pregnancy outcomes in women who have undergone an atrial switch repair for congenital d-transposition of the great arteries. Am J Obstet Gynecol 205(3):273 e1–5
22. Trigas V et al (2014) Pregnancy-related obstetric and cardiologic problems in women after atrial switch operation for transposition of the great arteries. Circ J 78(2):443–449
23. Cataldo S et al (2015) Pregnancy following Mustard or Senning correction of transposition of the great arteries: a retrospective study. BJOG 123(5):807–813
24. Tobler D et al (2010) Pregnancy outcomes in women with transposition of the great arteries and arterial switch operation. Am J Cardiol 106(3):417–420
25. Radford DJ, Stafford G (2005) Pregnancy and the Rastelli operation. Aust N Z J Obstet Gynaecol 45(3):243–247
26. Roche SL, Silversides CK, Oechslin EN (2011) Monitoring the patient with transposition of the great arteries: arterial switch versus atrial switch. Curr Cardiol Rep 13(4):336–346
27. Drenthen W et al (2007) Outcome of pregnancy in women with congenital heart disease: a literature review. J Am Coll Cardiol 49(24):2303–2311
28. Guedes A et al (2004) Impact of pregnancy on the systemic right ventricle after a Mustard operation for transposition of the great arteries. J Am Coll Cardiol 44(2):433–437
29. Siu SC et al (2001) Prospective multicenter study of pregnancy outcomes in women with heart disease. Circulation 104(5):515–521
30. Thorne S, MacGregor A, Nelson-Piercy C (2006) Risks of contraception and pregnancy in heart disease. Heart 92(10):1520–1525
31. European Society of, G et al (2011) ESC Guidelines on the management of cardiovascular diseases during pregnancy: the Task Force on the Management of Cardiovascular Diseases during Pregnancy of the European Society of Cardiology (ESC). Eur Heart J 32(24):3147–3197
32. Triulzi DJ et al (2009) The effect of previous pregnancy and transfusion on HLA alloimmunization in blood donors: implications for a transfusion-related acute lung injury risk reduction strategy. Transfusion 49(9):1825–1835
33. Roos-Hesselink JW et al (2004) Decline in ventricular function and clinical condition after Mustard repair for transposition of the great arteries (a prospective study of 22–29 years). Eur Heart J 25(14):1264–1270
34. Greutmann M et al (2015) Increasing mortality burden among adults with complex congenital heart disease. Congenit Heart Dis 10(2):117–127
35. Tanous D et al (2010) B-type natriuretic peptide in pregnant women with heart disease. J Am Coll Cardiol 56(15):1247–1253
36. Kampman MA et al (2014) N-terminal pro-B-type natriuretic peptide predicts cardiovascular complications in pregnant women with congenital heart disease. Eur Heart J 35(11):708–715
37. Grewal J, Silversides CK, Colman JM (2014) Pregnancy in women with heart disease: risk assessment and management of heart failure. Heart Fail Clin 10(1):117–129
38. Goldszmidt E et al (2010) Anesthetic management of a consecutive cohort of women with heart disease for labor and delivery. Int J Obstet Anesth 19(3):266–272

Shunt Lesions

9

Antonia Pijuan-Domenech and Maria Goya

Abbreviations

ASD	Atrial septal defect
AVSD	Atrioventricular septal defect
CHD	Congenital heart disease
C-section	Caesarean section
IUGR	Intrauterine growth retardation
LAVVR	Left AV-valvular regurgitation
mWHO	Modified World Health Organization
NYHA	New York Heart Association
PAH	Pulmonary arterial hypertension
PFO	Persistent foramen ovale
ROPAC	Registry of Pregnancy and Cardiac Disease
RS	Risk score
VSD	Ventricular septal defect

A. Pijuan-Domenech, MD (✉)
Integrated Hospital Vall d'Hebron-Sant Pau Adult Congenital Heart Disease Unit, Department of Cardiology, Hospital Universitari Vall d'Hebron, Barcelona, Spain
e-mail: tonyapijuan@hotmail.com

M. Goya, MD, PhD
Maternal-Fetal Medicine Unit, Department of Obstetrics and Gynecology, Hospital Universitari Vall d'Hebron, Barcelona, Spain

> **Key Facts**
> *Incidence*: VSD, 2.5 per 1,000 live births, and ASD, 1.5 per 1,000 live births.
> *Inheritance*: 5%. Occasionally autosomal dominant inheritance (50% Holt-Oram syndrome).
> *Medication*: Change anticoagulation to LMWH and possibly antiarrhythmic drugs; a beta-blocker is the first choice.
> *World Health Organization class*: Corrected class I and uncorrected class II.
> *Risk of pregnancy*: Atrial arrhythmias may occur and, in unrepaired lesions, thromboembolic events (paradoxical).
> *Life expectancy*: Normal.

> **Key Management**
> *Preconception*: ECG, echo and exercise test.
> *Pregnancy*: Consider thromboprophylaxis in unrepaired lesions if additional risk factors are present given risk of paradoxical embolism.
> *Labour*: Vaginal delivery.
> *Postpartum*: Consider thromboprophylaxis in unrepaired lesions.

9.1 The Condition

Despite increasing survival rates of adults with complex congenital heart disease CHD [1], simple shunt lesions are still the most common (CHD) lesions in the adult population [2]. Published data on pregnancy and CHD showed that atrial septal defects (ASD) and ventricular septal defects (VSD) were the first and third, respectively, most frequent lesions among pregnant patients with CHD [3]. In the European Society of Cardiology Registry of Pregnancy and Cardiac Disease (ROPAC), shunt lesions including ASD and VSD were also the most common cardiac lesion observed [4].

9.2 Pregnancy Outcomes

9.2.1 Pre-tricuspidic Left-to-Right Shunts

Atrial septal defects: Atrial septal defect (ASD), in the past, could go unnoticed until the first medical visit during pregnancy [5]. Due to the decline in systemic resistance and reduction in left-to-right shunt, the risk of cardiac decompensation remains low in comparison with other cardiac lesions even with a large left-to-right shunt, provided that there is no pulmonary arterial hypertension. Very few cases of urgent surgical or percutaneous treatment during pregnancy have been described [6].

Closure of an ostium secundum ASD during pregnancy is not usually necessary, but it is possible using transesophageal guidance [7].

The main cardiac complications described during pregnancy in patients with unrepaired ASD are atrial arrhythmias and thromboembolic events [3]. Patients that had ASD repaired as adult are still at risk of arrhythmias [8], particularly if the repair is done after 30 years of age [9].

Risk factors for thrombosis should be evaluated carefully in patients with unrepaired ASD during pregnancy. Thromboprophylaxis should be considered if additional risk factors are present, due to the risk of paradoxical embolism [10]. ESC guidelines, based on those of the Royal College of Obstetricians and Gynaecologists, consider the risk factors for venous thrombosis to be: maternal age greater than 35, obesity (BMI>30), parity>3, smoking, the presence of severe varicose veins, preeclampsia, assisted reproductive therapy, prolonged labour, small for gestational age, Caesarean section (C-section) and peripartum haemorrhage.

The rate of obstetric complications is higher in women with unrepaired ASD. Several studies have clearly demonstrated that small for gestational age, prematurity and fetal demise were significantly more common than in the general population [9, 11]. However, these figures are much better than in other CHD lesions in which cardiac output is limited [3].

Atrial septal defects (ASD) that have been repaired during childhood are normally associated with excellent long-term survival rates, similar to the general population. It has been reported that pregnancy in these patients has a similar rate of cardiac and obstetric complications as observed in healthy women. Consequently, after a thorough initial evaluation (before or in early pregnancy), these patients do not need to have intensive follow-up during pregnancy as long as they remain asymptomatic [9].

Since the transmission rate is about 5.5%, fetal assessment is recommended in all patients. There are some conditions that are inherited in an autosomal dominant fashion, such as an ASD associated with an atrioventricular conduction defect or Holt-Oram syndrome; in these circumstances, genetic counselling prior to pregnancy should be performed [10].

9.2.1.1 Patent Foramen Ovale
In an asymptomatic woman, closure of a persistent foramen ovale (PFO) to prevent paradoxical emboli during pregnancy is not necessary, despite the Valsalva manoeuvres performed during delivery. Twenty percent of the general population has a PFO, and the incidence of transient ischemic attack occurs only in 5 out of 100,000 [12]. If asymptomatic PFO has been diagnosed, prevention of paradoxal embolus should focus on preventing venous thrombosis. There is no indication for a Caesarean section as the risk of thrombosis is higher than after a vaginal delivery.

9.2.1.2 ASD in the Setting with Other Congenital Heart Diseases
An ASD can be associated with other cardiac lesions. The haemodynamic impact of an ASD can be completely different if other congenital heart lesions are present, especially when right atrial pressure is elevated. Shunt reversal has been described

in pregnant patients with a wide variety of lesions, like Ebstein's anomaly of the tricuspid valve [13] and in transposition of great arteries after atrial switch operation [14]; volume overload can modify the direction of shunt during pregnancy, causing a right-to-left shunt to appear or to worsen. Oxygen saturation should be routinely checked in all pregnant women with congenital heart disease.

9.2.2 Post-tricuspid Left-to-Right Shunts

9.2.2.1 Ventricular Septal Defect

It is unlikely that an isolated ventricular septal defect (VSD) would go undiagnosed until adulthood, but if a large VSD is diagnosed in adult life, pulmonary arterial hypertension (PAH) will be present. In the rare setting of a moderate VSD with left chamber dilatation, but without PAH, the risks of complications during pregnancy are presumed to be moderate, similar to those with significant left valve regurgitation.

No additional risk has been observed in women during pregnancy, with a small VSD or a repaired VSD, if there is no pulmonary arterial hypertension. Small perimembranous VSDs (without left chamber dilatation) have a low risk of complications during pregnancy. Corrected VSDs have a good prognosis during pregnancy, when left ventricular systolic function is preserved. However, at the time of preconception or early pregnancy evaluation, it is important to exclude the presence of pulmonary arterial hypertension and to confirm that left ventricular function is preserved.

Regarding obstetric complications, there is one study that shows pre-eclampsia being more frequent in women with unrepaired small VSD than in the general population and another which suggested that small for gestational age and premature delivery were also more prevalent in women with a repaired VSD than in the general population [15]. In a large meta-analysis of complications during pregnancy in patients with CHD, the patients with VSD showed a higher prevalence in pre-eclampsia and thromboembolic events than in general population, but no higher incidence of cardiac decompensation or arrhythmias were observed [3].

9.2.2.2 Ductus Arteriosus

The diagnosis of patent ductus arteriosus is rarely overlooked until adulthood. However, this may occur in a few possible clinical scenarios. The first is when a small PDA exists with an insignificant left-to-right shunt, in which the risk of complication is presumed to be very low. The second is when there is a large ductus with irreversible pulmonary arterial hypertension and shunt reversal; in this scenario, pregnancy carries a high risk of mortality [16]. A third possibility is when a moderate PDA exists with left-to-right shunt and no pulmonary arterial hypertension, but with left chamber enlargement; this is rare and there is no information in the literature. We presume that the risk of maternal complications is similar to the risk associated with aortic regurgitation. See Table 9.1.

9 Shunt Lesions

Table 9.1 You can see mean key point in shunt lesions and pregnancy

	Cardiac complications	Obstetric complications	Mode of delivery	Puerperium	Risk of transmission	WHO categories
Unrepaired ASD	Atrial arrhythmias Thromboembolic event	Prematurity SGA	Vaginal delivery Epidural	Thromboprophylaxis	5%	2
Repaired ASD	NO Atrial arrythmias[a]	General population	Vaginal delivery Epidural	–	5%	1
Small VSD or small PDA	NO	Pre-eclampsia	Vaginal delivery Epidural	–	3%	1
Repaired AVSD	Arrhythmia (10%) Cardiac decompensation (2%)	Pre-eclampsia Preterm labour SGA [1]	Vaginal delivery Epidural	24 h of maternal monitoring Thromboprophylaxis	8%	2 or 3
Eisenmenger syndrome	Right heart failure Thrombosis Death (30%)	Preterm labour Prematurity SGA	C-section Multidisciplinary team involvement	Intensive care monitoring	Depends on type of CHD	4

SGA small for gestational age
[a]IF ASD repaired in adult age

9.2.2.3 Atrioventricular Septal Defects

Patients with repaired atrioventricular septal defects (AVSD) are a separate population in terms of complications during pregnancy. In the large meta-analysis of pregnant patients with CHD [3], the risk of cardiac, obstetric, fetal and neonatal complications was higher than in other shunt lesions. The majority of patients with AVSD repaired in infancy are in excellent health and has a good New York Heart Association (NYHA) class, but residual lesions, mainly left AV-valvular regurgitation (LAVVR), are prevalent [17]. The risk of complications of an unrepaired partial AVSD is presumed to be similar to an unrepaired ostium secundum ASD, if no significant LAVVR is present. An unrepaired common AVSD in adult life is almost always associated with irreversible pulmonary arterial hypertension, and pregnancy in this situation carries a prohibitively high risk.

The most frequent cardiac complication observed during pregnancy in patients with repaired AVSD is arrhythmia [3] The larger the left atrial dimensions in relation to the degree of the LAVVR, then the greater the risk of arrhythmia, while those with arrhythmias outside pregnancy are also at a higher risk of occurrence during pregnancy [18]. Heterotaxy is prevalent in newborns with AVSD [19]. The risk of arrhythmias, both right and left atrial isomerism, is higher in adult patients than in patients with usual atrial arrangement [20]. Other complications described are persistence of pregnancy-related NYHA class deterioration as well as deterioration of pre-existing LAVVR [18]. Cardiac decompensation is described in 1–2 % of pregnancies [3, 18], usually managed medically, with urgent mitral valve replacement being exceptional in this setting. Obstetric and fetal complications are also higher in this population, especially when a maternal cardiac complication is present. Risk of transmission is described as high as 8 % (Fig. 9.1).

9.3 Management of Shunt Lesions During Pregnancy

Patients with repaired ASD during infancy do not need multidisciplinary team follow-up, provided that there has been a good preconception assessment and patients are in good condition without residual lesions, and pulmonary arterial hypertension is ruled out. However, the risk of transmission of congenital heart disease is higher than in the general population, and fetal echocardiography is recommended [21, 22]. See Fig. 9.1.

In contrast, patients with an ASD who had a late repair or whose ASD is unrepaired, and those with an AVSD, whether repaired or not, need multidisciplinary team follow-up.

Frequency of cardiac follow-up depends on residual lesions. In AVSD, cardiac decompensation is possible. If LAVV regurgitation is significant, clinical and echocardiographic close follow-up is required with frequent echocardiography. If significant atrial arrhythmias are detected, then anticoagulation and rhythm or rate control should be considered, depending on hemodynamic status; therapeutic low

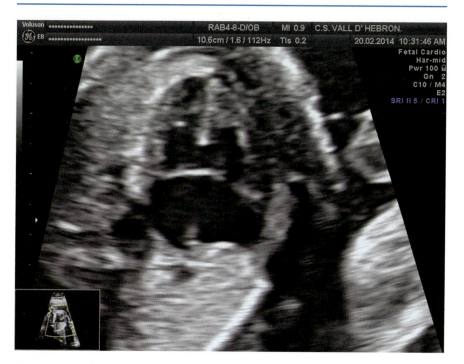

Fig. 9.1 You can see fetal echocardiography of an AVSD at 24 weeks (Courtesy of Dr Q Ferrer, Department of Pediatric Cardiology and Fetal-Maternal Medicine Department)

molecular heparin should be given twice or three times per day and be monitored with peak (3–4 h after injection) and trough anti-Xa levels. Metoprolol is the safest beta-blocker for the fetus.

In the presence of an unrepaired ASD, there is a high risk of paradoxical embolism; consequently, thromboprophylaxis should be given to all those with additional risk factors. The need for thromboprophylaxis should be assessed antepartum, postpartum and at any time the patient transitions from the outpatient to the inpatient setting.

In left-to-right shunts, maternal deterioration is not frequent, and spontaneous vaginal delivery is advised in most cases, with epidural anaesthesia. Cardiac indication of Caesarean section is rare in the setting of left-to-right shunt except if pulmonary hypertension is present. Recommendations for care during delivery and puerperium of a patient with repaired AVSD and significant LAVVR are showed in Fig. 9.2.

Labour can be conducted with the mother in the left lateral position to avoid inferior vena caval compression and maintain venous return. The second stage can be assisted with forceps or vacuum extraction if necessary. Prolonged labour should be avoided. In addition to fetal monitoring, maternal ECG monitoring should be performed to detect any arrhythmia during labour and the puerperium.

> **Mode of delivery:**
> Spontaneous vaginal delivery is indicated. C-section only due to obstetric reasons
> **Recommendations for first stage:**
> Maternal position: left lateral decubitus
> Continuous ECG and 02 saturation monitoring, diuresis and fluid balance
> Epidural anesthesia
> **Recommendations for second stage:**
> Shortage of expulsive using forceps
> **Puerperium:**
> Oxytocin to be administrated in perfusion during 1–2 h. Avoid bolus administration
> Control in high dependence obstetric Unit during 24 h, continue to ECG monitoring, 02 saturation and fluid administration.
> Start prophylactic low molecular heparin after 8 h of epidural catheter removal.

Fig. 9.2 You can see delivery plan of a patient with repaired AVSD and severe left atrioventricular valve regurgitation

9.3.1 Management of Patients with Eisenmenger Syndrome

PAH accompanies large left-to-right shunts; pulmonary vascular obstructive disease may develop in adults but occurs much later in pre-tricuspidic shunt than in high-pressure left-to-right shunts. In young women with unrepaired ostium secundum ASD or sinus venosus, the rate of pulmonary arterial hypertension is presumed to be low, around 5–10 % at maximum [23]. There is little information regarding cases of adult presentation of unrepaired partial AVSD and the rate of associated pulmonary arterial hypertension, but numbers are presumably similar to other pre-tricuspidic lesions. Small restrictive VSDs and small PDAs will not have associated PAH. In contrast, a large unrepaired VSD, a large PDA or unrepaired common AVSD at the childbearing age have a high probability of irreversible pulmonary arterial hypertension, shunt reversal and Eisenmenger syndrome.

For further information on haemodynamic impact of pregnancy in Eisenmenger syndrome, see Chaps. 16 and 17.

If the patient with Eisenmenger syndrome decided to continue with the pregnancy, a multidisciplinary team should be involved during the whole pregnancy, delivery and postpartum period. Due to low oxygen saturation, especially if below 85 %, a high risk of spontaneous abortion and fetal loss is present [24–26]. Maternal risk of decompensation is high, despite oxygen supplementation and strict balance of fluids [27]. Prostanoids (i.v. prostacyclin or inhaled iloprost) and inhibitors of phosphodiesterase type 5 are used, since there is no evidence of teratogenicity in animals. Endothelin receptor antagonists are generally avoided because of teratogenicity seen in animal testing [28].

Obstetric and fetal complications are common, as limited cardiac output and low oxygen saturation both contribute to placental insufficiency, causing intrauterine growth retardation (IUGR) and the need for early delivery [3, 27]. Thromboprophylaxis is usually prescribed, but full anticoagulation is controversial because of concerns about bleeding [10]. Avoiding possible paradoxical embolism through the care of peripheral lines and using air filters is wise during all admissions [29].

The majority of cases are delivered by Caesarean section as heart failure is usually present during the third trimester, despite good cardiac function prior to pregnancy. This has a class IIa recommendation in the ESC guidelines [10]. A multidisciplinary team involving an obstetrician, cardiologist and anaesthetist is mandatory. During delivery, pain and anxiety should be avoided, as well as hypotension due to drug administration. Small incremental doses must be given if epidural anaesthesia is used to avoid hypotension [30]. Invasive monitoring of systemic arterial pressure and a central venous pressure is probably indicated in all cases. Nitric oxide use may be helpful during anaesthesia.

During puerperium, there is an increase in venous return from the uterus and inferior vena caval decompression, resulting in additional overload to the already compromised right ventricle. For this reason, the puerperium is the highest risk period for mortality in Eisenmenger syndrome. Maternal ICU stay will be mandatory for more than 48 h and hospitalisation of at least 1 week postpartum. Fifty percent of mortality in pregnant patients with Eisenmenger syndrome has been observed during the puerperium [31].

9.4 Impact of Physiological Changes

During pregnancy, left-to-right shunt lesions are considered to be low risk. This is due to the decrease in systemic vascular resistance, which results in a reduced left-to-right shunt, counterbalancing the increase in plasma volume and cardiac output, provided there is no pulmonary arterial hypertension. Pulmonary pressures are presumed to stay at the basal level throughout pregnancy or even decrease to accommodate the increase in cardiac output during pregnancy [32]. This contrasts to the situation of PAH with a right-to-left shunt where the physiological changes of pregnancy can be detrimental (please see the PAH-CDH chapter 17).

9.5 Preconception Counselling

9.5.1 General Advice for Shunt Patients

Several risk scores have been developed in order to predict cardiac complications in patients with heart disease: the CARPREG risk score (RS) [33]; the modified World Health Organization (mWHO) [10] classification, proposed by Thorne et al. [34]; and, for CHD, the Khairy modified CARPREG RS (KRS) [35] and ZAHARA RS [36]. In the general population [37] and also in congenital heart disease population [38], mWHO has predicted complications with more accuracy than any other risk score.

In terms of shunts, the mWHO classification includes several categories: group I, successfully repaired simple lesions, like atrial or ventricular septal defect or patent ductus arteriosus, where only a small risk of complications is expected, and group II unoperated atrial or ventricular septal defect, where a small increase in maternal mortality and a moderate increase in maternal morbidity are expected. In the same conditions, if there is associated pulmonary arterial hypertension, lesions are considered group IV, and pregnancy is contraindicated due to a high risk of morbidity and mortality [10].

9.5.2 Atrioventricular Septal Defects

In the ZAHARA risk score, the presence of left or right AV regurgitation in the setting of repaired AVSD are risk factors to be added to the classical CARPREG risk classification [36]. In mWHO classification, AVSD repaired is considered to be in group II if no significant residual lesion is present [10] and higher (III) if residual lesions are present. Complete unrepaired AVSD, associated to severe pulmonary hypertension, is considered mWHO IV.

9.6 Contraception

In a repaired ASD/VSD with no residual lesions, none of the contraceptive options are contraindicated. In the situation of an unrepaired ASD/VSD in the presence or absence of PAH, the risk of thrombosis and paradoxical embolism precludes oestrogen-based contraceptives and limits the choice to progesterone-based contraceptives (high-dose oral, implant or IUCD), which are effective and safe in this context.

References

1. Khairy P, Ionescu-Ittu R, Mackie AS, Abrahamowicz M, Pilote L, Marelli AJ (2010) Changing mortality in congenital heart disease. J Am Coll Cardiol 56(14):1149–1157
2. Marelli A, Mackie A, Ionescu-Ittu R, Rahme E, Pilote L (2007) congenital heart disease in the general population changing prevalence and age distribution. Circulation 115:163–172
3. Drenthen W, Pieper PG, Roos-Hesselink JW, van Lottum WA, Voors AA, Mulder BJ, van Dijk AP, Vliegen HW, Yap SC, Moons P, Ebels T, van Veldhuisen DJ (2007) Outcome of pregnancy in women with congenital heart disease: a literature review. J Am Coll Cardiol 49(24):2303–2311
4. Ruys TP, Roos-Hesselink JW, Hall R, Subirana-Domènech MT, Grando-Ting J, Estensen M, Crepaz R, Fesslova V, Gurvitz M, De Backer J, Johnson MR, Pieper PG (2014) Heart failure in pregnant women with cardiac disease: data from the ROPAC. Heart 100(3):231–238
5. Warnes CA, Williams RG, Bashore TM, Child JS, Connolly HM, Dearani JA, del Nido P, Fasules JW, Graham TP Jr, Hijazi ZM, Hunt SA, King ME, Landzberg MJ, Miner PD, Radford MJ, Walsh EP, Webb GD, Smith SC Jr, Jacobs AK, Adams CD, Anderson JL, Antman EM, Buller CE, Creager MA, Ettinger SM, Halperin JL, Hunt SA, Krumholz HM, Kushner FG, Lytle BW, Nishimura RA, Page RL, Riegel B, Tarkington LG, Yancy CW (2008) ACC/AHA 2008 guidelines for the management of adults with congenital heart disease: a report of the American College of Cardiology/American Heart Association Task Force on Practice Guidelines (Writing Committee to Develop Guidelines on the Management of Adults With Congenital Heart Disease). J Am Coll Cardiol 52(23):143–263
6. Geva T, Martins JD, Wald RM (2014) Atrial septal defects. Lancet 383:1921–1932
7. Orchard EA, Wilson N, Ormerod OJM (2011) Device closure of atrial septal defect during pregnancy for recurrent cerebrovascular accidents. Int J Cardiol 148(2):240–241

8. Gatzoulis MA, Freeman MA, Siu SC, Webb GD, Harris L (1999) Atrial arrhythmia after surgical closure of atrial septal defects in adults. N Engl J Med 340(11):839–846
9. Yap SC, Drenthen W, Meijboom FJ, Moons P, Mulder BJ, Vliegen HW, van Dijk AP, Jaddoe VW, Steegers EA, Roos-Hesselink JW, Pieper PG, ZAHARA investigators (2009) Comparison of pregnancy outcomes in women with repaired versus unrepaired atrial septal defect. BJOG 116(12):1593–601
10. Regitz-Zagrosek V, Blomstrom Lundqvist C, Borghi C, Cifkova R, Ferreira R, Foidart J, Gibbs S, Gohlke-Baerwolf C, Gorenek B, Iung B, Kirby M, Maas A, Morais J, Nihoyannopoulos P, Pieper P, Presbitero P, Roos-Hesselink J, Schaufelberger M, Seeland U, Torracca L (2011) ESC guidelines on the management of cardiovascular diseases during pregnancy. Eur Heart J 32:3147–3197
11. Actis Dato GM, Rinaudo A, Revelli A, Actis Dato G, Punta G, Centofanti P, Cavaglia M, Barbato L, Massobrio M (1998) Atrial septal defect and pregnancy: a retrospective analysis of obstetrical outcome before and after surgical correction. Minerva Cardioangiol 46:63–68
12. Miller BR, Strbian D, Sundararajan S (2015) Stroke in the young. Patent foramen ovale and pregnancy. Stroke 46(8):181–183
13. Houser L, Zaragoza-Macias E, Jones TK, Aboulhosn J (2015) Transcatheter closure of atrial septal communication during pregnancy in women with Ebstein's anomaly of the tricuspid valve and cyanosis. Catheter Cardiovasc Interv 85(5):842–846
14. Canobbio MM, Morris CD, Graham TP, Landzberg MJ (2006) Pregnancy outcomes after atrial repair for transposition of the great arteries. Am J Cardiol 98(5):668–672
15. Yap SC, Drenthen W, Pieper PG, Moons P, Mulder BJ, Vliegen HW, van Dijk AP, Meijboom FJ, Jaddoe VW, Steegers EA, Boersma E, Roos-Hesselink JW (2010) Pregnancy outcome in women with repaired versus unrepaired isolated ventricular septal defect. BJOG 117(6):683–689
16. Baumgartner H, Bonhoeffer P, De Groot NM, de Haan F, Deanfield JE, Galie N, Gatzoulis MA, Gohlke-Baerwolf C, Kaemmerer H, Kilner P, Meijboom F, Mulder BJ, Oechslin E, Oliver JM, Serraf A, Szatmari A, Thaulow E, Vouhe PR, Walma E (2010) ESC guidelines for the management of grown-up congenital heart disease (new version 2010). Eur Heart J 23:2915–2957
17. Sojak V, Kooij M, Yazdanbakhsh A, Koolbergen DR, Bruggemans EF, Hazekamp MG (2015) A single-centre 37-year experience with reoperation after primary repair of atrioventricular septal defect. Eur J Cardiothorac Surg 2016;49(2):538–544
18. Drenthen W, Pieper PG, van der Tuuk K, Roos-Hesselink JW, Voors AA, Mostert B, Mulder BJ, Moons P, Ebels T, van Veldhuisen DJ (2005) Cardiac complications relating to pregnancy and recurrence of disease in the offspring of women with atrioventricular septal defects. Eur Heart J 26:2581–2587
19. Huggon IC, Cook AC, Smeeton NC, Magee AG, Sharland GK (2000) Atrioventricular septal defects diagnosed in fetal life: associated cardiac and extra-cardiac abnormalities and outcome. J Am Coll Cardiol 36(2):593–601
20. Loomba RS, Aggarwal S, Gupta N, Buelow M, Alla V, Arora RR, Anderson RH (2015) Arrhythmias in adult congenital patients with bodily isomerism. Pediatr Cardiol. published ahead of print.
21. Burn J, Brennan P, Little J, Holloway S, Coffey R, Somerville J, Dennis NR, Allan L, Arnold R, Deanfield JE (1998) Recurrence risks in offspring of adults with major heart defects: results from first cohort of British collaborative study. Lancet 351:311–316
22. Øyen N, Poulsen G, Boyd HA, Wohlfahrt J, Jensen PK, Melbye M (2009) Recurrence of congenital heart defects in families. Circulation 120:295–301
23. Steele PM, Fuster V, Cohen M et al (1987) Isolated atrial septal defect with pulmonary vascular obstructive disease—long-term follow-up and prediction of outcome after surgical correction. Circulation 76:1037–1042
24. Bédard E, Dimopoulos K, Gatzoulis MA (2009) Has there been any progress made on pregnancy outcomes among women with pulmonary arterial hypertension? Eur Heart J 30(3):256–265
25. Galiè N, Humbert M, Vachiery JL, Gibbs S, Lang I, Torbicki A, Simonneau G, Peacock A, Vonk Noordegraaf A, Beghetti M, Ghofrani A, Gomez Sanchez MA, Hansmann G, Klepetko

W, Lancellotti P, Matucci M, McDonagh T, Pierard LA, Trindade PT, Zompatori M, Hoeper M (2015) 2015 ESC/ERS guidelines for the diagnosis and treatment of pulmonary hypertension: the Joint Task Force for the Diagnosis and Treatment of Pulmonary Hypertension of the European Society of Cardiology (ESC) and the European Respiratory Society (ERS). Eur Respir J 46(4):903–975
26. Presbitero P, Somerville J, Stone S, Aruta E, Spiegelhalter D, Rabajoli F (1994) Pregnancy in cyanotic congenital heart disease. Outcome of mother and fetus. Circulation 89:2673–2676
27. Avila WS, Grinberg M, Snitcowsky R, Faccioli R, Da Luz PL, Bellotti G et al (1995) Maternal and fetal outcome in pregnant women with Eisenmenger's syndrome. Eur Heart J 16:460–464
28. Jaïs X, Olsson KM, Barbera JA, Blanco I, Torbicki A, Peacock A, Vizza CD, Macdonald P, Humbert M, Hoeper MM (2012) Pregnancy outcomes in pulmonary arterial hypertension in the modern management era. Eur Respir J 40(4):881–885
29. Oechslin E (2015) Management of adults with cyanotic congenital heart disease. Heart 101(6):485–494
30. Warnes CA (2015) Pregnancy and delivery in women with congenital heart disease. Circ J 79(7):1416–1421
31. Weiss BM, Zemp L, Seifert B, Hess OM (1998) Outcome of pulmonary vascular disease in pregnancy: a systematic overview from 1978 through 1996. J Am Coll Cardiol 31:1650–1657
32. Ouzounian J, Elkayam U (2012) Physiologic changes during normal pregnancy and delivery. Cardiol Clin 30(3):317–329
33. Siu S, Sermer MMD, Colman J, Alvarez AN, Mercier LA, Morton B, Kells C, Bergin L, Kiess M, Marcotte F, Taylor M, Gordon E, Spears J, Tam J, Amankwah K, Smallhorn K, Farine D, Sorensen S (2001) Prospective multicenter study of pregnancy outcomes in women with heart disease. Circulation 104:515–521
34. Thorne S, MacGregor A, Nelson-Piercy C (2006) Risks of contraception and pregnancy in heart disease. Heart 92:1520–1525
35. Khairy P, Ouyang DW, Fernandes SM, Lee-Parritz A, Economy KE, Landzberg MJ (2006) Pregnancy outcomes in women with congenital heart disease. Circulation 113:517–524
36. Drenthen W, Boersma E, Balci A, Moons P, Roos-Hesselink J, Mulder B, Vliegen H, van Dijk A, Voors A, Yap S, van Veldhuisen D, Pieper P (2010) Predictors of pregnancy complications in women with congenital heart disease. Eur Heart J 31:2124–2132
37. Pijuan-Domènech A, Galian L, Goya M, Casellas M, Merced C, Ferreira-Gonzalez I, Marsal-Mora JR, Dos-Subirà L, Subirana-Domènech MT, Pedrosa V, Baró-Marine F, Manrique S, Casaldàliga-Ferrer J, Tornos P, Cabero L, Garcia-Dorado D (2015) Cardiac complications during pregnancy are better predicted with the modified WHO risk score. Int J Cardiol 195:149–154
38. Balci A, Sollie-Szarynska KM, van der Bijl AG, Ruys TP, Mulder BJ, Roos-Hesselink JW, van Dijk AP, Wajon EM, Vliegen HW, Drenthen W, Hillege HL, Aarnoudse JG, van Veldhuisen DJ, Pieper PG (2014) Prospective validation and assessment of cardiovascular and offspring risk models for pregnant women with congenital heart disease. Heart 100(17):1373–1381

Aortic Stenosis

10

Stefan Orwat and Helmut Baumgartner

Abbreviations

AoV	Aortic valve
AS	Aortic stenosis
AVR	Aortic valve replacement
CO	Cardiac output
CW	Continuous wave
ECG	Electrocardiography
EF	Ejection fraction
ET	Exercise test
FU	Follow-up
Hb	Haemoglobin
HR	Heart rate
MV	Mitral valve
mWHO	Modified World Health Organization
ROPAC	Registry of Pregnancy and Cardiac Disease
SAX	Short-axis view
SV	Stroke volume
TTE	Transthoracic echocardiography
VR	Vascular resistance
WHO	World Health Organization

S. Orwat, MD • H. Baumgartner, MD (✉)
Department of Cardiovascular Medicine, Division of Adult Congenital and Valvular Heart Disease, University Hospital of Muenster, Münster, Germany
e-mail: helmut.baumgartner@ukmuenster.de

© Springer International Publishing Switzerland 2017
J.W. Roos-Hesselink, M.R. Johnson (eds.), *Pregnancy and Congenital Heart Disease*, Congenital Heart Disease in Adolescents and Adults,
DOI 10.1007/978-3-319-38913-4_10

> **Key Facts of Preconception**
> *Incidence*: 0.2 per 1,000 live births
> *Inheritance*: 8.0 % if the mother is affected and 3.8 % if the father is affected
> *Medication*:
> *World Health Organization class*: Severe symptomatic class IV, all other forms of classes II–III. Aortic dilatation 45–50 mm, without valve dysfunction class III, with valve dysfunction or >50 mm class IV
> *Risk of pregnancy*: Heart failure 6–30 %, some risk of arrhythmias
> *Life expectancy*: Reduced with severe stenosis and dilatation of the aorta

> **Key Management**
> *Preconception*: ECG, echo and exercise test. Pregnancy is contraindicated in severe symptomatic LVOTO.
> *Pregnancy*: 12 and 20 weeks with ECG and echo, thereafter depending on the severity of aortic stenosis, aortic dilatation and clinical status. Consider reduced activity with severe stenosis; in refractory heart failure, balloon valvuloplasty may be considered.
> *Labour*: Vaginal delivery is appropriate unless aortic dilatation >45 mm or heart failure is present.
> *Postpartum*: Close monitoring for signs of heart failure and echo in selected cases.

10.1 The Condition

Aortic stenosis (AS) is one of the most prevalent valvular diseases among young women and is typically encountered in the form of a congenitally bicuspid AS. Although the rate of progression of stenosis in this group is lower than in older patients, severe AS can occur. Rheumatic AS is a major health issue in developing countries and is usually associated with mitral valve disease. In addition to AS, women with bicuspid valves may have an associated aortopathy with or without aortic dilatation even in the absence of haemodynamically significant aortic stenosis. Left ventricular outflow obstruction can be valvular but also supravalvular or subvalvular. The pathophysiological consequences of fixed stenosis at any of these levels are the same. Dynamic subvalvular stenosis (i.e. hypertrophic obstructive cardiomyopathy) has to be separated from these entities and behaves differently during pregnancy.

Some women still asymptomatic prior to pregnancy may become symptomatic during pregnancy as a consequence of a limited ability to increase stroke volume across the stenosis resulting in increasing filling pressures. In addition, the increased heart rate and blood volume and the fall in the peripheral vascular resistance may promote heart failure in this patient group.

These women may in particular develop dyspnoea on exertion but also angina. Some circumstances seem to have an increased risk for acute decompensations. For example, the raised cardiac output and the elevated heart rate may be linked with an arrhythmia. In addition infection or anaemia may result in an acute decompensation from a combination of an increasing valve gradient and a shortened diastolic filling time.

10.2 Pregnancy Outcome

The risk of the mother with aortic stenosis during pregnancy depends on the severity of stenosis, comorbidities and symptoms. Generally speaking, asymptomatic women with mild or moderate aortic stenosis have a low risk and tolerate pregnancy well. Consistent with the current guidelines on valvular heart disease, severe symptomatic left ventricular outflow (independent on the location of obstruction) tract obstruction is a contraindication for pregnancy, and women should have an aortic valve replacement prior to pregnancy or should be advised against pregnancy [1, 2].

There are different studies that investigated the risk of pregnancy in women with aortic stenosis. The group of Silversides et al. reported on 49 pregnancies in women with congenital AS, of whom 59 % of patients had severe AS, and most of them were asymptomatic before pregnancy. In three pregnancies, early cardiac complications, including pulmonary oedema and atrial arrhythmias, occurred. One of them with severe AS required urgent percutaneous aortic valvuloplasty at 12 weeks of gestation. Six pregnancies were associated with adverse fetal events, which included prematurity, small for gestational age and neonatal respiratory distress syndrome [3].

Another study in this field reported on 12 pregnancies with predominant AS [4]. There was a higher incidence of maternal complications in women with more than mild AS compared with their matched healthy controls. Congestive heart failure was reported in 44 % of patients, arrhythmias in 25 % and hospitalizations in 33 %. Fetal outcome was also affected by the presence of more than mild AS with higher incidence of preterm birth, intrauterine growth retardation and low birth weight [4].

In a recent study of the ROPAC group, we investigated maternal and fetal adverse events in contemporary patients with moderate or severe AS based on a prospective observational study of a large number of pregnancies in patients with AS included in the Registry Of Pregnancy And Cardiac disease (ROPAC) [5]. Out of 2,966 pregnancies, we identified 99 pregnancies in women with AS, who had at least moderate AS (34 severe AS). No deaths were observed during pregnancy and the first week after delivery. However, 20.8 % of women required hospitalisation for cardiac reasons during pregnancy. This was significantly more common in severe AS compared to moderate AS (35.3 % vs. 12.9 %; $p=0.02$) and reached the highest rate (42.1 %) in severe, symptomatic AS. Pregnancy was complicated by heart failure in 6.7 % of asymptomatic and 26.3 % of symptomatic patients but could be managed medically except for one patient who was symptomatic prior to pregnancy and required balloon valvotomy. In addition, children of women with severe AS had a significantly higher percentage of low birth weight compared to women with moderate AS (35.0% vs. 6.0%; $p=0.006$). We concluded from our study that mortality in pregnant women with AS, including those with severe AS, appears to be close to zero in the current era. In addition, symptomatic and severe AS does, however, carry a substantial risk of heart failure and is associated with high rates of hospitalisation for cardiac reasons although heart failure can nearly always be managed medically.

There is only limited data on the risk or recurrent aortic valve disease in offspring of parents with aortic stenosis. In one study it is described as 8.0% if the mother is affected and 3.8% if the father is affected [6].

10.3 Management

The approach to women with aortic stenosis depends on the time of presentation (e.g. prior to pregnancy or during pregnancy). We attempt to give an overview about the management in the different phases (Fig. 10.1).

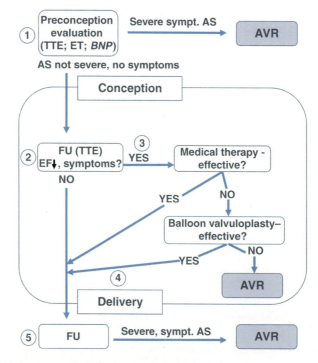

Fig. 10.1 Flow chart describing the management of women with aortic stenosis according to different phases (Phase 1–5). *AVR* aortic valve replacement, *TTE* transthoracic echocardiography, *ET* exercise test, *BNP* brain natriuretic peptide, *FU* follow-up, *EF* ejection fraction

10.3.1 Phase 1: Preconception Evaluation

All women with known aortic stenosis should have preconception evaluation. This evaluation should be done by an interdisciplinary team of obstetricians and cardiologists and should include careful history and family history, physical examination, electrocardiography and echocardiography. To assess the functional state, an exercise test in asymptomatic women may be helpful [7].

10.3.1.1 Echocardiography

Transthoracic echocardiography (TTE) is a safe and quick diagnostic tool and it is mandatory for the diagnosis of aortic stenosis. It allows morphological assessment of the valves and provides information on the aetiology of the disease. The morphological assessment of the aortic valve (AoV) is best performed in a parasternal short-axis view (SAX) (Fig. 10.2a). Congenital AS is typically encountered in the form of a bicuspid AoV. To establish the diagnosis, the valve has to be visualised in the SAX in systole where the orifice has a characteristic "fish-mouth" appearance (Fig. 10.2b).

In rheumatic valve disease, the valve is characterised by thickening at the edges of the cusps and commissural fusion, and in most cases, also the mitral valve (MV) is affected. The quantification of stenosis includes predominantly the measurement

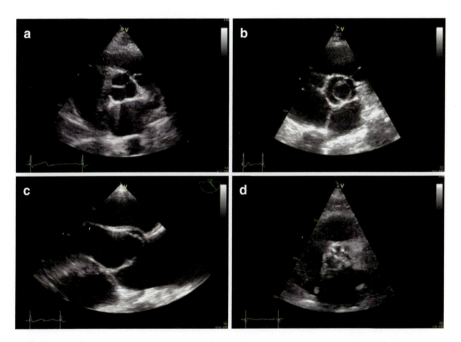

Fig. 10.2 (**a**) Normal tricuspid aortic valve in short axis. (**b**) Bicuspid aortic valve in short axis. (**c**) Transoesophageal echocardiography of a bicuspid aortic valve with typical "doming" of the cusps. (**d**) TTE of a severe aortic stenosis

of transaortic jet velocities and gradients as well the calculation of the aortic valve area, thus combining flow-dependent and relatively flow-independent variables.

The normal aortic valve area is in the range of 3–4 cm^2. Under normal conditions and also during pregnancy, the transvalvular flow has a peak flow velocity typically <2 m/s. With increasing narrowing of the AoV orifice, the transaortic jet velocities increase [1, 7]. Transaortic jet velocities are measured by recording of the maximal transaortic flow signal using continuous wave (CW) Doppler, and gradients can be derived from flow velocities using the simplified Bernoulli equation. The mean gradient can be determined by averaging the instantaneous gradients over the entire systole.

There are some pitfalls to watch for when measuring transaortic velocity and gradients. For an accurate measurement of the transaortic jet velocity, the Doppler beam needs to be aligned with the stenotic aortic jet. Alignment errors, which can frequently occur in pregnant women with atypical heart position or congenital aortic stenosis, lead to an underestimation of the true velocity and consequently of the calculated gradients resulting in underestimation of AS severity. As a consequence, a meticulous search of the highest transvalvular velocity is required. This necessitates a comprehensive Doppler study that is not only limited to the apical window but also includes right parasternal, suprasternal and sometimes (if possible in pregnant women) subcostal approaches using a small, dedicated CW Doppler transducer (pencil probe). It is not unusual that significantly higher aortic jet velocities can be recorded from these acoustic windows.

Transaortic jet velocities and gradients are highly flow dependent. In the presence of associated aortic regurgitation, high cardiac output states such as pregnancy, anaemia, hyperthyroidism, or transaortic flow velocities will further increase.

Aortic valve area, calculated using the continuity equation, is a relatively – although not entirely – flow-independent variable. Even if carefully performed, one major limitation of this method remains the LVOT area calculation from its diameter. Since the LVOT shape is rather elliptical than circular, this will result in flow underestimation and therefore valve area underestimation [8, 9]. Any discrepancy in the measurement of the LVOT diameter will be squared, leading to errors in the calculation of the AVA.

Planimetry of the valve area, primarily by 2D TEE, has also been proposed. However, the orifice of a stenotic aortic valve, especially in a doming bicuspid aortic valve (Fig. 10.2c), frequently represents a complex three-dimensional structure that cannot be reliably assessed with a planar 2D image.

As stenosis severity encompasses a continuous spectrum of disease, its assessment needs to be viewed in a continuous way. In clinical practice, peak transaortic jet velocities, mean gradients and valve areas (calculated by the continuity equation) should be estimated and the findings are ideally concordant (Table 10.1).

Classification of AS severity is not difficult when measurements of velocity, gradient and valve area are concordant but becomes challenging when conflicting values of these indices are found. Because pressure gradients are flow dependent, gradients by itself may provide misleading information about the severity of aortic stenosis during pregnancy. The situation of a peak velocity >4 m/s and mean gradient

10 Aortic Stenosis

Table 10.1 Quantification of aortic stenosis severity

	Mild aortic stenosis	Moderate aortic stenosis	Severe aortic stenosis
Peak aortic jet velocity (m/s)	2.5–2.9[a]	3.0–3.9[a]	≥4.0[a]
Mean gradient (mmHg)	<20[a]	20–39[a]	≥40[a]
Aortic valve area (cm^2)	>1.5	1.0–1.5	≤1.0
Indexed valve area (cm^2/m^2 BSA)			≤0.6 cm^2/m^2

[a]In the presence of normal transvalvular flow, not evaluated in pregnancy. According to current ESC guidelines and AHA/ACC guidelines

>40 mmHg despite a valve area greater than 1.0 cm^2 can be found in the presence of a high transvalvular flow, especially in pregnancy. The increased heart rate during pregnancy may also influence the peak and mean systolic gradients (as calculated from the Bernoulli equation) but should not affect the calculated valve area as calculated by the continuity equation. Until now it is unclear which parameter during pregnancy, gradient or valve orifice, describes best the haemodynamic situation.

The ascending aorta should be routinely assessed in women with AS since a dilation of the ascending aorta is frequently observed especially in patients with bicuspid valves. The assessment is performed in a PLAX view at early systole and includes measurements at the levels of the aortic annulus, the sinuses of Valsalva, the sinotubular junction and the ascending aorta. In case of an aortic diameter greater than 50 mm (or >27 mm/m^2 BSA), surgery before pregnancy should be considered [2].

Supravalvular AS is a rare congenital lesion (e.g. in Williams-Beuren syndrome) in which the ascending aorta is narrowed. Subvalvular AS consists of a fixed obstruction below the aortic valve level in the left ventricular outflow tract and can be due to a thin fibrous membrane or a fibromuscular narrowing. Both forms are fixed stenosis with similar pathophysiological consequences as in valvular stenosis. Hypertrophic obstructive cardiomyopathy represents a dynamic obstruction of the left ventricular outflow tract and is usually well tolerated during pregnancy [10, 11].

10.3.1.2 Other Tests

Exercise testing is recommended in asymptomatic patients before pregnancy to confirm asymptomatic status and evaluate exercise tolerance, blood pressure response and arrhythmias [2]. In addition, electrocardiography (ECG) is recommended to exclude, among other findings, arrhythmias. To what extent an elevated brain natriuretic peptide adds prognostic information in this setting remains unclear.

10.3.2 Pre-pregnancy Counselling/Risk Estimation

Pre-pregnancy counselling has to address how pregnancy may affect not just the mother but also the fetus. This means women should be given information on maternal and fetal morbidity and mortality associated with pregnancy. This allows women to make an informed choice whether to accept the risk associated with pregnancy.

Several risk scores for predicting cardiac complications in patients with acquired or valvular heart disease have been proposed. They try to predict cardiac and obstetric complications in different forms of heart disease and are therefore not specific for women with aortic stenosis.

The CARPREG risk score is the most popular one [12]. It classifies the different heart conditions in three risk categories [13]. To categorise these women, the study identifies four predictors of primary cardiac events (each one point):

- Prior cardiac event (heart failure, transient ischaemic attack or stroke before pregnancy) or arrhythmia
- Baseline NYHA class >II or cyanosis
- Left heart obstruction (mitral valve area <2 cm^2, aortic valve area <1.5 cm^2 or peak left ventricular outflow tract gradient >30 mmHg by echocardiography)
- Reduced systemic ventricular systolic function (ejection fraction <40%)

The estimated risk of a cardiac event in pregnancies with 0, 1 and >1 points was reported to be 5%, 27% and 75%, respectively.

The current European Heart Society guidelines have extended the modified World Health Organization (mWHO) score to assess maternal risk. The score classifies patients in four categories indicating the risk of cardiovascular complications and the consequences for management during pregnancy. Women in mWHO class I have a low risk; class II, small risk of complications; and class III, significant risk of complications. Women in class IV have such a high risk of morbidity and mortality that they should be advised against pregnancy [2].

According to the modified WHO classification of maternal cardiovascular risk, patients with severe symptomatic aortic stenosis are assigned to class IV, whereas all other forms of aortic stenosis are assigned to classes II–III. Aortic dilatation between 45 and 50 mm associated with a bicuspid aortic valve (without significant dysfunction of the valve) is assigned to class III, aortic dilatation >50 mm to class IV.

Patients with a low- or moderate-risk condition (WHO I–III) should be seen by the end of the first trimester and a follow-up plan with time intervals for review and investigations such as echocardiograms defined. The follow-up plan should be individualised taking into account the severity of aortic stenosis, aortic dilatation and clinical status of the patient.

10.3.3 Phase 2: Care During Pregnancy

As many general cardiologists or obstetricians will see only a few women with aortic stenosis, referral to a specialist centre for counselling is advisable. Management of pregnant patients with aortic stenosis should be ensured by experienced multidisciplinary teams. The follow-up frequencies depend on the severity of stenosis with at least monthly visits and echocardiographic assessments in patients with severe stenosis.

Symptoms due to severe aortic stenosis such as dyspnoea, angina pectoris, dizziness or syncope on exertion usually become apparent in the second trimester or early third trimester when the haemodynamic load on the heart significantly increases. Onset of symptoms related to AS before this stage seems to be a poor prognostic sign. It could be a diagnostic challenge to decide if shortness of breath is related to an aggravation of aortic stenosis or just to physiological changes during pregnancy [14].

10.3.4 Echocardiography During Pregnancy

TTE should be done regularly during pregnancy. The frequency depends on symptoms and severity of stenosis. Particular attention should be given to the evaluation of left ventricular function, accompanying valvular lesions and changes of aortic stenosis severity. In women with more than mild AS, an increase in pressure gradients over the stenotic valve is usual [15]. In contrast to that, aortic valve area, which is less flow dependent, should stay constant throughout pregnancy. Concerning left ventricular function, ejection fraction should not show significant changes unlike longitudinal strain, which decreases during normal pregnancy [16]. Any drop in ejection fraction during pregnancy in women with AS should be a warning sign.

10.3.5 Laboratory Assessment During Pregnancy

During pregnancy laboratory tests could be helpful. Troponin I is normally not elevated in pregnancy in women without heart disease and could therefore indicate an acute decompensation or myocardial ischaemia in women with aortic stenosis [17]. In many pregnant women with different heart diseases, an elevated B-type natriuretic peptide (BNP) level could be found. In a study by Tanous et al., BNP levels <100 picograms per millilitre had a negative predictive value of 100% for identifying events during pregnancy. Although studies with pregnant women and aortic stenosis do not exist, serial B-type natriuretic peptide levels may be helpful in predicting outcome and in differentiating between pregnancy and aortic stenosis-related shortness of breath, thus diagnosing heart failure [18].

10.3.6 Phase 3: Treatment During Pregnancy

Symptomatic patients with severe AS should be advised to reduce their activity which is in most cases the mainstay of antepartum care [19]. Some patients may benefit from hospitalisation during the third trimester for bed rest and closer monitoring. These women should receive thromboprophylaxis with low molecular weight heparin. In the case of persistent symptoms, medical treatment may be indicated. If medical treatment, mainly with diuretics, is insufficient, invasive procedures should be considered. Percutaneous aortic balloon valvuloplasty can be considered during pregnancy as a palliative procedure, allowing delay of valve replacement until after birth [20]. A higher success rate in non-calcified valves with only minimal or absent regurgitation can be expected.

In case of persistent symptomatic severe AS after valvuloplasty or contraindication for valvuloplasty, cardiac surgery must be considered. High fetal mortality rates are described for surgery between the 13th and 28th week [21]. Maternal mortality seems to be comparable to that of non-pregnant women undergoing the same procedure [21]. During cardiac surgery, the objectives for anaesthetic induction are to maintain sinus rhythm, preload and cardiac contractility and to avoid decreased left ventricular afterload.

10.3.7 Arrhythmias

The available literature on supraventricular arrhythmias in valvular heart disease and pregnancy is limited to case series. The incidence described varies from 2% to 17.5% [22–24].

Maintenance of normal sinus rhythm is critical, as the atrial contraction may account for up to 40% of ventricular filling in this patient group [25]. A recent study could show that left-sided lesions are a predictor of atrial fibrillation and/or atrial flutter and that these arrhythmias are associated with higher rates of maternal mortality and lower fetal birth weight [26]. In patients with atrial fibrillation, beta-blocker or a non-dihydropyridine for rate control should be administered [27].

10.3.8 Phase 4: Labour and Delivery

When women with AS remain asymptomatic during pregnancy, the final haemodynamic challenge occurs during the time of delivery and the immediate postpartum period. For women with aortic stenosis, this stage should be a team approach of cardiologists, obstetricians and anaesthesiologists ("delivery team"). In asymptomatic women in good condition and normal cardiac function, spontaneous onset of labour is appropriate and is preferable to induce labour [2]. Spontaneous labour is commonly quicker and carries a higher chance of a successful delivery than induced labour [28]. There is no consensus with regard to the recommended mode of delivery in symptomatic patients, but vaginal delivery carries a lower risk of complications for both the mother and fetus. Compared with Caesarean section, it causes smaller shifts in blood volume, less haemorrhage, the absence of abdominal surgery, decreased thrombogenic risk and fewer infections.

The hypertrophied ventricle that accompanies AS is sensitive to abrupt changes in preload so vasodilation from anaesthetic agents or haemorrhage around the time of labour and delivery can destabilise cardiac function more profoundly. To manage the stress of labour, early epidural analgesia is important. Good regional analgesia helps to avoid further increases in cardiac output associated with contractions. Caesarean section should be reserved mainly for obstetric indications or in the case of aortic problems or severe heart failure [2]. Nevertheless in some centres, Caesarean delivery is advocated for women with severe AS or acute heart failure [2].

10.3.9 Phase 5: After Delivery/Postpartum Period

Care should be given with intravenous bolus of oxytocin in the third stage of labour, as it might cause a sudden fall in cardiac output, and controlled intravenous infusion might be more appropriate [29].

The early postpartum period carries some potential risks. Uterine contraction permanently returns some 500 ml of blood to the circulation, which can have a deleterious effect on patients with diminished left ventricular function or severe aortic stenosis. After delivery, most haemodynamic changes are rapidly reversed in the first 2 weeks with further normalisation towards preconception values after 3–12 months [29]. Several days of close monitoring for signs of heart failure and echocardiographic examinations are recommended in selected cases [2].

10.4 The Impact of the Physiological Changes of Pregnancy

Several studies have extended our understanding of the haemodynamic changes during pregnancy [16, 30, 31]. The increased cardiovascular demand in the setting of pregnancy is accomplished by numerous haemodynamic changes (also see Fig. 10.3):

- Increase in plasma volume (40%)
- Increase in stroke volume
- Increase in heart rate
- Increase in cardiac output (30–50%)
- Decrease in systemic vascular resistance
- Decrease in pulmonary vascular resistance
- Increase in lower-extremity venous pressure

Delivery and the postpartum period are associated with additional haemodynamic changes, and adjustment to these changes can be problematic in the setting of a fixed left ventricular outflow tract obstruction. It is well known that stenotic lesions are less well tolerated and carry a higher pregnancy risk than regurgitant valvular lesions as the increase in circulating blood volume aggravates the haemodynamic consequences of the stenosis.

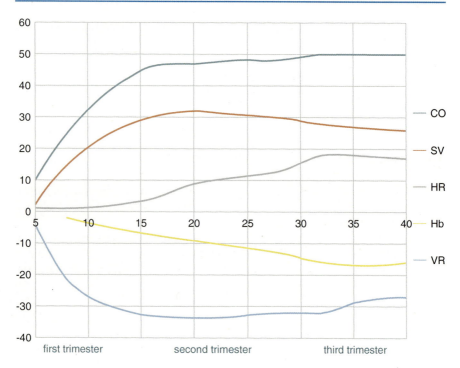

Fig. 10.3 Normal cardiovascular changes in pregnancy in women without aortic stenosis (Adapted from [29, 32]). Heart rate (*HR*) increases steadily until the beginning of the third trimester, when cardiac output (CO) and stroke volume (SV) reach a plateau at the beginning of the second trimester. (*Hb* haemoglobin, *VR* vascular resistance)

> **Conclusion**
>
> In patients with AS, appropriate preconceptional patient evaluation and counselling are essential. Most women with a mild or moderate AS and normal left ventricular ejection fraction tolerate pregnancy well. Severe AS is associated with increased maternal morbidity and unfavourable fetal outcome, but maternal mortality seems to be unlikely with appropriate patient care during pregnancy and delivery in expert hands.

References

1. Vahanian A, Alfieri O, Andreotti F et al (2012) Guidelines on the management of valvular heart disease (version 2012). Eur Heart J 33:2451–2496. doi:10.1093/eurheartj/ehs109
2. European Society of Gynecology, Association for European Paediatric Cardiology, German Society for Gender Medicine et al (2011) ESC Guidelines on the management of cardiovascular diseases during pregnancy: the Task Force on the Management of Cardiovascular Diseases during Pregnancy of the European Society of Cardiology (ESC). Eur Heart J 32:3147–3197. doi:10.1093/eurheartj/ehr218
3. Silversides CK, Colman JM, Sermer M et al (2003) Early and intermediate-term outcomes of pregnancy with congenital aortic stenosis. Am J Cardiol 91:1386–1389

4. Hameed A, Karaalp IS, Tummala PP (2001) The effect of valvular heart disease on maternal and fetal outcome of pregnancy. J Am Coll Cardiol 37:893–899. doi:10.1016/S0735-1097(00)01198-0
5. Orwat S, Diller GP, Van Hagen IM et al (2015) The risk of pregnancy in aortic stenosis: results from the ROPAC registry. Eur Heart J 36:5
6. Nora JJ (1994) From generational studies to a multilevel genetic-environmental interaction. JAC 23:1468–1471
7. Baumgartner H, Hung J, Bermejo J et al (2009) Echocardiographic assessment of valve stenosis: EAE/ASE recommendations for clinical practice. J Am Soc Echocardiogr 22:1–23. doi:10.1016/j.echo.2008.11.029; quiz 101–102
8. Rosenhek R, Klaar U, Schemper M et al (2004) Mild and moderate aortic stenosis. Natural history and risk stratification by echocardiography. Eur Heart J 25:199–205. doi:10.1016/j.ehj.2003.12.002
9. Baumgartner H, Kratzer H, Helmreich G, Kuehn P (1990) Determination of aortic valve area by Doppler echocardiography using the continuity equation: a critical evaluation. Cardiology 77:101–111
10. Sikka P, Suri V, Aggarwal N et al (2014) Are we missing hypertrophic cardiomyopathy in pregnancy? Experience of a tertiary care hospital. J Clin Diagn Res 8:OC13–OC15. doi:10.7860/JCDR/2014/9924.4803
11. Ashikhmina E, Farber MK, Mizuguchi KA (2015) Parturients with hypertrophic cardiomyopathy: case series and review of pregnancy outcomes and anesthetic management of labor and delivery. Int J Obstet Anesth 24:344–355. doi:10.1016/j.ijoa.2015.07.002
12. Drenthen W, Boersma E, Balci A et al (2010) Predictors of pregnancy complications in women with congenital heart disease. Eur Heart J 31:2124–2132. doi:10.1093/eurheartj/ehq200
13. Siu SC, Sermer M, Colman JM et al (2001) Prospective multicenter study of pregnancy outcomes in women with heart disease. Circulation 104:515–521
14. Baumgartner H, Bonhoeffer P, De Groot NMS et al (2010) ESC guidelines for the management of grown-up congenital heart disease (new version 2010). Eur Heart J 31:2915–2957. doi:10.1093/eurheartj/ehq249
15. Yuan S-M (2014) Bicuspid aortic valve in pregnancy. Taiwan J Obstet Gynecol 53:476–480. doi:10.1016/j.tjog.2013.06.018
16. Savu O, Jurcut R, Giusca S et al (2012) Morphological and functional adaptation of the maternal heart during pregnancy. Circ Cardiovasc Imaging 5:CIRCIMAGING.111.970012–297. doi:10.1161/CIRCIMAGING.111.970012
17. Roth A, Elkayam U (2008) Acute myocardial infarction associated with pregnancy. J Am Coll Cardiol 52:171–180. doi:10.1016/j.jacc.2008.03.049
18. Tanous D, Siu SC, Mason J et al (2010) B-type natriuretic peptide in pregnant women with heart disease. J Am Coll Cardiol 56:1247–1253. doi:10.1016/j.jacc.2010.02.076
19. Easterling TR, Chadwick HS, Otto CM (1988) Aortic stenosis in pregnancy. Obstetrics and Gynecology 72(1):113–118
20. Myerson SG, Mitchell ARJ, Ormerod OJM, Banning AP (2005) What is the role of balloon dilatation for severe aortic stenosis during pregnancy? J Heart Valve Dis 14:147–150
21. Elassy SMR, Elmidany AA, Elbawab HY (2014) Urgent cardiac surgery during pregnancy: a continuous challenge. Ann Thorac Surg 97:1624–1629. doi:10.1016/j.athoracsur.2013.10.067
22. Ayhan A, Yapar EG, Yüce K et al (1991) Pregnancy and its complications after cardiac valve replacement. Int J Gynaecol Obstet 35:117–122
23. Suri V, Sawhney H, Vasishta K et al (1999) Pregnancy following cardiac valve replacement surgery. Int J Gynaecol Obstet 64:239–246
24. Leśniak-Sobelga A, Tracz W, KostKiewicz M et al (2004) Clinical and echocardiographic assessment of pregnant women with valvular heart diseases—maternal and fetal outcome. Int J Cardiol 94:15–23. doi:10.1016/j.ijcard.2003.03.017
25. Stott DK, Marpole DGF, Bristow JD et al (1970) The role of left atrial transport in aortic and mitral stenosis. Circulation 41:1031–1041. doi:10.1161/01.CIR.41.6.1031
26. Salam AM, Ertekin E, van Hagen IM et al (2015) Atrial fibrillation or flutter during pregnancy in patients with structural heart disease: data from the ROPAC. JACC: Clin Electrophysiol. doi:10.1016/j.jacep.2015.04.013

27. Sliwa K, Johnson MR, Zilla P, Roos-Hesselink JW (2015) Management of valvular disease in pregnancy: a global perspective. Eur Heart J 36:1078–1089. doi:10.1093/eurheartj/ehv050
28. Uebing A, Steer PJ, Yentis SM, Gatzoulis MA (2006) Pregnancy and congenital heart disease. BMJ 332:401–406. doi:10.1136/bmj.332.7538.401
29. Ruys TPE, Cornette J, Roos-Hesselink JW (2013) Pregnancy and delivery in cardiac disease. J Cardiol 61:107–112. doi:10.1016/j.jjcc.2012.11.001
30. Hunter S, Robson SC (1992) Adaptation of the maternal heart in pregnancy. Br Heart J 68:540–543
31. Kaleschke G, Baumgartner H (2011) Pregnancy in congenital and valvular heart disease. Heart 97:1803–1809. doi:10.1136/heartjnl-2011-300369
32. Robson SC, Hunter S, Boys RJ, Dunlop W (1989) Serial study of factors influencing changes in cardiac output during human pregnancy. Am J Physiol 256:H1060–H1065

Pregnancy in Hypertrophic Cardiomyopathy

11

Michelle Michels

Abbreviations

ACE	Angiotensin converting enzyme
ARBs	Angiotensin receptor blockers
FDA	Food and Drug Administration
G+	Genotype positive
HCM	Hypertrophic cardiomyopathy
ICD	Implantable cardioverter defibrillator
LV	Left ventricular
LVOT	Left ventricular outflow tract
NYHA	New York Heart Association
SCD	Sudden cardiac death
VKA	Vitamin K antagonist
WHO	World Health Organization

> **Key Facts**
> *Incidence and inheritance*: Most common autosomal dominant inherited cardiac disease. Affects 1/500 people.
> *World Health Organization class*: Range from class I (for genotype-positive, HCM-negative subjects) to class IV (severe, symptomatic LVOT obstruction or severe systolic LV dysfunction).

M. Michels, MD, PhD
Thoraxcenter, Center for Inherited Cardiovascular Diseases,
Erasmus University Medical Center, Rotterdam, The Netherlands
e-mail: m.michels@erasmusmc.nl

> *Risk of pregnancy*: Usually tolerated well and major complications limited to high-risk and/or symptomatic women. Typically II–III.
> *Medication*: Antiarrhythmic and anticoagulation medication may need to be changed.
> *Life expectancy*: Reduced in high-risk women with evidence of heart failure and an increased risk of sudden death.

> **Key Management Principles**
> *Preconception*: Genetic counseling is indicated for both women and men. Full risk assessment, functional status, echocardiography (specific assessment of provocable LVOT obstruction), exercise testing, and Holter monitoring.
> *Pregnancy*: The frequency of follow-up determined by WHO class and family history of sudden death. Fetal echo should be offered. Most common problems: LVOT obstruction, arrhythmias, and diastolic dysfunction.
> *Delivery*: Vaginal delivery, monitoring determined by WHO grade. Hemodynamic stability key, particularly in those with a provocable gradient. Avoid volume overload with ventricular dysfunction.
> *Postpartum*: Close observation for 24–48 h.

11.1 The Condition

Hypertrophic cardiomyopathy (HCM) is the most common autosomal inherited cardiac disease typically caused by mutations in cardiac sarcomere protein genes. It is defined by an increased left ventricular (LV) wall thickness of 15 mm or more, which is not solely explained by abnormal loading conditions. The prevalence in adults is between 1/200 and 1/500 and disease penetrance is age related [1, 2].

HCM is characterized by great genetic and clinical heterogeneity; even in a family with the same pathological mutation, the phenotype can vary widely (Fig. 11.1). Currently, we know that the phenotype can vary from genotype-positive/HCM-negative (G+/HCM−) subjects at advanced age to patients first presenting with sudden death (SD) at young age (Patient A and D in Fig. 11.1) [3, 4]. The precise proportion of the G+/HCM− subjects that will develop overt disease is currently unknown, and while some patients remain asymptomatic throughout their lives, the disease generally progresses slowly with time [5, 6]. The symptoms in HCM are mainly caused by diastolic LV dysfunction, left ventricular outflow tract (LVOT) obstruction, and supraventricular and ventricular arrhythmias [3]. About a third of the HCM patients will experience heart failure-related symptoms based on a significant LVOT obstruction, caused by the hypertrophied septum and the systolic anterior movement of the mitral valve in systole (Fig. 11.2). LVOT obstruction is thought to be hemodynamically significant when the gradient exceeds 50 mmHg and is

11 Pregnancy in Hypertrophic Cardiomyopathy

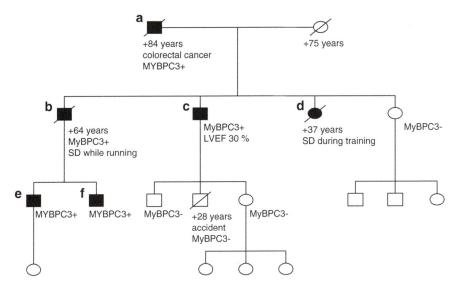

Fig. 11.1 Pedigree of a HCM family showing extensive phenotypic heterogeneity. Family member *A* = G+/HCM− at advanced age, noncardiac cause of death. Family member *B* = G+/HCM+ SD during exercise. Family member *C* = G+/HCM+ severe systolic dysfunction. Family member *D* = index patient of the family, first presentation with SD. Family member *E* and *F* = G+/HCM− (*HCM* hypertrophic cardiomyopathy, *MYBPC3* myosin-binding protein C, *G+* genotype positive, *SD* sudden death)

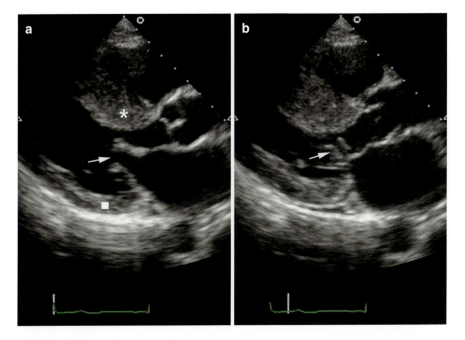

Fig. 11.2 Parasternal long-axis echocardiography of hypertrophic cardiomyopathy patient. (**a**) Diastolic frame: *asterix* interventricular septum; *square* left ventricular posterior wall; *arrow* mitral valve. (**b**) Systolic frame: *arrow* systolic anterior movement of mitral valve

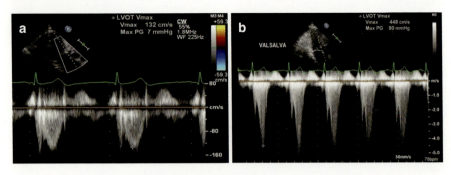

Fig. 11.3 Provocation of left ventricular outflow tract obstruction (LVOT) with Valsalva. (**a**) LVOT gradient 7 mmHg at rest. (**b**) LVOT gradient 80 mmHg during Valsalva

associated with sudden cardiac death (SCD) and heart failure-related complications [7, 8]. While HCM may be associated with a normal life expectancy and stable clinical course, about 5–15 % of patients progress to either the restrictive or the dilated-hypokinetic stage of HCM with progression of heart failure-related symptoms, eventually leading to end-stage heart failure [4].

Both supraventricular and ventricular arrhythmias are prevalent in HCM patients. Atrial fibrillation is the most frequent, affecting more than 20 % of patients and associated with an unfavorable outcome [9]. In all HCM patients, it is important to estimate the risk of SCD caused by ventricular arrhythmias and to select patients for prophylactic implantable cardioverter defibrillator (ICD) implantation. The implantation of an ICD for secondary prevention is universally accepted [1, 10]. The selection of patients for primary prevention of SCD with ICD implantation differs between Europe and America. The recent European Society of Cardiology guidelines promote the use of the HCM risk score, in which age, maximal wall thickness, LVOT gradient, left atrial dimension, the presence of ventricular tachycardia on Holter monitoring, unexplained syncope, and family history are used to calculate the SCD risk. A high risk is defined as the risk of SCD $\geq 6\%$ at 5 years, warranting ICD implantation [1, 8]. The American guidelines favor evaluation of major risk factors (family history, maximal wall thickness, unexplained syncope, the presence of ventricular tachycardia on Holter monitoring, and an abnormal blood pressure response to exercise) to estimate the SCD risk in order to select high-risk patients [10].

Echocardiography is the cornerstone of diagnosis in HCM. It is important to assess maximal LV wall thickness, LV systolic and diastolic function, left atrial dimension, and the presence of LVOT obstruction both at rest and during provocation. LVOT obstruction is present at rest in about a third of the patients; this increases to two thirds of the patients with exercise echocardiography [11]. By convention, LVOT obstruction is defined as the presence of a LVOT gradient ≥ 30 mmHg. LVOT gradient ≥ 50 mmHg is considered as threshold at which LVOT obstruction becomes hemodynamically important and is generally accepted as the threshold for invasive therapies in symptomatic HCM patients on optimal medical therapy [1, 12]. Provocation of LVOT obstruction with the Valsalva maneuver in different positions (sitting, semi-supine, and in some cases standing) is recommended in all patients (Fig. 11.3). Exercise echocardiography is recommended in symptomatic HCM patients with LVOT gradients <50 mmHg after bedside manoeuvre. The presence and magnitude of LVOT obstruction are important for the management of symptoms and the assessment of the SCD risk [1].

11.2 Pregnancy Outcomes

The most common causes of complications are caused by diastolic dysfunction of the hypertrophied noncompliant LV, LVOT obstruction, and arrhythmias [13]. The maternal mortality rate is very low and limited to those patients with HCM who were significantly symptomatic before pregnancy, had significant impaired LV function before pregnancy, and/or had high LVOT gradient [14]. Most women who experience symptoms during pregnancy are already known with similar symptoms before pregnancy [15]. In pregnant HCM patients, the New York Heart Association (NYHA) class > II and the presence of LVOT obstruction are related with maternal and neonatal events [14, 16, 17]. Patients known with structural heart disease and arrhythmias are more likely to experience complaints during pregnancy [18].

11.3 Management

11.3.1 Antenatal Considerations

Current cardiac medication and its use during pregnancy should be discussed with the patient, as some medications might need to be adjusted to prevent adverse fetal events. The US Food and Drug Administration (FDA) classifies drugs used during pregnancy and breastfeeding from category A (=safest) to X (=known danger) [13]. The medications that are most widely used in HCM patient include beta-blockers, calcium antagonists, disopyramide, amiodarone, diuretics, angiotensin-converting enzyme (ACE) inhibitors, angiotensin receptor blockers (ARBs), and vitamin K antagonists (VKA). In HCM patients whose symptoms are controlled by beta-blockers, the medication should be continued during pregnancy (class IIa, level C recommendation) [1]. The fetal events are usually not severe and manageable, including growth retardation, neonatal bradycardia, and hypoglycemia. Monitoring of fetal growth and of neonatal condition is recommended in all pregnant patients on beta-blockers. The use of metoprolol (FDA class C) is preferred over atenolol (FDA class D), because the latter has been associated with more growth retardation. The calcium antagonists verapamil and diltiazem (both FDA class C) can be used during pregnancy when their benefits outweigh the potential risk as it can cause AV block in the fetus. Disopyramide (FDA class C) should be used with caution since it can cause uterine contractions. Amiodarone (FDA class D) is used in HCM for rhythm control in atrial fibrillation and for the treatment of ventricular arrhythmias. Amiodarone can cause growth retardation, fetal thyroid toxicity, bradycardia, and premature birth and should only be used when absolutely necessary. ACE inhibitors and ARBs are contraindicated in women who are pregnant or wish to become pregnant, because of the teratogenic effects on the fetal kidney. Loop diuretics can be used during pregnancy, but aldosterone antagonist should be avoided. All HCM patients with atrial fibrillation have an indication for oral anticoagulants; the use of the CHA2DS2-VASc score is not recommended to calculate the stroke risk (class I, level C recommendation) [1]. In the first trimester, low molecular weight heparin is recommended, because of the risk of embryopathy of VKA. In the second and third trimester, VKA (FDA class D) is recommended. After the 36th week of gestation, low molecular weight heparin is recommended because of the bleeding risk during delivery. The new oral anticoagulants are contraindicated because of proven toxicity in animals and lack of data in humans.

11.3.2 Follow-Up During Pregnancy

Development of heart failure symptoms is relatively uncommon during pregnancy, occurring in <5% of previously asymptomatic HCM patients and in 15% of the overall cohort. Clinical deterioration is twice as common in patients with LVOT obstruction compared to those without [14]. Beta-blockers (metoprolol) should be started in women who develop symptoms during pregnancy (class I, level C recommendation). Loop diuretics may be necessary to limit fluid retention [1]. The 2011 ESC guidelines on the management of cardiovascular disease during pregnancy also advise to consider beta-blockers in all HCM patients with more than mild LVOT obstruction or a maximal wall thickness exceeding 15 mm, but this is not recommended in the more recent ESC HCM guideline [1, 13]. The latter recommends starting beta-blockers in women who develop symptoms during pregnancy [1]. Women with arrhythmias before pregnancy are more likely to experience arrhythmias during pregnancy, but pregnancy alone does not seem to significantly increase the risk of arrhythmia [16, 17]. Cardioversion for poorly tolerated atrial fibrillation should be considered during pregnancy; this should be performed in centers with the ability for cardiac monitoring and emergency caesarean section (class IIa, level C recommendation) [1].

G+/HCM− women are in WHO class I and don't need specific cardiac follow-up during their pregnancy after HCM is excluded by ECG and echocardiography before or shortly after conception.

Pregnant HCM patients who are in WHO class II are at low to moderate risk and should be assessed each trimester. Those in WHO class III have a high risk of complications and should be followed twice a month in specialized centers, by a multidisciplinary team. This team should consist of cardiologists, obstetricians, and anesthesiologists in experienced maternal-fetal medicine units. HCM patients that are in WHO class IV should be advised against pregnancy, but if they are pregnant and don't consider termination follow-up should be arranged according to those women who are in class III [13].

During follow-up, special attention should be paid to symptoms and signs of heart failure and arrhythmias, LV function, and LVOT obstruction. Echocardiography should be performed each trimester and when new symptoms occur.

11.3.3 Management During Labor and Delivery

By the end of the second trimester, the multidisciplinary team should make a delivery plan. During labor cardiac output is increased by catecholamine-induced increase in heart rate and stroke volume. Tachycardia will shorten the LV diastolic filling period, decreasing preload and increasing LVOT obstruction. Venous return is impaired by the performance of the Valsalva manoeuvre with maternal pushing during labor and delivery and this might also increase LVOT obstruction. During labor the patient should be positioned in a lateral decubitus position in order to attenuate the hemodynamic impact of uterine contractions.

Substantial blood loss during delivery can lead to reduction of venous return and a relative increase in LVOT obstruction. In a recent paper describing the association of cardiomyopathy with adverse cardiac events during delivery, one fifth of the HCM patients experienced either heart failure or arrhythmias at delivery [19].

Asymptomatic women with mild disease may go into spontaneous labor; for others, a planned vaginal delivery is generally preferred (class I, level C recommendation) [1]. Compared to caesarean section, vaginal delivery is associated with less blood loss and lower infection risk. A caesarean section in general should be performed for obstetric indications. There is no consensus on absolute contraindications for vaginal delivery, but in HCM patients with severe LVOT obstruction, severe heart failure, or preterm labor while on vitamin K antagonist, a caesarean section should be considered [1, 13]. To avoid the provocation of significant LVOT obstruction caused by maternal pushing during delivery, vaginal delivery may be assisted by low forceps or vacuum extraction. In HCM patients with a high risk of arrhythmias, monitoring of the heart rate and rhythm should be considered.

Epidural or spinal anesthesia should be used with caution, since vasodilatation and hypotension can induce or increase preexistent LVOT obstruction. Single-shot spinal anesthesia should be avoided [1, 13].

Post partum, the use of prostaglandins is acceptable, but oxytocin should only be given as a slow infusion, to avoid hypotension and tachycardia [13].

In the case of severe blood loss or hypotension, fluids should be used for volume replacement; inotropes are relatively contraindicated in HCM because of the potential induction or aggravation of LVOT obstruction. When necessary, pure alpha-antagonists like phenylephrine are preferred.

Clinical observation after delivery should be continued for 24–48 h because of the increased risk of pulmonary edema due to fluid shifts post-delivery [1, 10, 13].

11.4 The Effect of Pregnancy Adaptations

The physiological changes during pregnancy are mostly tolerated well by asymptomatic or mildly symptomatic women with HCM. The hypertrophied LV can accommodate the rise in blood volume, cardiac output, and the reduction of systemic vascular resistance and blood pressure without a significant rise in LV filling pressures.

11.5 Preconception Counseling

Since HCM is a hereditary disease in the fast majority of patients, genetic counseling by a geneticist is recommended in HCM patients, and genetic testing is recommended to enable cascade screening of their relatives (class I, level C recommendation) [1, 10, 13]. All HCM patients (men and women) should be informed about the possibility of transferring the hereditary predisposition to their offspring. Children of parents with HCM have an inheritance risk of 50 %, regardless of the gender of the affected parent. Special attention should be paid to HCM patients and G+/HCM− family members with questions about family planning regarding the risk of transmission of the disease to their offspring. When the pathological mutation is known, prenatal screening or preimplantation genetic testing is theoretically possible. These are not routinely performed due to phenotypic heterogeneity, age-related disease manifestation, the availability of treatment options, and the fact that longevity is maintained in these patients when viewed as a group [20].

11.5.1 Preconception Risk Assessment

In known HCM patients, the risk of pregnancy should ideally be assessed and discussed with the patient before conception. Alternatively, the risk assessment should be performed early after conception. Different classifications and risk scores have been developed to estimate maternal risk; most studies indicated the presence of LVOT obstruction as a risk factor for maternal and neonatal events. The modified World Health Organization (WHO) classification is the best available risk assessment model for estimating cardiovascular risk and should be used to assess the risk [1, 13, 21]. Risk assessment should include a detailed history (including NYHA functional class), physical examination, electrocardiogram, echocardiography, exercise testing, and Holter monitoring [22]. The echocardiography should focus on LV function, LVOT obstruction in rest, and, after provocation, mitral regurgitation and filling pressures. Exercise testing is used to assess functional capacity, heart rate response, and exercise-induced arrhythmias. In pregnant women submaximal exercise testing to reach 80 % of predicted maximal heart rate is recommended [13]. Holter monitoring (preferably for 48 h) is performed to evaluate the presence of ventricular or supraventricular arrhythmias [1]. In Table 11.1, the modified WHO classification and its applicability to HCM are described.

The clinical use of genetic testing has revealed a new subset within the HCM spectrum: the G+/HCM− family members. The reported risk of adverse cardiac events in G+/HCM− is very low, and in the largest study thus far, no SCD occurred in mutation carriers without hypertrophy [23]. G+/HCM− subjects with normal ECG and normal echocardiography are allowed to participate in competitive sports [1, 24], and based on the current literature describing the virtual absence of any cardiovascular events in G+/HCM− subjects, our HCM program considers G+/HCM− subjects to be in WHO class I during pregnancy.

Table 11.1 Modified WHO classification of maternal cardiovascular risk: principles and application on HCM

Risk class	Risk of pregnancy	Application to HCM
I	No detectable increased risk of maternal mortality and no/mild risk of morbidity	Genotype-positive/HCM-negative subjects
II	Small increased risk of maternal mortality or severe morbidity	Mild to moderate LVOTO
		Asymptomatic with or without medication
		Normal or mild systolic LV dysfunction
		Well-controlled arrhythmia
III	Significantly increased risk of maternal mortality or severe morbidity	Severe LVOTO
		Symptomatic with medication
		Moderate LV dysfunction
		Arrhythmias despite medication
IV	Extremely high risk of maternal mortality or severe morbidity; pregnancy contraindicated	Severe symptomatic LVOTO
		Severe systolic LV dysfunction

Adapted from Elliott et al. [1]
WHO World Health Organization, *HCM* hypertrophic cardiomyopathy, *LVOTO* left ventricular outflow tract obstruction, *LV* left ventricular

Asymptomatic HCM patients with mild to moderate LVOT obstruction with or without medication, well-controlled arrhythmias, and maximal mildly reduced LV dysfunction are in WHO class II. Those women with severe LVOT obstruction and symptoms despite medical therapy, poorly controlled arrhythmias, or moderate LV dysfunction are in WHO class III. A small minority of HCM patients, those with end-stage disease with severe systolic LV dysfunction and those with severe symptomatic LVOT obstruction, will be in WHO class IV. HCM patients with LVOT obstruction who are in NYHA class III despite optimal medical therapy are candidates for septal reduction therapy. After successful septal reduction therapy with relief of the LVOT gradient and a significant reduction in symptomatology, patients will move from WHO class IV to II or III, and pregnancy will be safer for both the mother and baby ([1, 13], Table 11.1).

References

1. Elliott PM, Anastasakis A, Borger MA et al (2014) 2014 ESC guidelines on diagnosis and management of hypertrophic cardiomyopathy. Eur Heart J 35:2733–2779
2. Semsarian C, Ingles J, Maron MS et al (2015) New perspectives on the prevalence of hypertrophic cardiomyopathy. J Am Coll Cardiol 65:1249–1254
3. Maron BJ, Ommen SR, Semsarian C et al (2014) Hypertrophic cardiomyopathy: present and future, with translation into contemporary cardiovascular medicine. J Am Coll Cardiol 64:83–99
4. Olivotto I, Cecchi F, Poggesi C et al (2012) Patterns of disease progression in hypertrophic cardiomyopathy: an individualized approach to clinical staging. Circ Heart Fail 5:535–546

5. Jensen MK, Havndrup O, Christiaensen M, Andersen PS, Diness B, Axelsson A et al (2013) Penetrance of hypertrophic cardiomyopathy in children and adolescents. Circulation 127:48–54
6. Michels M, Soliman OI, Kofflard MJ, Hoedemaekers YM, Dooijes D, Majoor-Krakauer D et al (2009) Diastolic abnormalities as the first feature of hypertrophic cardiomyopathy in Dutch myosin-binding protein C founder mutations. JACC Cardiovasc Imaging 2:58–64
7. Maron MS, Olivotto I, Betocchi et al (2003) Effect of left ventricular outflow tract obstruction on clinical outcome in hypertrophic cardiomyopathy. N Engl Med 348:295–303
8. O'Mahony C, Jichi F, Pavlou M et al (2014) A novel clinical risk prediction model for sudden cardiac death in hypertrophic cardiomyopathy (HCM risk-SCD). Eur Heart J 35:2010–2020
9. Guttmann OP, Rahman MS, O'Mahony C et al (2014) Atrial fibrillation and thromboembolism in patients with hypertrophic cardiomyopathy: systematic review. Heart 100:465–472
10. Gersh BJ, Maron BJ, Bonow RO et al (2011) 2011 ACCF/AHA guideline for the diagnosis and treatment of hypertrophic cardiomyopathy: a report of the American College of Cardiology Foundation/American Heart Association Task Force on Practice Guidelines. Circulation 124(24):e783–e831
11. Maron MS, Olivotto I, Zenovich A et al (2006) Hypertrophic cardiomyopathy is predominantly a disease of left ventricular outflow tract obstruction. Circulation 114(21):2232–2239
12. Wigle ED, Sasson Z, Henderson MA et al (1985) Hypertrophic cardiomyopathy. The importance of the site and the extent of hypertrophy. A review. Prog Cardiovasc Dis 28:1–83
13. Regitz-Zagrosek V, Blomstrom LC, Borghi C et al (2011) ESC Guidelines on the management of cardiovascular diseases during pregnancy: the Task Force on the Management of Cardiovascular Diseases during Pregnancy of the European Society of Cardiology (ESC). Eur Heart J 32:3147–3197
14. Autore C, Conte MR, Piccininno (2002) Risk associated with pregnancy in hypertrophic cardiomyopathy. J Am Coll Cardiol 40:1864–1869
15. Thaman R, Varnava A, Hamid MS et al (2003) Pregnancy related complications in women with hypertrophic cardiomyopathy. Heart 89:752–756
16. Siu SC, Sermer M, Colman JM et al (2001) Prospective multicenter study of pregnancy outcomes in women with heart disease. Circulation 104(5):515–521
17. Drenthen W, Boersma E, Balci A et al (2010) Predictors of pregnancy complications in women with congenital heart disease. Eur Heart J 31:2124–2132
18. Silversides CK, Harris L, Haberer K et al (2006) Recurrence rates of arrhythmias during pregnancy in women with previous tachyarrhythmias and impact on fetal and neonatal outcomes. Am J Cardiol 97(8):1206–1212
19. Lima V, Parikh P, Zhu J et al (2015) Association of cardiomyopathy with adverse cardiac events in pregnant women at the time of delivery. J Am Coll Cardiol HF 3:257–266
20. Krul SPJ, van der Smagt JJ, van de Berg MP, Sollie KM, Pieper PG, van Spaendonck-Zwarts (2011) Systematic review of pregnancy in women with inherited cardiomyopathies. Eur J Heart Fail 13:584–594
21. Balci A, Sollie-Szarynska KM, van der Bijl et al (2014) Prospective validation and assessment of cardiovascular and offspring risk models for pregnant women with congenital heart disease. Heart 100:1373–1381
22. Stergiopoulous K, Shiang E, Bench T (2011) Pregnancy in patients with pre-existing cardiomyopathies. J Am Coll Cardiol 58:337–350
23. Christiaans I, Birnie E, Bonsel GJ, Mannens MM, Michels M, Majoor-Krakauer D et al (2011) Manifest disease, risk factors for sudden cardiac death, and cardiac events in a large nationwide cohort of predictively tested hypertrophic cardiomyopathy mutation carriers: determining the best cardiological screening strategy. Eur Heart J 32:1161–1170
24. Maron BJ, Zipes DP (2005) 36th Bethesda conference: eligibility recommendations for competitive athletes with cardiovascular abnormalities. J Am Coll Cardiol 45:1312–1375

Aortopathy

12

Julie De Backer, Laura Muiño-Mosquera, and Laurent Demulier

Abbreviations

ACE	Angiotensin converting enzyme
ART	Assisted reproductive technologies
ASI	Aortic size index
ASRM	American Society for Reproductive Medicine
BAV	Bicuspid aortic valve
BSA	Body surface area
C-	Caesarean
ESC	European Society of Cardiology
FBN1	Fibrillin 1 gene
HTAD	Heritable thoracic aortic disorders
IRAD	International Registry of Aortic Dissections
IUGR	Intrauterine growth retardation
LDS	Loeys–Dietz syndrome
MAC	Montalcino Aortic Consortium
MFS	Marfan syndrome
PGD	Preimplantation diagnosis
PND	Prenatal diagnosis

J. De Backer, MD, PhD (✉)
Department of Cardiology and Center for Medical Genetics,
Ghent University Hospital, Ghent, Belgium
e-mail: Julie.DeBacker@UGent.be

L. Muiño-Mosquera, MD
Department of Pediatric Cardiology and Center for Medical Genetics,
Ghent University Hospital, Ghent, Belgium

L. Demulier, MD
Department of Cardiology, Ghent University Hospital, Ghent, Belgium

TAAD   Thoracic aortic aneurysms and dissections
TAAs   Thoracic aortic aneurysms
TAD   Thoracic aortic dissection
TS   Turner syndrome
vEDS   Vascular Ehlers–Danlos syndrome
VSMC   Vascular Smooth Muscle Cells

> **Key Facts**
>
> *Incidence*: Aortic aneurysm occurs in 9 per 100,000 patient-years and acute aortic dissection in 2.6–4.7 per 100,000 person-years.
>
> *Inheritance*: Monogenetic aortic diseases are most commonly transmitted in an autosomal dominant way. Multifactorial disorders, such as atherosclerosis and hypertension, may also be involved.
>
> *Medication*: ACE inhibitors and angiotensin receptor blockers should be stopped or changed to α methyldopa or beta-blockers.
>
> *World Health Organization class*: II/III when the aortic root diameter is <40 mm and class IV, when the aortic root diameter is >45 mm.
>
> *Risk of pregnancy*: Elevated risk of dissection.
>
> *Life expectancy*: Improved dramatically with appropriate follow-up and prophylactic aortic root surgery for aortic dilatation, but it is still reduced. The role of prophylactic surgery before pregnancy is uncertain.

> **Key Management**
>
> *Preconception*: Transthoracic echocardiography for assessment of valvular function and aortic root diameters. CT or MRI of the aorta with prophylactic surgery for women with Marfan syndrome and an aortic root diameter >45 mm and for women with Loeys–Dietz syndrome and an aortic root diameter >40 mm. Genetic counseling in all monogenetic aortopathies.
>
> *FU during pregnancy*: Known gene mutation, but normal aortic diameters: check at 20 weeks with echo. Known gene mutation and dilated aorta or history of dissection four to eight weekly imaging of aorta during pregnancy and up to 6 months postpartum. CMR is safe after 12 weeks (gadolinium contraindicated during pregnancy). Careful blood pressure monitoring and aggressive treatment of hypertension are mandatory.
>
> *Delivery*: Aortic diameter <40 mm or <20 mm/m^2 in Turner syndrome: vaginal; between 40 and 45 mm class IIa indication for vaginal delivery and IIb for Caesarean (C-) section; aortic diameter >45 mm or >20 mm/m^2 in Turner syndrome: C-section.
>
> *Postpartum*: Image of aorta before discharge and at 6 weeks post-delivery. Increased risk until 6 months post-delivery; continue close surveillance until then. Beta-blockers and calcium channel blockers can be used safely during breastfeeding.

12 Aortopathy

12.1 The Condition

This chapter will cover disease related to aortic aneurysms and dissections. Aortic coarctation and aortic valve disease (including bicuspid aortic valve (BAV)) will be covered elsewhere. For a correct understanding and interpretation of the disease, we will start with a description of the normal aorta.

12.1.1 The Normal Aorta

The aorta (Fig. 12.1) is the largest artery of the body, extending from the aortic valve to the bifurcation into the common iliac arteries. The aorta has two main functions: a conduit function, distributing oxygenated blood to the systemic circulation, and a pressure control function, regulating systemic vascular resistance and cardiac output through baroreceptors located in the ascending aorta and aortic arch. Through its elasticity, the aorta functions as a passive pump creating an almost continuous peripheral blood flow, commonly known as "the Windkessel effect" [1].

Anatomically, the aorta is subdivided into four major segments: the *ascending aorta* – comprising the aortic root (including the annulus, sinuses of Valsalva, and sinotubular junction) – and the tubular ascending aorta, the *aortic arch* (segment of the aorta between the brachiocephalic artery and left subclavian artery), the *descending thoracic aorta* (extending from the isthmus between the origin of the left subclavian artery and ligamentum arteriosum to the diaphragm), and the *descending abdominal aorta* (extending from the diaphragm to the iliac bifurcation) [2] (Fig. 12.1).

Normal diameters of the aorta vary according to the location (tapering down going from the ascending to the descending part) and according to the individual's gender and body surface area (BSA). Irrespective of BSA, women tend to have smaller aortas than men [3, 4]. With age, the aortic diameter increases at all segments with an average increase of 1 mm per decade for the ascending and descending thoracic aorta [5].

The aortic wall is histologically composed of three layers: a thin inner tunica intima lined by the endothelium; a thick tunica media characterized by smooth muscle cells embedded in an extracellular matrix and concentric sheets of elastic and collagen fibers, bordered by a lamina elastica interna and externa; and the outer tunica adventitia containing mainly fibroblasts, collagen, vasa vasorum, and lymphatics [6].

The composition of the vessel wall varies according to the location: the abdominal aortic wall consists of fewer elastic lamellae, contains less structural proteins and has a lower elastin to collagen ratio when compared to the thoracic aorta [7].

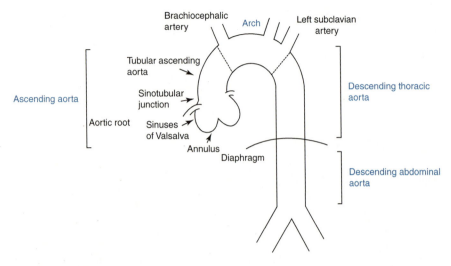

Fig. 12.1 Aortic anatomy

12.1.2 The Diseased Aorta

Although more diseases are recognized, the two main conditions that we will consider in the scope of this chapter include aortic aneurysm and aortic dissection/rupture – the latter being consequences of preceding aortic aneurysm in many cases. Aortic aneurysm is defined as a permanent localized or diffuse dilatation of the aorta to at least 1.5 times its normal caliber and may affect the aortic root, tubular ascending aorta, aortic arch, and descending thoracic or abdominal aorta [2, 8]. Since pregnancy-related aortopathy is most commonly located in the thoracic aortic segments [9], we will further focus on thoracic aortic aneurysms and dissections (TAAD).

Aortic aneurysms will only occasionally lead to symptoms, related to local pressure, such as coughing, hoarseness, or swallowing difficulties. In most cases, however, thoracic aortic aneurysms (TAAs) will have an asymptomatic course and – if left undiagnosed or untreated – they can lead to dissection, an acute life-threatening event that is still associated with high mortality and morbidity rates. In thoracic aortic dissection (TAD), blood is diverted from its usual location within the lumen of the aorta into a false lumen within the media through a tear in the intima. The dissection can subsequently propagate both proximal and distal to the tear, hence affecting vital branching arteries and leading to coronary, cerebral, spinal, and/or visceral ischemia. Several classification systems for TAD exist, of which the Stanford classification is the most widely used. In Stanford type A dissection, the ascending aorta is involved, whereas type B dissection is typically located distally from the left subclavian artery. The distinction between both subtypes is relevant in view of important differences in prognosis and management. In aortic rupture, the tear in the aortic wall extends through all vessel layers, leading to life-threatening intrathoracic hemorrhage.

Due to its asymptomatic course, the exact incidence of thoracic aortic aneurysms is largely unknown. A recent contemporary, prospective cohort study of middle-aged individuals in Sweden reported an incidence rate of 9 per 100,000 patient-years (95% CI 6.8–12.6) [10]. Estimating the incidence of acute aortic dissection is somewhat easier and has been studied more widely, but one has to bear in mind that a substantial proportion of aortic dissections may be left undiagnosed due to the high acute mortality rate of the disease. The incidence in the general population ranges from 2.6 to 4.7 per 100,000 person-years [11, 12]. The mortality rate associated with TAD reported a decade ago from the large International Registry of Aortic Dissections (IRAD) indicated that without urgent surgical intervention, type A dissection is associated with mortality rates as high as 20% by 24 h and 40% by day 7 [13]. Type B aortic dissections generally have a better outcome with a 30-day mortality rate of 10%. Uncomplicated type B dissections are conventionally treated medically, whereas complicated type B dissections are treated using endovascular techniques or open surgery – results being comparable according to recent studies [14]. Despite advances in medical and surgical treatment options, mortality rates remain high, as demonstrated in a more recent prospective cohort study where the acute and in-hospital mortality was 39% for aortic dissection and 41% for ruptured TAD [10]. Women with aortic dissection typically present at an older age compared to men and display a higher hospital mortality and worse surgical outcome [15]. Etiological factors underlying TAAD include conventional cardiovascular risk factors although the lack of any significant association of TAA or AD with trends in smoking prevalence in a recent epidemiological study may suggest a difference in etiology compared with abdominal aortic aneurysms [8]. Differences in the pathogenesis of thoracic and abdominal aortic aneurysms may result from differences in aortic structures, biochemical properties, and origin of the vascular smooth muscle cells (VSMC) [16].

The underlying pathophysiology of TAAD has been widely studied, and many new insights have emerged from the study of monogenetic aortic diseases. These disease entities will be discussed in more detail below. Through human and mouse studies of monogenetic aortic diseases, it is now increasingly clear that aneurysms and dissections may result from alterations in structural, functional, and signal transduction properties in the wall of the aorta. The ensemble of these processes is referred to as altered mechanobiology and is illustrated in Fig. 12.2 and nicely reviewed by Humphrey and colleagues [46]. Based on these concepts, it is easy to conceive that dissections can be triggered by abnormalities in any of these processes: altered mechanical factors (hypertension, increased cardiac output, increased wall shear stress), alterations in structural components of the aortic wall (genetic defects in components of the elastic fibers), alterations in the signaling pathway (genetic defects in any component such as the TGFβ pathway), or altered signal transduction (genetic defects in extracellular matrix components, intracellular receptors, modulators).

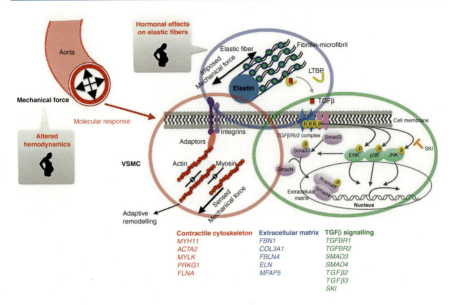

Fig. 12.2 Concept of mechanobiology underlying homeostasis in the thoracic aorta and the possible effects of pregnancy. Mechanical force is sensed in the aortic wall and transmitted through the extracellular matrix to the intracellular molecular level. The signal is sensed by the smooth muscle cell contractile apparatus as well as by components of the TGFβ signaling pathway. Pregnancy affects the mechanical stimulus on the one hand and the elastic fibers in the extracellular matrix on the other hand. Alterations, either due to higher imposed forces (hypertension) or due to (genetic) alterations in the various components required for proper sensing and/or transduction of the signal, may lead to aneurysms/dissections. Genes involved in these pathways are listed at the bottom of the figure and are reported in Table 12.1 with their respective disorders

12.2 Pregnancy Outcomes

Since the first report on pregnancy-related aortic dissection in 1944 [47], over 80 additional reports have been published, most of them being case reports. A limited number of population-based studies and surgical series on the occurrence of aortic dissection have also been published, but caution is warranted when interpreting these results because of their heterogeneity with regard to design, study population, and diseases under study (type A vs. type B dissection).

Although the estimated incidence of aortic dissection during pregnancy is relatively low (0.05–1.39 per 100,000 person-years [48, 49] or 0.6 % per pregnancy [15]), the high maternal mortality rates (between 21 and 53 %) account for the high ranking in the list of maternal death causes [48, 50–52]. The reported figures show some variation according to the country they are issued from. Aortic dissection ranks first on the list of mortality causes in the UK and the Netherlands, but is only the third cause of cardiovascular death in the French registry where three fatal dissections are reported during the period of 2007–2009, two out of these three being in women with Turner syndrome [53].

Table 12.1 Overview of the syndromic forms of H-TAD with their respective genes and main clinical features. Genes are grouped according to the categories presented in Fig. 12.1

	Disorder	Gene(s)	Main cardiovascular features	Additional clinical features
ECM associated	Marfan [17–20]	*FBN1*	Aortic root aneurysm, aortic dissection, mitral valve prolapse, main pulmonary artery dilatation, ventricular dysfunction, arrhythmia	*Lens luxation*, skeletal features (arachnodactyly, pectus deformity, scoliosis, flat feet, increased arm span, dolichocephalia)
	Vascular Ehlers–Danlos [21]	*COL3A1*	Arterial dissections, middle-sized artery aneurysm	*Translucent skin, dystrophic scars*, facial characteristics
	MFAP5 [22]	*MFAP5*	Aortic root dilatation, atrial fibrillation, mitral valve prolapse	Pectus deformities
	Cutis laxa syndromes [23, 24]	*FBLN4, ELN*	Arterial aneurysms and dissections, arterial tortuosity, arterial stenoses, BAV	Hyperlax skin and joints, lung emphysema, craniofacial anomalies, bone fragility
TGFβ associated	Loeys–Dietz [25, 26]	*TGFBR1/TGFBR2*	Aneurysms and dissections of the aorta and middle-sized arteries, arterial tortuosity, mitral valve prolapse, congenital cardiac malformations	*Bifid uvula/cleft palate, hypertelorism*, marfanoid skeletal features
	Aneurysm–osteoarthritis syndrome [27–30]	*SMAD3*	Aneurysms and dissections of the aorta and middle-sized arteries, intracranial aneurysms, visceral and iliac artery aneurysms, arterial tortuosity, mitral valve prolapse, congenital cardiac malformations	*Osteoarthritis*, hypertelorism, marfanoid skeletal features
	TGFB2 [31–33]	*TGFB2*	Aortic root aneurysms and dissections, mitral valve prolapse, cerebrovascular disease	Marfanoid skeletal features
	TGFB3 [34–36]	*TGFB3*	Aortic root aneurysms	Marfanoid skeletal features, hypertelorism, muscle hypotonia, and congenital joint contractures
	Shprintzen–Goldberg [37, 38]	*SKI*	Mild aortic root dilatation, mitral valve prolapse	*Craniosynostosis*, distinct craniofacial features, marfanoid skeletal features, mild-to-moderate intellectual disability
	Juvenile polyposis [39]	*SMAD4*	Aortic root aneurysms, mitral valve prolapse, hereditary hemorrhagic telangiectasia	*Juvenile polyposis, periventricular nodular heterotopia* with seizures and joint hypermobility

(continued)

Table 12.1 (continued)

	Disorder	Gene(s)	Main cardiovascular features	Additional clinical features
Contractile unit associated	EDS-PH [40]	FLNA	Aneurysms of the aorta, pulmonary artery, and middle-sized arteries	Periventricular nodular heterotopia with seizures, joint hypermobility
	ACTA2 [41, 42]	ACTA2	Thoracic aortic aneurysms and dissection, BAV, PDA, cerebrovascular disease, coronary artery disease	Livedo reticularis, iris flocculi
	PRKG1 [43]	PRKG1	Aneurysms and dissection of the aorta and middle-sized arteries, arterial tortuosity	
	MYH11 [41, 44]	MYH11	PDA	
	MYLK [45]	MYLK	Thoracic aortic aneurysms and dissection	Gastrointestinal tract involvement

BAV bicuspid aortic valve, *PDA* patent ductus arteriosus

In women younger than 40 years of age, pregnancy has reportedly been associated with a significant increase in the risk for acute aortic dissection (with odds ratios for pregnancy up to 23 in one study [49]. Other studies however could not demonstrate a direct link between dissection and pregnancy [48]. A selective reporting bias may be invoked as a possible explanation for these discrepancies [54]. These data should be interpreted carefully, especially in women with underlying conditions, until large prospective studies assessing all aspects of a direct link are published. Data on aortic disease extracted from the large international registry on the outcome of pregnancy in patients with congenital heart disease are expected to be very valuable (the ROPAC study, see for more information at http://www.escardio.org/Guidelines-&-Education/Trials-and-Registries/Observational-registries-programme/Registry-Of-Pregnancy-And-Cardiac-disease-ROPAC).

The risk for aortic dissection during pregnancy increases with gestational age, with most of the events occurring during the third trimester (55–78 %) [51, 55]. The majority of reported aortic dissections occurring during pregnancy (70 %) are type A aortic dissections [9], although type B aortic dissections seem to be more commonly reported in women with Marfan syndrome (see below).

In addition to the hemodynamic and hormonal changes occurring during pregnancy, the process of labor imposes substantial stress on the aorta and, hence, increases the risk for dissection. Uterine contractions, pain, stress, exertion, and bleeding, all impose an extra demand on the cardiovascular system [56]. The correct management of women at increased risk for dissection during labor in an experienced fetomaternal unit is, therefore, mandatory [57]. Follow-up of the aortic diameter and awareness of a possibly higher risk of aortic dissection should be considered until 6 months postpartum [51].

12.2.1 Predisposing Conditions

Several diseases are associated with increased aortic vulnerability, and affected women will therefore require special multidisciplinary care starting before pregnancy and extending well after delivery.

12.2.2 Heritable Thoracic Aortic Disorders: H-TAD

H-TAD is a heterogeneous group of disorders characterized by the common denominator of thoracic aortic disease (TAD) [58]. The presentation of aortic involvement varies widely from an incidental finding on an imaging study to fatal aortic dissection. The term "heritable" does not necessarily imply that all these disorders have a known genetic cause – despite significant advances in the genetic background of TAD, many patients and families do not harbor mutations in the genes identified so far. Based on the presence of additional clinical features in other organ systems, H-TAD can be further subdivided into syndromic and nonsyndromic forms. The spectrum of genes identified in these various clinical entities is highly variable.

Genes can be grouped in those encoding components of the extracellular matrix, genes encoding components of the TGFβ signaling pathway, and genes encoding components of the VSMC contractile apparatus. An overview of the clinical conditions according to the currently known genetic defects with their respective typical clinical characteristics is provided in Table 12.1. Nearly all genes listed in this table can also be identified in patients with nonsyndromic forms of H-TAD.

12.2.3 Marfan Syndrome

Marfan syndrome (MFS) is the prototype of syndromic H-TAD. MFS is caused by mutations in the fibrillin 1 gene (*FBN1*) and typically affects a myriad of organ systems including the ocular, the skeletal, and the cardiovascular systems. The clinical presentation is highly variable, both within and between families [17–19, 59]. When considering the cardiovascular system, aortic aneurysms and dissections are the most common and life-threatening problems related to MFS. The risk for aortic dissection in MFS is significantly increased to 170 per 100,000 individuals per year (compared to 6 per 100,00 per year in the general population) [60]. Other cardiovascular manifestations related to MFS include mitral valve prolapse, subclinical cardiomyopathy, and arrhythmias [20, 61–65].

The intrinsic aortic wall fragility associated with MFS along with the hemodynamic and hormonal changes occurring during pregnancy, as described above, gives rise to a higher risk for (fatal) dissection and aortic rupture in pregnant MFS women. Early publications, mostly case reports, on pregnancy in MFS showed a grim outcome with more than half of the cases ending with (fatal) aortic dissection. Most of the women in these earlier publications had preexistent severe cardiovascular disease, but based on these reports, patients were generally counseled against pregnancy [66]. A systematic assessment of pregnancy in MFS women was undertaken for the first time in 1981. Pyeritz and colleagues reviewed pregnancy-related cardiovascular risks in 26 patients with MFS and compared these to non-MFS women. Cardiovascular complications were not significantly different between both groups, but MFS women showed a higher rate of spontaneous abortion. Although no aortic diameters are reported in this study, the authors proposed an aortic root diameter of 40 mm before pregnancy as a threshold for stratifying women as having low risk (1%) or increased risk (10%) for dissection. Since then this stratification has been widely applied and debated in the literature [9, 67–71], but remains a reference value in the current European guidelines for the management of cardiovascular diseases during pregnancy [55]. In these guidelines the modified WHO classification is applied to determine maternal risk, where MFS patients may fall under class II to IV: women with no aortic dilation are classified as WHO II, women with an aortic dilation between 40 and 45 mm are classified as WHO III, and women with an aortic diameter above 45 mm are classified as WHO IV.

The risk of aortic complications in MFS is not only present during pregnancy and delivery but also during the puerperium and even beyond pregnancy. Indeed the concerns about the long-term effect of pregnancy on aortic root growth, the

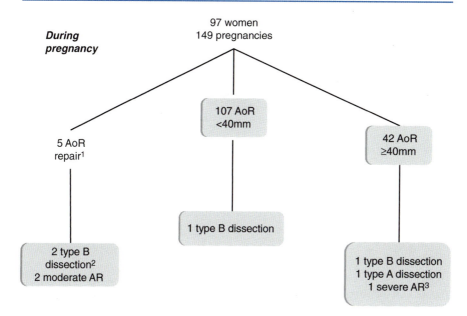

Fig. 12.3 Cardiovascular outcome in MFS women during pregnancy (Data pooled from [72, 74–76]). [1]Two women with valve sparing surgery, three women with Bentall of which two after acute type A dissection, and [2]two women with previous type A dissection [3]needing AoR replacement 6 months after pregnancy

incidence of dissection, and the need for elective aortic root replacement have been raised and need further assessment [72, 73].

Between 1995 and 2013, four prospective trials addressing pregnancy-related cardiovascular complications in MFS patients have been conducted – the main findings on pregnancy outcome in these women are illustrated in Fig. 12.3. A total of 97 women undergoing 149 pregnancies have been followed prospectively. Forty-two women in this combined cohort had an aortic root exceeding 40 mm prior to pregnancy, and five had undergone aortic root surgery prior to pregnancy [72, 74–76].

Three out of these four studies not only assessed the immediate effect of pregnancy but also looked at cardiovascular effects on the longer term [72, 74, 75]. A significant aortic root growth associated with pregnancy was observed in only one study (3 mm per pregnancy – interquartile range 0–7 mm). Aortic dissection was reported in a small subset of five women (Fig. 12.3). Type B aortic dissection was seen in four out of five cases. Although the latter observation warrants caution when advising patients to undergo elective surgery prior to pregnancy, large-scale studies are needed to confirm these findings. Also of note when interpreting these data is that in older cohorts (two out of these four studies [74, 75]), patients with other, more aggressive aortic disorders may have been included.

On the long-term adverse aortic outcome, defined as increased aortic root growth, the need for aortic surgery and aortic dissection was observed in two studies [72, 74]. Increased aortic root growth seemed more pronounced when the initial aortic root diameter equaled or exceeded 40 mm. Additionally, the study by Donnelly and colleagues showed increased adverse aortic outcome (defined as a composite of death, aortic dissection, the need for acute aortic surgery, and a severe symptomatic aortic regurgitation) in the parous versus nulliparous group. In multivariate analysis the initial aortic root diameter and the rate of aortic root growth during pregnancy were the principal predictors of long-term adverse outcome [72].

Some aspects in the interpretation of these data need consideration:

1. Some women included in these studies may actually have a genetically different diagnosis from MFS, as reflected by some unusual clinical features (carotid artery dissection is an uncommon feature in MFS, and type B aortic dissection occurs more frequently in other H-TAD entities).
2. The "comparison" group cannot be strictly considered a "control" group, because of occult biases in why those patients may have elected not to have any pregnancy.

Reports on pregnancy-related complications in MFS have obviously mainly focused on the aorta, but other notable risks include cardiac arrhythmias and venous thromboembolism (with respective OR of 10.64 and 5.25) and as reported in a retrospective analysis in 339 deliveries to women with MFS [77].

Overall, these studies indicate that in women known with a diagnosis of MFS and undergoing appropriate multidisciplinary care before, during, and after pregnancy, outcome of pregnancy on the short term is acceptable. Women contemplating pregnancy should be properly counseled about the associated risks before pregnancy.

12.2.4 Loeys–Dietz Syndrome

Loeys–Dietz syndrome (LDS) is caused by mutations in the genes encoding receptors for TGFβ (*TGFBR1* and *TGFBR2*) and is clinically characterized by more generalized aortic aneurysms and involvement of branching vessels in association with some distinctive dysmorphic features (hypertelorism, bifid uvula) along with some systemic features that show overlap with MFS (pectus deformities, scoliosis)[25]. The first retrospective study of 21 pregnancies reported four aortic dissections and two uterine ruptures in patients with LDS. These women were not diagnosed with LDS prior to pregnancy and, hence, did not receive proper management [26]. A subsequent report by Attias and colleagues comparing patients with *TGFBR2* mutations to patients with *FBN1* mutations did not find significant differences between the two cohorts. Of the 39 pregnancies occurring among 17 women in the *TGFBR2* cohort, one patient experienced sudden death in the immediate postpartum period (no diagnosis was made at that time). No aortic complications were reported during pregnancy or postpartum in the others. Among 87 women in the *FBN1* cohort, 217 pregnancies occurred. Four of these patients presented with aortic dissection or death during pregnancy ($p = 1$) [78].

Prospective studies are currently ongoing, one of which is the data collection by the Montalcino Aortic Consortium (MAC) – data on 316 pregnancies in 122 women indicate that the risk for aortic dissection is low (five dissections reported) and mainly occurred in women who were unaware of the diagnosis and hence did not receive proper care at the time of their pregnancy. Women with more pronounced systemic features seem to be at an increased risk (G. Jondeau et al. 2016 unpublished data).

12.2.5 Aneurysm Osteoarthritis Syndrome

So far, no data on pregnancy-related complications in patients harboring mutations in the *SMAD3* gene have been reported. In 1 retrospective series of 23 pregnancies in 13 women harboring a mutation in the *SMAD3* gene, no vascular complications or uterine ruptures were reported. One patient suffered a postpartum hemorrhage [29]. As is the case with LDS, prospective data collection is ongoing and results are awaited.

12.2.6 Vascular Ehlers–Danlos Syndrome

Patients with vascular Ehlers–Danlos syndrome (vEDS) are characterized by extensive vascular fragility and may present arterial dissection without preceding dilatation. Management is challenging since imaging studies may not predict events. Results from a randomized trial with celiprolol showed a significant reduction in vascular events in the treated group [79]. vEDS is caused by mutations in the *COL3A1* gene. Although the disease primarily affects major branching vessels of the aorta, the aorta itself may also be involved. In addition to these vascular complications, vEDS patients are also at risk for developing uterine rupture during pregnancy. Initial reports mentioned increased maternal mortality per pregnancy, ranging from 4.3% to 25% [21, 80, 81]. A more recent study, however, indicated that women with previous pregnancies did not have increased long-term mortality when compared to nulliparous women with vEDS [82]. The pregnancy-related death rate observed in this study covering 256 pregnancies in vEDS was 5.3%. Based on these recent observations, counseling policies in women with vEDS have shifted from strongly discouraging pregnancy to a more nuanced vision with careful prepregnancy counseling of the couple addressing the risks as well as long-term prognosis in vEDS. In case of an affected child, there is an increased risk for premature rupture of the membranes due to their intrinsic fragility [83].

12.2.7 Other H-TADs

The outcome of pregnancy in women harboring mutations in the *ACTA2* gene has been reported in one study [84]. Fifty-three women having a total of 137 pregnancies were included. Of these, eight had aortic dissections in the third trimester or the postpartum period (6% of pregnancies). Notably, one woman also had a myocardial infarct during pregnancy that was independent of her aortic dissection, indicating that patients with *ACTA2* mutations are also prone to cardiovascular disease outside the aorta. Assuming a population-based frequency of peripartum aortic dissections of 0.6%, the rate of peripartum aortic dissections in women with ACTA2 mutations is significantly increased (8 out of 39; 20%). Six of these reported dissections were Stanford type A dissections; three were fatal. Three women had ascending aortic dissections at diameters less that 5.0 cm (range 3.8–4.7 cm). Importantly, five out of the six women presenting with aortic dissection had hypertension, either during or before their pregnancy, indicating the importance of proper treatment.

In most of the other syndromic as well as in the vast majority of nonsyndromic H-TAD entities, very little or no data specifically related to pregnancy are available, and therefore, the recommendations are largely based on the knowledge obtained in MFS.

12.2.8 Turner Syndrome

Turner syndrome (TS) is a genetic sex chromosome disorder affecting approximately 1 in 2,000 live-born females, resulting from complete or partial absence of the X chromosome. The phenotype is highly variable and includes short stature, dysmorphic features, cardiovascular malformations, premature ovarian failure, and predisposition to autoimmune diseases. Different karyotype anomalies may lead to development of the syndrome, with or without cell line mosaicism, explaining part of the heterogeneity of clinical features. Monosomy X (45,X) has been associated with an increased risk of cardiac congenital anomalies [85].

Congenital cardiovascular anomalies can be divided into two main categories: aortic valve (mainly BAV) and thoracic vascular abnormalities (aortic coarctation and other arch anomalies) [85, 86].

With increasing age, the importance and impact of acquired cardiovascular disease on morbidity and mortality in Turner patients increase exponentially. A significant proportion will develop aortic dilation, ranging from 13 to 37% in MRI studies, depending on the age group and measurement level along the aorta [85, 87]. Due to the short stature of Turner women, aortic diameters should be interpreted after correction for BSA. The BSA-normalized aortic diameter is termed aortic size index (ASI). An ASI above 20 mm/m^2 is considered abnormal [88]. Excess cardiovascular mortality in TS is mainly due to ischemic heart disease, cerebrovascular disease, and aortic disease [85]. Aortic dissection is an important cause of early mortality, affecting Turner women mostly during the third and fourth decade of life (median age 35). The incidence is up to 100-fold increased compared to the general population, with a lifelong risk estimated at 1.4% [88, 89]. Stanford type A aortic dissection is seen in about two-third of cases, compared to one-third of type B. Risk factors for aortic dissection in Turner patients are not well defined. The current acknowledged risk markers are mainly based on case reports and a registry-based surveys: aortic dilation, bicuspid aortic valve, aortic coarctation, karyotype 45,X, and hypertension [85, 90]. One prospective MRI-based study confirmed the predictive value of aortic dilation, with a high dissection rate in those with an ASI above 25 mm/m^2 [88].

More recently, pregnancy has been recognized as a predisposing condition for aortic dissection in TS women, especially in the context of assisted reproductive technologies (ART) [91]. This aspect is important given the low rate of spontaneous pregnancy in TS women (2–7%), mainly occurring in women with a mosaic karyotype [92, 93]. Most of the other pregnancies in TS are achieved through oocyte donation. Pregnancy-associated hypertensive disorders, including preeclampsia and gestational hypertension, are a major concern after oocyte donation in the general population (general incidence 16–40%). This figure may rise up to 35–38% in TS women [94, 95].

Since the late 1990s, several worrying case reports have been published on unexpected acute aortic dissection in pregnant TS women with a high maternal mortality rate (75%) [94]. Aortic dissections occurred mainly during the third trimester and the early postpartum period, probably associated with the higher hemodynamic impact of pregnancy. Underlying congenital and acquired cardiovascular anomalies including BAV, coarctation of the aorta, or aortic dilation were present in the majority of published cases. However, aortic dissection may also occur in the absence of any of these. Half of the affected patients were known to have hypertension. Following these reports several national and international multicenter retrospective surveys were conducted in ART centers to determine the pregnancy outcome after oocyte donation in Turner patients, revealing an increased maternal mortality rate around 2% related to acute aortic syndromes [94–96]. Strikingly, less than half of Turner patients underwent cardiovascular screening before entering the OD program and only a quarter of them received echocardiographic follow-up during pregnancy.

12.3 Management

Management of women at risk for aortic complications during pregnancy requires a multidisciplinary approach at a tertiary center involving cardiologists, obstetricians, anesthesiologists, and medical geneticists.

Management of patients known to have aortic disease mainly consists of strict follow-up with aortic imaging, medical treatment aimed at reducing aortic wall stress, and prophylactic aortic surgery when indicated. Essentially, these strategies do not change in case of pregnancy, with the exception of the frequency of imaging and adjustment of the medical treatment in some cases.

Adequate and timely diagnosis of predisposing conditions, as well as prepregnancy counseling, and appropriate follow-up of patients at risk for an aortic event are essential to prevent fatal maternal and fetal outcome. In this section, we will discuss the different aspects of prevention of aortic dissection and rupture during pregnancy.

Strict and frequent follow-up of women with aortic aneurysms during pregnancy is the cornerstone of prevention of aortic dissection. Women with known aortopathy should be referred to a tertiary center for follow-up during pregnancy and management of delivery [97]. Regular echocardiographic follow-up should be scheduled every 4–8 weeks during pregnancy and up to 6 months' postpartum. For those women with a dilated distal ascending aorta, aortic arch, or descending aorta, follow-up with MRI without gadolinium is recommended during pregnancy [55]. Careful blood pressure monitoring and treatment of hypertension is mandatory in all of these women.

12.3.1 Medical Treatment

No randomized drug trials in pregnant women with aortic disease has been performed, and nor does it seem likely that one would ever be performed; hence, treatment recommendations have been extrapolated from nonpregnant cohorts. Much, if not most, evidence for medical treatment of aortic disease is derived from studies in MFS. Finding a drug capable of arresting aortic root growth is considered the ultimate goal in the medical management of aortic disease in MFS, and for a while, hopes were raised for losartan, based on spectacular results in a mouse model for MFS [98]. Unfortunately, similar results could not be reproduced in humans, as has been demonstrated by several large-scale trials published recently [99–101]. Based on these results, slowing the rate of growth is the best we can offer, and beta-blockade remains the mainstay of treatment in MFS. Losartan can be considered as an alternative for those intolerant for beta-blockers, but not in pregnancy!

In the prospective studies of pregnancy in MFS, mentioned in more detail above, the use of beta-blockers varied with about one-third of the patients being treated in the studies from Rossiter, Donnelly, and Meijboom, and all but one patient receiving treatment in the French study. That one patient not receiving treatment presented with aortic dissection [72, 74–76]. These data provide the evidence that supports the recommendation that beta-blockade should be used throughout pregnancy in patients with aortic disease. Issues with birth defects occurring more frequently with the use of certain beta-blockers (Table 12.2) led us to avoid those agents and start or switch patients to either metoprolol or labetalol, but fetal growth restriction has been demonstrated with the use of beta-blockers in MFS [72] as well as in hypertension [102] and congenital heart disease [103], and, therefore, patients should be counseled about this risk before conception. Celiprolol, used for the prevention of vascular complications in vEDS, is not reported to affect fetal outcome [104]. In women with ACTA2 mutations, blood pressure should be carefully monitored, and treatment with beta-blockers considered [84].

An overview of the effect of drugs on pregnancy and lactation of the various drugs mentioned is provided in Table 12.2.

12.3.2 Aortic Surgery

As is the case outside pregnancy, the operative risk associated with thoracic aortic surgery is highly dependent on the setting, being much higher in emergency settings when compared to elective procedures [105, 106]. In well-prepared circumstances,

Table 12.2 Effect of drugs used during pregnancy in women with aortic disease

Drug	Risk cat. (FDA)	Placental passage	Breast milk passage	Fetal risks
Atenolol	D	Yes	Yes	Suggested association with hypospadias and retroperitoneal fibromatosis
			Saver alternative recommended	IUGR
				Fetal bradycardia
Bisoprolol	C	Yes	Yes	IUGR as a beta-blocker although the use in pregnancy has not been studied
			Unknown long-term effect	Fetal bradycardia
Labetalol	C	Yes	Yes	Suggested association with congenital anomalies
			Compatible with breastfeeding	IUGR
				Fetal bradycardia
Metoprolol	C	Yes	Yes	Not teratogenic but causes fetal loss at high doses
			Compatible with breastfeeding	No association with congenital malformations
				IUGR
				Fetal bradycardia
Propranolol	C	Yes	Yes	Suggested association with cardiovascular defects and hypospadias
			Compatible with breastfeeding	IUGR
				Fetal bradycardia, hypoglycemia, polycythemia, thrombocytopenia, and hyperbilirubinemia
Celiprolol	NA[a]	Yes[b]	Yes	Safety in humans has not been established
			Unknown effect	Data from animal studies do not indicate harmful direct or indirect effects[c]

FDA US Food and Drug Administration, *IUGR* intrauterine growth retardation
[a]Currently not approved by the FDA. Under revision for treatment of vEDS
[b]Kofahl *Eur J Clin Pharmacol* 1993
[c]www.medicines.org.uk

with optimal perioperative care, including both maternal and fetal monitoring, the maternal risk may be reduced to a minimum [107], but the risk of fetal demise remains high. Aortic surgery during pregnancy is not only associated with a high fetal mortality but also with late neurological impairment in 3–6% of the children [108]; therefore, it should only be considered if medical treatment cannot control progression of aortic dilation and/or the life of the mother is in danger. The optimal period for surgery is between the 13th and 28th week of pregnancy. When the gestational age reaches 28 weeks, it may be better to deliver the baby by C-section, and arrange the aortic surgery afterwards [55].

12.3.3 Delivery

Delivery in women with aortic disease should take place at a tertiary center with a cardiothoracic surgery unit available. The decision on the most appropriate location for the delivery should be made on an individual basis. In a woman at high risk of complications, the delivery should be performed in the cardiothoracic operating room [97].

Cervical ripening using either prostaglandins or mechanical methods and induction of labor with oxytocin are relatively safe in most women with cardiac disease, although there are no specific data on patients with aortic disease [103]. Vaginal delivery is restricted to low-risk patients with an aortic diameter below 40 mm. To reduce hemodynamic stress, adequate pain relief through epidural anesthesia is required, the second stage of labor should be reduced, and vacuum extraction or a low-forceps delivery may be required [109, 110]. Regarding epidural anesthesia, prior scoliosis surgery and dural ectasia should be taken into account, especially in MFS patients. Up to 70 % of patients with MFS have spinal deformations and should be assessed by anesthetist in the combined clinic [111]. Higher doses of anesthetics may be needed and extra care should be taken to avoid dural taps. If difficulties in siting the epidural catheter are anticipated, then an elective C-section should be considered [112]. A small retrospective study on the anesthetic management of MFS women did not show that general anesthesia was superior to spinal/epidural anesthesia. Vasoactive drugs (ephedrine, noradrenaline) as well as potentially hypertensive drugs (e.g., Methergine) should be avoided [109]. Predelivery counseling by an experienced anesthetist is strongly recommended in these patients [112]. There are no large-scale trials on the optimal mode of delivery in women with aortic diameters >40 mm. Expert consensus, as reported in the European guidelines, gives a class IIa indication for vaginal delivery and IIb for C-section when the aorta is between 40 and 45 mm. C-section is recommended if the aortic diameter is >45 mm [55].

12.3.4 Breastfeeding and Postdelivery Care

The risk for aortic dissection remains increased up to 6 months after delivery, and women should remain under strict surveillance during that period. Imaging of the aorta 6 weeks after delivery is recommended. Beta-blockers, angiotensin-converting enzyme (ACE) inhibitors, and angiotensin receptor blockers can be used safely during breastfeeding.

12.3.5 Obstetrical and Fetal Outcome

In addition to the cardiovascular risks associated with pregnancy in H-TAD and TS, obstetric complications and impaired neonatal outcome also need to be taken into account in the counseling and management of these patients.

Obstetric complications in patients with MFS are widely reported, mostly in retrospective series. Initial reports on pregnancy in MFS patients by Pyeritz and colleagues described a higher rate of spontaneous abortion (21%) and preterm labor (12%) when compared to controls [66]. The reported rate of spontaneous abortions in MFS patients in subsequent studies varies between 12 and 18%, which does not seem to be much higher than the average population risk of 13% [69, 75, 113, 114]. Preterm labor, related to premature rupture of membranes and cervical incompetence, does appear to occur more frequently in MFS women in some studies, with figures varying between 5 and 12% [66, 113, 114] and an odds ratio of 2.15 reported in one series [77]. Other studies however did not confirm an increased risk for preterm labor [70, 75], once again indicating the need for prospective large-scale trials.

Adverse neonatal outcomes are related to prematurity and fetal growth restrictions in 5–11% of newborns [66, 70, 72, 113]. The latter observation was shown to be associated with a higher rate of beta-blocker usage in the study by Donnelly and colleagues (28% vs. 7%, $p=0.002$) [72]. Similar observations with the use of beta-blockers during pregnancy have been reported in women with hypertension and congenital heart disease and are thought to be related to a decreased mean arterial blood pressure [102, 103, 115]. On the other hand, small-for-gestational-age babies were reported with a higher frequency in one study in MFS patients that were not treated with beta-blockers [70], indicating that factors other than the beta-blockers could also contribute to this finding.

Reports on obstetric complications and fetal outcome in other H-TAD entities are scarce. A higher incidence of fatal uterine rupture in patients with LDS and vEDS has been reported in initial studies [21, 26], but this seemed to occur less frequently in subsequent series of both diseases with two nonfatal uterine ruptures in the large vEDS series reported by Murray [82] and no cases of uterine rupture in the large series of 316 pregnancies in LDS by Jondeau (G. Jondeau et al. 2016 unpublished data). Women pregnant with a child affected with vEDS have a higher risk of premature rupture of the membranes due to its intrinsic fragility [83].

Delivery through C-section is needed in the majority of TS pregnancies, due to cephalopelvic disproportion or hypertensive complications. A recent study in three Nordic countries showed reassuring data on neonatal outcome in singletons, with reported incidences of low birthweight (8,8%), preterm birth (8%), and major birth defects (3.8%) comparable to conventional in vitro fertilization results. A nationwide French study including all ART centers however reported a higher percentage of prematurity (38%) [94]. Twin pregnancies seem to carry a higher risk, and therefore single embryo transfer is currently recommended. A review of the literature found up to 36% fetal death (spontaneous abortions or perinatal death) and 20% rate of malformations (either TS or Down syndrome) [92].

12.4 The Effect of Pregnancy Adaptations

Two major concerns arise when addressing the effect of pregnancy on the aorta:

1. Growth of a known aneurysm
2. Risk of aortic dissection

The effect of pregnancy on the aorta is conventionally considered to be threefold [116–118]:

(1) Due to the increased cardiac output required for adequate placental perfusion, wall shear stress in the aorta will increase; (2) the hormonal changes inherent to pregnancy and aimed at softening tissues in preparation for delivery will also affect the elastic fibers in the aortic wall, leading to increased fragility; (3) in later stages of pregnancy, compression of the lower aorta and iliac arteries by the uterus will induce increased outflow resistance in the arterial tree.

The exact contribution and final impact of these changes on the aorta is however not fully elucidated, and some features remain to be confirmed in the clinical setting. For example, the impact of 17β-estradiol and progesterone has only been demonstrated in vitro, showing an increase of elastin and fibrillin 1 and a decrease in collagen deposition in aortic VSMC when exposed to these hormones [119]. Clinical studies show contradictory results, and the effect of estrogens and progesterone on arterial stiffness, especially during the third trimester, still needs to be clarified [120, 121]. What has been established is that the diameter of the aortic root increases significantly (1.2 mm on average) over the course of normal pregnancy and remains enlarged up to 6 weeks after pregnancy, even in normotensive women [122]. It is assumed that while these effects are largely ignorable in healthy women, their impact on an underlying diseased aorta may have severe consequences as is reflected, for example, in an adverse immediate and long-term aortic outcome in patients with Marfan syndrome [72, 74] (see below).

12.5 Preconception Counseling

As already mentioned, pregnancy may increase the risk of aortic dissection and progression of aortic disease in women with predisposing condition affecting the aorta. Counseling of women with these disorders should tackle the cardiovascular and obstetric risks associated with pregnancy and should also address the risk of transmission of the disease to the offspring. Cardiovascular and genetic counseling should take place during adolescence, ideally during the transition process from pediatric to adult cardiology care.

The risk of aortic dissection and the advice towards pregnancy should be discussed on an individual basis. Since the aorta in most of these women will grow over time, postponing pregnancy should be discouraged in some cases. A thorough cardiovascular evaluation with careful measurement of aortic diameters prior to pregnancy is recommended in all women with underlying aortic conditions. In addition to cardiac ultrasound, also evaluating valvular and myocardial function, we recommend imaging of the entire aorta and branching vessels with CT or MRI scan prior to pregnancy [55]. According to the ESC guidelines on the management of pregnancy in women with congenital heart disease, an aortic root diameter above 45 mm in patients with MFS is considered as high risk for dissection during pregnancy, and therefore, these women should be strongly advised to avoid pregnancy [55]. In addition to the aortic diameter, other factors including aortic growth rate prior to pregnancy and family history of dissection should be taken into account [9, 72]. In case of vEDS, pregnancy has been regarded as a high-risk situation both for cardiovascular and obstetric complications, and therefore, women were counseled against pregnancy. However, after the recent publication from Murray et al. in which pregnancy in itself did not add further risk of death on the long term [82], the current recommendation is to carefully discuss the risk pertaining to pregnancy as well as the long-term outcome of the disease on an individual basis. The couple needs to be informed of the fact that life expectancy in vEDS is significantly reduced, implying that they may not see their child grow into adulthood. Women with TS should also undergo detailed cardiovascular evaluation before pregnancy, independent of the conception mode (with or without ART), the karyotype, or the presence of mosaicism. The check-up should also include accurate blood pressure measurement (ideally by ambulatory blood pressure monitoring). As far as contraindications to pregnancy in TS are concerned, the American Society for Reproductive Medicine (ASRM) recommendations are the most stringent. Any significant cardiovascular abnormality on MRI or an aortic dilation of more than 20 mm/m^2 BSA are regarded as absolute contraindications for attempting pregnancy [91]. They also state that all TS patients should be encouraged to seek alternatives, such as gestational surrogacy or adoption, as TS itself should be seen as a relative contraindication. The French recommendations include the following listing of contraindications: history of aortic surgery or aortic dissection, aortic dilation above 35 mm or 25 mm/m^2 BSA, an increase in aortic diameter of more than 10% confirmed on MRI, and the presence of aortic coarctation or uncontrolled hypertension despite treatment. Isolated BAV (without aortic dilation) is not considered a contraindication but a risk factor [123]. The European Society of Cardiology (ESC) guidelines on the management of cardiovascular diseases during pregnancy acknowledge the increased risk for aortic dissection in TS pregnancies and state that those with aortic dilation are at the highest risk [55].

Medical treatment needs to be adjusted prior to conception as some agents, including ACE inhibitors and angiotensin receptor blockers, can cause severe embryopathy. Ideally, these agents would be switched to safer drugs in the preconception clinic as stopping the treatment as soon as conception takes place risks exposing the embryo to teratogenic agents. Beta-blockers are the most commonly used drugs in this setting, but may not be entirely safe as their use has been associated with an increase in fetal malformations. Atenolol can cause fetal malformations and hypospadias if used during the first trimester and should therefore be avoided. Other beta-blockers such as metoprolol, labetalol, and bisoprolol may be used safely during pregnancy, although caution with regard to fetal growth is warranted (see above, Table 12.2) [55].

The safety of prophylactic aortic root surgery is a matter of debate. Only five cases in women with MFS have been reported so far. No long-term prospective trials have taken place so far, and data from studies conducted in MFS patients indicate that (type B) aortic dissection still occurred in the two women with prior aortic root replacement (albeit in the setting of acute dissection) and that two women with prior valve sparing aortic root replacement in an elective setting developed significant aortic valve regurgitation through the course of their pregnancy [73]. According to the ESC guidelines on pregnancy, prophylactic aortic root surgery is recommended in women with MFS when the aortic root diameter exceeds 45 mm; the most recent Canadian guidelines on thoracic aortic disease recommend earlier prepregnancy surgery at a diameter above 40 mm [55, 124]. This lower threshold is also applied in patients with Loeys–Dietz syndrome. Clear guidelines for other H-TAD entities are lacking, and the general recommendations are to perform surgery at an aortic root diameter >45 mm. In women with Turner syndrome, an indexed aortic diameter of 27 mm/m^2 BSA is suggested as a threshold to consider prophylactic surgery. It is obvious from these knowledge gaps and discrepancies that there is a clear need for more prospective data in larger patient cohorts in order to establish the indications and safety of prophylactic aortic root surgery.

Genetic counseling addressing the transmission risk of the disease depends on the underlying condition. In this respect, an aspect that tends to be neglected in clinical practice is that affected males can equally transmit the disease and should also receive proper genetic counseling. MFS and most of the other H-TAD as well as vEDS are transmitted as an autosomal dominant trait, resulting in a 50 % chance of having an affected child. Inheritance of TS is less well studied. Spontaneous pregnancy occurs in only 2 % of the patients with TS [92]. Generally, a transmission risk of 25 %, with a higher rate of spontaneous abortions due to monosomy Y, is quoted.

Currently, prenatal diagnosis (PND) and preimplantation diagnosis (PGD) can be offered to those patients with a known mutation in most countries. A French study indicated that a majority of MFS patients (74 %) was in favor of prenatal testing. The opinion of caregivers varied, but most of them agreed that these issues should be addressed in a multidisciplinary team [125].

12.6 Conclusion

In disorders associated with aortic fragility, pregnancy increases the risk of complications including increased aneurysmal growth, aortic regurgitation, and aortic dissection. Key to preventing these complications is the delivery of multidisciplinary care by an experienced and knowledgeable team. Prior to pregnancy, appropriate counseling should be given, including genetic counseling, and the cardiovascular status of the patient examined, allowing treatment to be optimized and changed where appropriate.

Data regarding risks, management, and treatment in aortic disease related to pregnancy are based on case studies and retrospective analyses; the data are often inconsistent possibly because the genetic basis of many of these disorders is only now becoming clear, meaning that many of the earlier cohorts were heterogeneous.

Large prospective studies in well-defined cohorts are needed and efforts such as the ROPAC study are therefore crucial and very welcome. Future research should be focused on the above-mentioned key knowledge gaps in the pathophysiology, management, and treatment of pregnant patients with aortic disease, including but not limited to:

- Prospective assessment of aortic and obstetric outcome in well-defined homogenous cohorts of patients with different types of H-TAD and TS
- Study of the correlation between beta-blocker use and aortic outcome and fetal growth in patients with various types of H-TAD
- Prospective assessment of the safety of prepregnancy aortic root replacement

Key Messages
- Pregnancy may increase the risk of aortic dissection in women with underlying aortic disease.
- Management of pregnancy in women with aortic disease requires a multidisciplinary approach, involving cardiologists, obstetricians, anesthetists, and clinical geneticists.
- Individualized prepregnancy counseling on a case-by-case basis addressing cardiovascular and obstetric risks is essential.
- Genetic counseling addressing the transmission risk is equally important (in women and men).
- Appropriate follow-up with cardiovascular imaging before and during pregnancy is the cornerstone of prevention of aortic dissection in pregnant women with aneurysms. Follow-up intervals depend on the underlying condition and prepregnancy status and should also cover a 6-month postpartum period.
- In patients with MFS, it is safe to consider pregnancy when the aortic diameter is 40 mm or less.
- Medical treatment with beta-blockers during pregnancy should be encouraged in patients with MFS and in all other conditions if hypertension is present. The patient should be informed about the potential fetal impact.
- Medical treatment with angiotensin receptor blockers and ACE inhibitor is contraindicated during pregnancy.
- Recommendations regarding prophylactic aortic root surgery are inconsistent. Surgical replacement before pregnancy is generally recommended if the aortic root is above 45 mm in patients with MFS and above 27 mm/m^2 in patients with TS. Lower thresholds of 400–45 mm may be considered in women with LDS or in women with MFS and a positive family history for dissection or a rapid growth rate. Very limited data regarding safety of pregnancy after this procedure are available.
- In women with aortic diameters between 40 and 45 mm, delivery with C-section should be considered, and in women with aortic diameters >45 mm, C-section is advised.
- In patients with short stature, thoracic aortic diameters must be evaluated in relation to body surface area.
- Surgical treatment during pregnancy carries an important risk for the mother and fetus and should only be performed in life-threatening circumstances. C-section is recommended after 28th week of pregnancy before aortic surgical treatment.

Disclosures J. De Backer holds a grant as Senior Clinical Investigator from the Fund for Scientific Research (FWO), Flanders (Belgium). L. Muino Mosquera is supported by a doctoral fellowship from the Special Research Fund (BOF) of the University of Ghent (Belgium).

References

1. Westerhof N, Lankhaar J-W, Westerhof BE (2009) The arterial Windkessel. Med Biol Eng Comput 47(2):131–141
2. Hiratzka LF, Bakris GL, Beckman JA, Bersin RM, Carr VF, Casey DE et al (2010) 2010 ACCF/AHA/AATS/ACR/ASA/SCA/SCAI/SIR/STS/SVM guidelines for the diagnosis and management of patients with thoracic aortic disease: a report of the American College of Cardiology Foundation/American Heart Association Task Force on Practice Guidelines, American Association for Thoracic Surgery, American College of Radiology, American Stroke Association, Society of Cardiovascular Anesthesiologists, Society for Cardiovascular Angiography and Interventions, Society of Interventional Radiology, Society of Thoracic Surgeons, and Society for Vascular Medicine. Circulation 121:e266–e369
3. Devereux RB, de Simone G, Arnett DK, Best LG, Boerwinkle E, Howard BV et al (2012) Normal limits in relation to age, body size and gender of two-dimensional echocardiographic aortic root dimensions in persons ≥15 years of age. Am J Cardiol 110(8):1189–1194
4. Campens L, Demulier L, De Groote K, Vandekerckhove K, De Wolf D, Roman MJ et al (2014) Reference values for echocardiographic assessment of the diameter of the aortic root and ascending aorta spanning all age categories. Am J Cardiol 114(6):914–920
5. Hannuksela M, Lundqvist S, Carlberg B (2006) Thoracic aorta – dilated or not? Scand Cardiovasc J 40(3):175–178
6. Braverman AC, Thompson RW, Sanchez LA (2012) Diseases of the aorta. In: Mann DL, Zipes DP, Libby P (eds) Braunwald's heart disease, 9th edn. Elsevier Saunders, Philadelphia, pp 1309–1337
7. Halloran BG, Davis VA, McManus BM, Lynch TG, Baxter BT (1995) Localization of aortic disease is associated with intrinsic differences in aortic structure. J Surg Res 59(1):17–22
8. Sidloff D, Choke E, Stather P, Bown M, Thompson J, Sayers R (2014) Mortality from thoracic aortic diseases and associations with cardiovascular risk factors. Circulation 130(25):2287–2294
9. Immer FF, Bansi AG, Immer-Bansi AS, McDougall J, Zehr KJ, Schaff HV et al (2003) Aortic dissection in pregnancy: analysis of risk factors and outcome. Ann Thorac Surg 76(1):309–314
10. Landenhed M, Engström G, Gottsäter A, Caulfield MP, Hedblad B, Newton-Cheh C et al (2015) Risk profiles for aortic dissection and ruptured or surgically treated aneurysms: a prospective cohort study. J Am Heart Assoc 4(1):e001513
11. Nienaber CA (2003) Aortic dissection: new frontiers in diagnosis and management: part II: therapeutic management and follow-up. Circulation 108(6):772–778
12. Pacini D, Di Marco L, Fortuna D, Belotti LMB, Gabbieri D, Zussa C et al (2013) Acute aortic dissection: epidemiology and outcomes. Int J Cardiol 167(6):2806–2812
13. Nienaber CA (2003) Aortic dissection: new frontiers in diagnosis and management: part I: from etiology to diagnostic strategies. Circulation [Internet] 108(5):628–635
14. Hanna JM, Andersen ND, Ganapathi AM, McCann RL, Hughes GC (2014) Five-year results for endovascular repair of acute complicated type B aortic dissection. J Vasc Surg 59(1):96–106
15. Nienaber CA, Fattori R, Mehta RH, Richartz BM, Evangelista A, Petzsch M et al (2004) Gender-related differences in acute aortic dissection. Circulation 109(24):3014–3021
16. Guo D-C, Papke CL, He R, Milewicz DM (2006) Pathogenesis of thoracic and abdominal aortic aneurysms. Ann N Y Acad Sci 1085:339–352

17. Loeys BL, Dietz HC, Braverman AC, Callewaert BL, De Backer J, Devereux RB et al (2010) The revised Ghent nosology for the Marfan syndrome. J Med Genet 47(7):476–485
18. Judge DP, Dietz HC (2005) Marfan's syndrome. Lancet 366(9501):1965–1976
19. Dietz HC, Cutting GR, Pyeritz RE, Maslen CL, Sakai LY, Corson GM et al (1991) Marfan syndrome caused by a recurrent de novo missense mutation in the fibrillin gene. Nature 352(6333):337–339
20. Yetman AT, Bornemeier RA, McCrindle BW (2003) Long-term outcome in patients with Marfan syndrome: is aortic dissection the only cause of sudden death? JAC 41(2):329–332
21. Pepin M, Schwarze U, Superti-Furga A, Byers PH (2000) Clinical and genetic features of Ehlers-Danlos syndrome type IV, the vascular type. N Engl J Med 342(10):673–680
22. Barbier M, Gross M-S, Aubart M, Hanna N, Kessler K, Guo D-C et al (2014) MFAP5 loss-of-function mutations underscore the involvement of matrix alteration in the pathogenesis of familial thoracic aortic aneurysms and dissections. Am J Hum Genet 95(6):736–743
23. Renard M, Holm T, Veith R, Callewaert BL, s LCAE, Baspinar O et al (2010) Altered TGF & beta; signaling and cardiovascular manifestations in patients with autosomal recessive cutis laxa type I caused by fibulin-4 deficiency. Eur J Hum Genet 18(8):895–901
24. Callewaert B, Renard M, Hucthagowder V, Albrecht B, Hausser I, Blair E et al (2011) New insights into the pathogenesis of autosomal-dominant cutis laxa with report of five ELN mutations. Hum Mutat 32(4):445–455
25. Loeys BL, Chen J, Neptune ER, Judge DP, Podowski M, Holm T et al (2005) A syndrome of altered cardiovascular, craniofacial, neurocognitive and skeletal development caused by mutations in TGFBR1 or TGFBR2. Nat Genet 37(3):275–281
26. Loeys BL, Schwarze U, Holm T, Callewaert BL, Thomas GH, Pannu H et al (2006) Aneurysm syndromes caused by mutations in the TGF-beta receptor. N Engl J Med 355(8):788–798
27. van der Linde D, van de Laar IMBH, Bertoli-Avella AM, Oldenburg RA, Bekkers JA, Mattace-Raso FUS et al (2012) Aggressive cardiovascular phenotype of aneurysms-osteoarthritis syndrome caused by pathogenic SMAD3 variants. JAC [Internet] Elsevier Inc 60(5):397–403
28. van de Laar IMBH, Oldenburg RA, Pals G, Roos-Hesselink JW, de Graaf BM, Verhagen JMA et al (2011) Mutations in SMAD3 cause a syndromic form of aortic aneurysms and dissections with early-onset osteoarthritis. Nat Genet 43(2):121–126
29. van de Laar IMBH, van der Linde D, Oei EHG, Bos PK, Bessems JH, Bierma-Zeinstra SM et al (2011) Phenotypic spectrum of the SMAD3-related aneurysms-osteoarthritis syndrome. J Med Genet [Internet] 49(1):47–57
30. van der Linde D, Verhagen HJM, Moelker A, van de Laar IMBH, Van Herzeele I, De Backer J et al (2012) Aneurysm-osteoarthritis syndrome with visceral and iliac artery aneurysms. YMVA [Internet] Elsevier Inc 57(1):96–102
31. Guo D-C, Hanna N, Regalado ES, Detaint D, Gong L, Varret M et al (2012) TGFB2 mutations cause familial thoracic aortic aneurysms and dissections associated with mild systemic features of Marfan syndrome. Nat Genet. Nature Publishing Group, p 1–8
32. Lindsay ME, Schepers D, Bolar NA, Doyle JJ, Gallo E, Fert-Bober J et al (2012) Loss-of-function mutations in TGFB2 cause a syndromic presentation of thoracic aortic aneurysm. Nat Genet [Internet]. Nature Publishing Group, p 1–7
33. Renard M, Callewaert B, Malfait F, Campens L, Sharif S, Del Campo M et al (2012) Thoracic aortic-aneurysm and dissection in association with significant mitral valve disease caused by mutations in TGFB2. Int J Cardiol [Internet] Elsevier Ireland Ltd 165(3):584–587
34. Bertoli-Avella AM, Gillis E, Morisaki H, Verhagen JMA, de Graaf BM, van de Beek G et al (2015) Mutations in a TGF-β Ligand, TGFB3, cause syndromic aortic aneurysms and dissections. J Am Coll Cardiol 65(13):1324–1336
35. Morisaki H, Akiko Y, Itaru Y, Razia S, Tatsuya O, Hiroshu T (2014) Pathogenic mutations found in 3 Japanese families with MFS/LDS-like disorder. Presented at the biannual meeting on Marfan syndrome and related disorders. Paris, Fr

36. Matyas G, Naef P, Oexle K (2014) De novo TGFB3 mutation in a patient with overgrowth and Loeys-Dietz syndrome features. Presented at the biannual meeting on Marfan syndrome and related disorders, Paris, Fr, Paris
37. Doyle AJ, Doyle JJ, Bessling SL, Maragh S, Lindsay ME, Schepers D et al (2012) Mutations in the TGF-β repressor SKI cause Shprintzen-Goldberg syndrome with aortic aneurysm. Nat Genet 44(11):1249–1254
38. Carmignac V, Thevenon J, Adès L, Callewaert B, Julia S, Thauvin-Robinet C et al (2012) In-frame mutations in exon 1 of SKI cause dominant Shprintzen-Goldberg syndrome. Am J Hum Genet [Internet] Am Soc Hum Genet 91(5):950–957
39. Andrabi S, Bekheirnia MR, Robbins-Furman P, Lewis RA, Prior TW, Potocki L (2011) SMAD4 mutation segregating in a family with juvenile polyposis, aortopathy, and mitral valve dysfunction. Am J Med Genet A 155A(5):1165–1169
40. Reinstein E, Frentz S, Morgan T, García-Miñaúr S, Leventer RJ, McGillivray G et al (2013) Vascular and connective tissue anomalies associated with X-linked periventricular heterotopia due to mutations in Filamin A. Eur J Hum Genet 21(5):494–502
41. Renard M, Callewaert B, Baetens M, Campens L, Macdermot K, Fryns J-P et al (2011) Novel MYH11 and ACTA2 mutations reveal a role for enhanced TGFbeta signaling in FTAAD. Int J Cardiol [Internet] 165(2):314–321
42. Guo D-C, Pannu H, Tran-Fadulu V, Papke CL, Yu RK, Avidan N et al (2007) Mutations in smooth muscle α-actin (ACTA2) lead to thoracic aortic aneurysms and dissections. Nat Genet 39(12):1488–1493
43. Guo D-C, Regalado E, Casteel DE, Santos-Cortez RL, Gong L, Kim JJ et al (2013) Recurrent gain-of-function mutation in PRKG1 causes thoracic aortic aneurysms and acute aortic dissections. Am J Hum Genet 93(2):398–404
44. Pannu H, Tran-Fadulu V, Papke CL, Scherer S, Liu Y, Presley C et al (2007) MYH11 mutations result in a distinct vascular pathology driven by insulin-like growth factor 1 and angiotensin II. Hum Mol Genet 16(20):2453–2462
45. Wang L, Guo D-C, Cao J, Gong L, Kamm KE, Regalado E et al (2010) Mutations in myosin light chain kinase cause familial aortic dissections. Am J Hum Genet Am Soc Hum Genet 87(5):701–707
46. Humphrey JD, Milewicz DM, Tellides G, Schwartz MA (2014) Cell biology. Dysfunctional mechanosensing in aneurysms. Science 344(6183):477–479
47. Schnitker M, Bayer C (1944) Dissecting aneurysm of the aorta in young individuals, particularly in association with pregnancy: with report of a case. Ann Intern Med 20:486–511
48. Thalmann M, Sodeck GH, Domanovits H, Grassberger M, Loewe C, Grimm M et al (2011) Acute type A aortic dissection and pregnancy: a population-based study. Eur J Cardiothorac Surg [Internet] Eur Assoc Cardio-Thorac Surg 39(6):e159–e163
49. Nasiell J, Lindqvist PG (2010) Aortic dissection in pregnancy: the incidence of a life-threatening disease. Eur J Obstet Gynecol Reprod Biol 149(1):120–121
50. Wilkinson H, Trustees and Medical Advisers (2011) Saving mothers' lives. Reviewing maternal deaths to make motherhood safer: 2006–2008. BJOG: Int J Obstet Gynecol 118(11):1402–1403; discussion1403–1404
51. Rajagopalan S, Nwazota N, Chandrasekhar S (2014) Outcomes in pregnant women with acute aortic dissections: a review of the literature from 2003 to 2013. Int J Obstet Anesth 23(4):348–356
52. Huisman CM, Zwart JJ, Roos-Hesselink JW, Duvekot JJ, van Roosmalen J (2013) Incidence and predictors of maternal cardiovascular mortality and severe morbidity in The Netherlands: a prospective cohort study. PLoS One 8(2):e56494
53. Bouvier-Colle M-H, Deneux-Tharaux C, del Carmen Saucedo M (2013) Les Morts Maternelles en France. Mieux comprendre pour mieux prévenir. www.inserm.fr, p 1–120
54. Oskoui R, Lindsay J (1994) Aortic dissection in women. AJC 73(11):821–823
55. European Society of Gynecology (ESG), Association for European Paediatric Cardiology (AEPC), German Society for Gender Medicine (DGesGM), Regitz-Zagrosek V, Blomstrom

Lundqvist C, Borghi C et al (2011) ESC guidelines on the management of cardiovascular diseases during pregnancy: the Task Force on the Management of Cardiovascular Diseases during Pregnancy of the European Society of Cardiology (ESC). Eur Heart J 32:3147–3197
56. Sanghavi M, Rutherford JD (2014) Cardiovascular physiology of pregnancy. Circulation 130(12):1003–1008
57. Regitz-Zagrosek V, Gohlke-Bärwolf C, Iung B, Pieper PG (2014) Management of cardiovascular diseases during pregnancy. Curr Probl Cardiol 39(4–5):85–151
58. Pyeritz RE (2014) Heritable thoracic aortic disorders. Curr Opin Cardiol 29(1):97–102
59. De Backer J, Loeys B, Leroy B, Coucke P, DIETZ H, de Paepe A (2007) Utility of molecular analyses in the exploration of extreme intrafamilial variability in the Marfan syndrome. Clin Genet 72(3):188–198
60. Jondeau G, Detaint D, Tubach F, Arnoult F, Milleron O, Raoux F et al (2012) Aortic event rate in the Marfan population: a cohort study. Circulation 125(2):226–232
61. de Backer JF, Devos D, Segers P, Matthys D, François K, Gillebert TC et al (2006) Primary impairment of left ventricular function in Marfan syndrome. Int J Cardiol [Internet] 112(3):353–358
62. Alpendurada F, Wong J, Kiotsekoglou A, Banya W, Child A, Prasad SK et al (2010) Evidence for Marfan cardiomyopathy. Eur J Heart Fail 12(10):1085–1091
63. Kiotsekoglou A, Bajpai A, Bijnens BH, Kapetanakis V, Athanassopoulos G, Moggridge JC et al (2008) Early impairment of left ventricular long-axis systolic function demonstrated by reduced atrioventricular plane displacement in patients with Marfan syndrome. Eur J Echocardiogr 9(5):605–613
64. Rybczynski M, Mir TS, Sheikhzadeh S, Bernhardt AMJ, Schad C, Treede H et al (2010) Frequency and age-related course of mitral valve dysfunction in the Marfan syndrome. AJC [Internet] Elsevier Inc 106(7):1048–1053
65. Hoffmann BA, Rybczynski M, Rostock T, Servatius H, Drewitz I, Steven D et al (2012) Prospective risk stratification of sudden cardiac death in Marfan's syndrome. Int J Cardiol [Internet]. Elsevier Ireland Ltd, p 1–7. Available from: http://eutils.ncbi.nlm.nih.gov/entrez/eutils/elink.fcgi?dbfrom=pubmed&id=22738784&retmode=ref&cmd=prlinks
66. Pyeritz RE (1981) Maternal and fetal complications of pregnancy in the Marfan syndrome. Am J Med 71(5):784–790
67. Elkayam U, Ostrzega E, Shotan A, Mehra A (1995) Cardiovascular problems in pregnant women with the Marfan syndrome. Ann Intern Med 123(2):117–122
68. Goland S, Elkayam U (2009) Cardiovascular problems in pregnant women with Marfan syndrome. Circulation 119(4):619–623
69. Lalchandani S, Wingfield M (2003) Pregnancy in women with Marfan's syndrome. Eur J Obstet Gynecol 110(2):125–130
70. Lind J, Wallenburg HC (2001) The Marfan syndrome and pregnancy: a retrospective study in a Dutch population. Eur J Obstet Gynecol 98(1):28–35
71. Pacini L, Digne F, Boumendil A, Muti C, Detaint D, Boileau C et al (2009) Maternal complication of pregnancy in Marfan syndrome. Int J Cardiol 136(2):156–161
72. Donnelly RT, Pinto NM, Kocolas I, Yetman AT (2012) The immediate and long-term impact of pregnancy on aortic growth rate and mortality in women with Marfan syndrome. JAC Elsevier Inc 60(3):224–229
73. Mulder BJM, Meijboom LJ (2012) Pregnancy and Marfan syndrome. JAC Elsevier Inc 60(3):230–231
74. Meijboom LJ (2005) Pregnancy and aortic root growth in the Marfan syndrome: a prospective study. Eur Heart J 26(9):914–920
75. Rossiter JP, Repke JT, Morales AJ, Murphy EA, Pyeritz RE (1995) A prospective longitudinal evaluation of pregnancy in the Marfan syndrome. Am J Obstet Gynecol 173(5):1599–1606
76. Omnes S, Jondeau G, Detaint D, Dumont A, Yazbeck C, Guglielminotti J et al (2013) Pregnancy outcomes among women with Marfan syndrome Int J Gynecol Obstet 122(3):219–223

77. Hassan N, Patenaude V, Oddy L, Abenhaim HA (2015) Pregnancy outcomes in Marfan syndrome: a retrospective study. Am J Perinatol 30(2):123–302
78. Attias D, Stheneur C, Roy C, Collod-Beroud G, Detaint D, Faivre L et al (2009) Comparison of clinical presentations and outcomes between patients with TGFBR2 and FBN1 mutations in Marfan syndrome and related disorders. Circulation 120(25):2541–2549
79. Ong K-T, Perdu J, De Backer J, Bozec E, Collignon P, Emmerich J et al (2010) Effect of celiprolol on prevention of cardiovascular events in vascular Ehlers-Danlos syndrome: a prospective randomised, open, blinded-endpoints trial. Lancet 376(9751):1476–1484
80. Lurie S, Manor M, Hagay ZJ (1998) The threat of type IV Ehlers-Danlos syndrome on maternal well-being during pregnancy: early delivery may make the difference. J Obstet Gynaecol 18(3):245–248
81. Rudd NL, Nimrod C, Holbrook KA, Byers PH (1983) Pregnancy complications in type IV Ehlers-Danlos syndrome. Lancet 1(8314–5):50–53
82. Murray ML, Pepin M, Peterson S, Byers PH (2014) Pregnancy-related deaths and complications in women with vascular Ehlers-Danlos syndrome. Genet Med 16(12):874–880
83. Lind J, Wallenburg HCS (2002) Pregnancy and the Ehlers-Danlos syndrome: a retrospective study in a Dutch population. Acta Obstet Gynecol Scand 81(4):293–300
84. Regalado ES, Guo D-C, Estrera AL, Buja LM, Milewicz DM (2013) Acute aortic dissections with pregnancy in women with ACTA2 mutations. Am J Med Genet A. Nov 15
85. Mortensen KH, Andersen NH, Gravholt CH (2012) Cardiovascular phenotype in Turner syndrome – integrating cardiology, genetics, and endocrinology. Endocr Rev 33(5):677–714
86. Sachdev V, Matura LA, Sidenko S, Ho VB, Arai AE, Rosing DR et al (2008) Aortic valve disease in Turner syndrome. J Am Coll Cardiol 51(19):1904–1909
87. Mortensen KH, Hjerrild BE, Stochholm K, Andersen NH, Sørensen KE, Lundorf E et al (2011) Dilation of the ascending aorta in Turner syndrome – a prospective cardiovascular magnetic resonance study. J Cardiovasc Magn Reson 13:24
88. Matura LA, Ho VB, Rosing DR, Bondy CA (2007) Aortic dilatation and dissection in Turner syndrome. Circulation 116(15):1663–1670
89. Gravholt CH, Landin-Wilhelmsen K, Stochholm K, Hjerrild BE, Ledet T, Djurhuus CB et al (2006) Clinical and epidemiological description of aortic dissection in Turner's syndrome. Cardiol Young 16(5):430–436
90. Carlson M, Silberbach M (2007) Dissection of the aorta in Turner syndrome: two cases and review of 85 cases in the literature. J Med Genet 44(12):745–749
91. Practice Committee of American Society For Reproductive Medicine (2012) Increased maternal cardiovascular mortality associated with pregnancy in women with Turner syndrome. Fertil Steril 97(2):282–284
92. Tarani L, Lampariello S, Raguso G, Colloridi F, Pucarelli I, Pasquino AM et al (1998) Pregnancy in patients with Turner's syndrome: six new cases and review of literature. Gynecol Endocrinol 12(2):83–87
93. Birkebaek NH, Cruger D, Hansen J, Nielsen J, Bruun-Petersen G (2002) Fertility and pregnancy outcome in Danish women with Turner syndrome. Clin Genet 61(1):35–39
94. Chevalier N, Letur H, Lelannou D, Ohl J, Cornet D, Chalas-Boissonnas C et al (2011) Materno-fetal cardiovascular complications in Turner syndrome after oocyte donation: insufficient prepregnancy screening and pregnancy follow-up are associated with poor outcome. J Clin Endocrinol Metab 96(2):E260–E267
95. Hagman A, Källén K, Bryman I, Landin-Wilhelmsen K, Barrenäs M-L, Wennerholm U-B (2013) Morbidity and mortality after childbirth in women with Turner karyotype. Hum Reprod 28(7):1961–1973
96. Hagman A, Loft A, Wennerholm U-B, Pinborg A, Bergh C, Aittomäki K et al (2013) Obstetric and neonatal outcome after oocyte donation in 106 women with Turner syndrome: a Nordic cohort study. Hum Reprod 28(6):1598–1609
97. van Hagen IM, Roos-Hesselink JW (2014) Aorta pathology and pregnancy. Best Pract Res Clin Obstet Gynaecol 28:537

98. Habashi JP, Judge DP, Holm TM, Cohn RD, Loeys BL, Cooper TK et al (2006) Losartan, an AT1 antagonist, prevents aortic aneurysm in a mouse model of Marfan syndrome. Science 312(5770):117–121
99. Forteza A, Evangelista A, Sánchez V, Teixido-Tura G, Sanz P, Gutiérrez L et al (2015) Efficacy of losartan vs. atenolol for the prevention of aortic dilation in Marfan syndrome: a randomized clinical trial. Eur Heart J. Oct 29
100. Lacro RV, Dietz HC, Sleeper LA, Yetman AT, Bradley TJ, Colan SD et al (2014) Atenolol versus losartan in children and young adults with Marfan's syndrome. N Engl J Med 371(22):2061–2071
101. Milleron O, Arnoult F, Ropers J, Aegerter P, Detaint D, Delorme G et al (2015) Marfan Sartan: a randomized, double-blind, placebo-controlled trial. Eur Heart J. May 2
102. Magee LA, Duley L (2000) Oral beta-blockers for mild to moderate hypertension during pregnancy. Cochrane Database Syst Rev (4):CD002863
103. Ruys TPE, Maggioni A, Johnson MR, Sliwa K, Tavazzi L, Schwerzmann M et al (2014) Cardiac medication during pregnancy, data from the ROPAC. Int J Cardiol 177(1):124–128
104. Kofahl B, Henke D, Hettenbach A, Mutschler E (1993) Studies on placental transfer of celiprolol. Eur J Clin Pharmacol 44(4):381–382, Springer
105. Gott VL, Greene PS, Alejo DE, Cameron DE, Naftel DC, Miller DC et al (1999) Replacement of the aortic root in patients with Marfan's syndrome. N Engl J Med 340(17):1307–1313
106. John AS, Gurley F, Schaff HV, Warnes CA, Phillips SD, Arendt KW et al (2011) Cardiopulmonary bypass during pregnancy. Ann Thorac Surg 91(4):1191–1196
107. Yates MT, Soppa G, Smelt J, Fletcher N, van Besouw J-P, Thilaganathan B et al (2015) Perioperative management and outcomes of aortic surgery during pregnancy. J Thorac Cardiovasc Surg 149(2):607–610
108. Chambers CE, Clark SL (1994) Cardiac surgery during pregnancy. Clin Obstet Gynecol 37(2):316–323
109. Gordon CF, Johnson MD (1993) Anesthetic management of the pregnant patient with Marfan syndrome. J Clin Anesth 5(3):248–251
110. Ruys TPE, Cornette J, Roos-Hesselink JW (2013) Pregnancy and delivery in cardiac disease. J Cardiol 61(2):107–112
111. Simpson LL, Athanassious AM, D'Alton ME (1997) Marfan syndrome in pregnancy. Curr Opin Obstet Gynecol 9(5):337–341
112. Allyn J, Guglielminotti J, Omnes S, Guezouli L, Egan M, Jondeau G et al (2013) Marfan's syndrome during pregnancy: anesthetic management of delivery in 16 consecutive patients. Anesth Analg 116(2):392–398
113. Meijboom LJ, Drenthen W, Pieper PG, Groenink M, van der Post JAM, Timmermans J et al (2006) Obstetric complications in Marfan syndrome. Int J Cardiol 110(1):53–59
114. Lipscomb KJ, Smith JC, Clarke B, Donnai P, Harris R (1997) Outcome of pregnancy in women with Marfan's syndrome. Br J Obstet Gynaecol 104(2):201–206
115. von Dadelszen P, Ornstein MP, Bull SB, Logan AG, Koren G, Magee LA (2000) Fall in mean arterial pressure and fetal growth restriction in pregnancy hypertension: a meta-analysis. Lancet 355(9198):87–92
116. Hunter S, Robson SC (1992) Adaptation of the maternal heart in pregnancy. Heart 68(6):540–543
117. Robson SC, Dunlop W, Hunter S (1987) Haemodynamic changes during the early puerperium. Br Med J (Clin Res Ed) 294(6579):1065
118. Roos-Hesselink JW, Ruys PTE, Johnson MR (2013) Pregnancy in adult congenital heart disease. Curr Cardiol Rep 15(9):401
119. Natoli AK, Medley TL, Ahimastos AA, Drew BG, Thearle DJ, Dilley RJ et al (2005) Sex steroids modulate human aortic smooth muscle cell matrix protein deposition and matrix metalloproteinase expression. Hypertension 46(5):1129–1134

120. Robb AO, Mills NL, Din JN, Smith IBJ, Paterson F, Newby DE et al (2009) Influence of the menstrual cycle, pregnancy, and preeclampsia on arterial stiffness. Hypertension 53(6):952–958
121. Ulusoy RE, Demiralp E, Kirilmaz A, Kilicaslan F, Ozmen N, Kucukarslan N et al (2006) Aortic elastic properties in young pregnant women. Heart Vessels 21(1):38–41
122. Easterling TR, Benedetti TJ, Schmucker BC, Carlson K, Millard SP (1991) Maternal hemodynamics and aortic diameter in normal and hypertensive pregnancies. Obstet Gynecol 78(6):1073–1077
123. Cabanes L, Chalas C, Christin-Maitre S, Donadille B, Felten ML, Gaxotte V et al (2010) Turner syndrome and pregnancy: clinical practice. Recommendations for the management of patients with Turner syndrome before and during pregnancy. Eur J Obstet Gynecol Reprod Biol 152(1):18–24
124. Boodhwani M, Andelfinger G, Leipsic J, Lindsay T, McMurtry MS, Therrien J et al (2014) Canadian Cardiovascular Society position statement on the management of thoracic aortic disease. Can J Cardiol 30:577–589
125. Coron F, Rousseau T, Jondeau G, Gautier E, Binquet C, Gouya L et al (2012) What do French patients and geneticists think about prenatal and preimplantation diagnoses in Marfan syndrome? Prenat Diagn 32(13):1318–1323

Aortic Coarctation

13

Margarita Brida and Gerhard-Paul Diller

Abbreviations

ACE   Angiotensin-converting enzyme
MRI   Magnetic resonance imaging
WHO   World Health Organization

> **Key Facts**
> Incidence: 5–8 % of all congenital heart defects.
> Inheritance: Multifactorial, overall 3 % risk.
> Medication: ACE and AT1-antagonists replaced with α-methyldopa and beta-blockers.
> World Health Organization class: Repaired coarctation, WHO II–III; severe native coarctation, WHO IV.
> Risk of pregnancy: Hypertension occurs in 30 %. Pregnancy increases risk of aortic complications.
> Life expectancy: Reduced in native severe coarctation and nearly normal in well repaired.

M. Brida, MD, PhD
Department of Cardiovascular Disease, University of Zagreb School of Medicine, University Hospital Centre, Zagreb, Croatia

Division of Adult Congenital and Valvular Disease, University Hospital Muenster, Münster, Germany

G.-P. Diller, MD, PhD (✉)
Department of Cardiovascular Disease, Division of Adult Congenital and Valvular Disease, University Hospital, Münster, Germany

Imperial College London, London, UK
e-mail: Gerhard.Diller@ukmuenster.de

> **Key Management**
> Preconception: Imaging (CT or cMR) to assess aortic structure and ECG, echo and exercise test for ventricular function
> Pregnancy: Normal aorta – 20 weeks with echo only. Abnormal: four to eight weekly depending on the degree of abnormality. Aggressive treatment of hypertension
> Labour: Vaginal delivery, with an effective epidural. Caesarean section with aortic dilatation of >45 mm
> Postpartum: Maintenance of effective antihypertensive therapy and re-image if structurally abnormal aorta prior to discharge

13.1 The Condition

Due to the greater availability of corrective surgery, we are seeing more pregnancies in women with a repaired aortic coarctation (CoA). Those with a good repair are generally low risk, but occasionally, we see pregnant women with an unrecognised and therefore unrepaired "native" CoA; these women have a much higher risk during pregnancy. CoA is a complex cardiovascular disorder, involving not only a circumscribed narrowing of the aorta but also a generalised arteriopathy. The narrowing is typically located in the area of insertion of the ductus arteriosus, just below the origin of left subclavian artery, and only in rare cases occurs in other parts of the aorta. CoA is the fifth most common congenital heart defect and accounts for 5–8 % of all congenital heart defects. There is a male predominance, with a male to female ratio of up to 2:1. CoA is often accompanied by other cardiac lesions, most commonly a bicuspid aortic valve (up to 85 %), mitral valve abnormalities, ventricular septal defects and may be part of a syndrome (Turner, Williams-Beuren or Noonan syndromes [1–3]).

Patients with significant CoA exhibit signs early in life, while those remaining undiagnosed until adulthood typically have milder forms and are often asymptomatic. These patients may remain asymptomatic for a long time and sometimes present for the first time in pregnancy [4, 5]. The classic presenting sign in adult patients with CoA is arterial hypertension. Symptoms, if present, arise from arterial hypertension proximal to the obstruction, in the upper body, and from hypotension distal to the obstruction, in the abdomen and legs. Key symptoms are headache, tinnitus, nosebleeds, dizziness, abdominal angina, cold feet, exertional leg fatigue or claudication.

13.1.1 Native Coarctation

Occasionally, the diagnosis of CoA is made during pregnancy when previously unknown hypertension is discovered. Arterial hypertension, especially systolic, should alert medical practitioners to the possibility of CoA. Other key clinical findings are isolated hypertension in the upper extremities, delayed and weak femoral pulses, and palpable collateral arteries or a systolic murmur. In many cases, a diagnosis can be made with these findings. In everyday clinical practice, it is important to measure blood pressure in both arms and to assess peripheral pulses in all four limbs.

Key findings on examination in CoA include:

- A higher systolic blood pressure in the right arm compared with the right leg, but similar diastolic blood pressure levels. Differences in pressures, however, depend not only on the severity of the coarctation but also on the presence and the flow through collaterals as well as on the cardiac output.
- Pulses are delayed and less intense over the right femoral artery compared with the right radial or brachial artery. Also, the right and left brachial artery pulsations should be compared to determine if the coarctation is proximal (decreased or absent left brachial pulsation), distal (no difference in brachial pulsations) or distal with anomalous right subclavian artery after the coarctation (decreased or absent right brachial pulsation) [15, 16].
- Ankle-brachial pressure index will show significantly lower systolic pressures in legs when compared to the arms.
- Palpable collaterals may develop from subclavian, axillary, internal thoracic, scapular and intercostal arteries and can occasionally be seen over the lateral chest wall.
- A systolic murmur, sometimes associated with a thrill, is often present along the left sternal border and the mid-back between the left scapula and spine. The murmur radiates to the neck. A delayed-onset, continuous crescendo-decrescendo murmur can also sometimes be heard over the back due to the enlargement of the collateral circulation. Moreover patient may have one additional murmur at the upper right sternal border if bicuspid aortic valve is present with components of stenosis or insufficiency [17].

Continuous wave Doppler echocardiography from a standard suprasternal position is generally used to confirm the diagnosis. The most characteristic echocardiographic sign of CoA is the presence of diastolic "runoff" phenomenon, in combination with high peak systolic velocity (Fig. 13.1). However, factors such as cross-sectional area, length of the narrowed segment, presence of collateral circulation, patent ductus arteriosus and cardiac output can influence the flow across the descending aorta. As a consequence, maximum and mean Doppler echocardiographic measurements are generally considered unreliable in determining the severity of CoA. These parameters can underestimate the severity of the obstruction if significant collateral vessels are present or alternatively overestimate the severity if there is increased aortic stiffness [18, 19]. Alternatively, magnetic resonance imaging (MRI) is a non-invasive technique which is safe in pregnancy and can be used to visualise the entire aorta (Fig. 13.2). It can assess (i) the anatomy of the aorta, particularly of the coarctation site (extent and degree of aortic narrowing), (ii) the

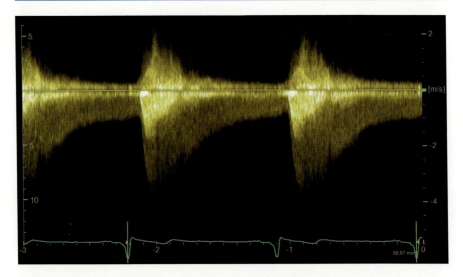

Fig. 13.1 Example of a diastolic runoff or tailing phenomenon (*arrow*) in a patient with severe aortic coarctation on transthoracic echocardiography from a standard suprasternal position

collateral circulation and, consequently, (iii) the hemodynamic impact of the CoA. However, the use of gadolinium in pregnancy is currently contraindicated. Computed tomography and cardiac catheterization are also generally avoided during pregnancy due to radiation exposition.

13.2 Pregnancy Outcomes

Major complications during pregnancy are uncommon in the context of an uncorrected CoA, but can be fatal. Haemodynamic changes, hormonal alterations and hypertension affect the aortic wall during pregnancy and increase the risk of aortic rupture or dissection at the site of the narrowing or in the ascending aorta in patients with coexisting bicuspid aortic valves. Maternal and neonatal mortalities are reported to be 0–9% and 8–19%, respectively in previous series [20, 21].

13.2.1 Repaired Coarctation

While in the past patients who had undergone coarctation repair were considered to be cured, it is now recognised that even a well-repaired CoA is frequently associated with premature morbidity and mortality. Surprisingly, despite improvements in repair techniques, better medical management of hypertension, comorbidity surveillance for cardiovascular disease and monitoring for aortic complications, this seems to have had a limited impact on late mortality. In early studies, reporting in 1989, survival at 30 years was 72%; a more recent study by Brown et al. reporting

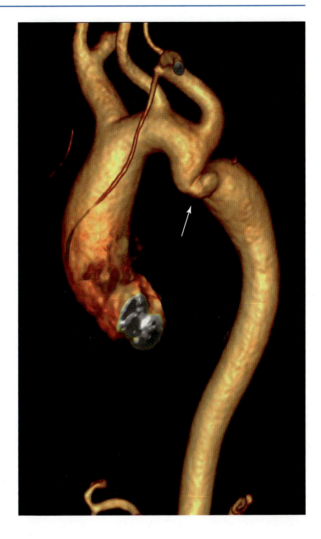

Fig. 13.2 Magnetic resonance imaging of severe aortic coarctation (*arrow*)

in 2013 showed an almost identical survival of 74 % during long-term follow-up [27, 28]. Older age at the time of the initial repair (>20 years) has been associated with decreased survival, but patients younger than 5 years at the time of the initial operation had the greatest risk of reoperation, while patients older than 9 years had a greater prevalence of residual hypertension [28]. As a consequence, lifelong follow-up care after CoA treatment is required, ideally on an annual basis. Patients with a repaired CoA do not have impaired fertility. The largest study to date on the outcome of pregnancy after repair of aortic coarctation showed that, overall, maternal and neonatal outcome of pregnancy is excellent and without major cardiovascular complications. On the other hand, the rate of miscarriage and preeclampsia was higher than experienced by the general population [29]. Women planning a family should be thoroughly investigated before conception to exclude late problems including systemic hypertension, residual coarctation and re-coarctation and aortic aneurysm formation. Also the physician should investigate for potential clinical signs of premature coronary and cerebrovascular disease [30].

13.3 Management

When CoA is first diagnosed, the choice of treatment depends on the haemodynamic impact of the coarctation, the patient's symptoms, the degree of upper limb arterial hypertension, the gestational age and the potential for fetal compromise due to restricted uteroplacental perfusion. If there is only mild to moderate obstruction and without signs of hypertension, no treatment is generally necessary. Regular blood pressure monitoring is, however, indicated throughout pregnancy. Beta-blocker therapy should be initiated if the blood pressure is abnormal (e.g. above 130/90 mmHg before 20 weeks of gestation). It is important to maintain a good balance between blood pressure control (vital for maternal wellbeing) and adequate fetal perfusion and growth [22]. In the case of severe coarctation, treatment is challenging. Women who are in an early stage of pregnancy should be consulted about the risks of further continuation of pregnancy and the availability of options such as elective abortion. If blood pressure can be controlled with medication, it is generally recommended to carry the pregnancy to term and aim for repair of the coarctation after delivery [21, 22]. The biggest concern is that hypertension is refractory to drug therapy and is accompanied by underperfusion of the placenta. If the blood pressure cannot be adequately controlled by medication, intervention is recommended. Both surgery and stent placement with the fetus in situ can be considered, and a multidisciplinary team should make the decision. In the current ESC guidelines for the management of grown-up CHD, stenting has become the treatment of first choice in adults and is adopted in many centres for native CoA with appropriate anatomy. However there are limited data on CoA stenting in pregnancy [24, 25]. Potentially teratogen exposure to radiation can be limited by performing the procedure with the use of minimum radiation necessary and after the second trimester. Moreover, an abdominal lead shielding can be used. Aneurysm formation and a higher rate of reinterventions are associated with angioplasty, especially after ballooning in comparison to stenting [23, 24]. Surgery, on the other hand, seems to be associated with increased fetal mortality, higher risk of dissection or aortic rupture when compared to the non-pregnant state [46].

13.3.1 Systemic Hypertension

Hypertension is seen in more than 30% of cases after CoA repair in early childhood and in the absence of restenosis [31]. In general, pregnancy is tolerated well by mother and fetus as long as hypertension is well controlled. Ambulatory blood pressure monitoring (in the right arm) and exercise testing should be performed before pregnancy, and regular blood pressure monitoring is important throughout pregnancy due to the risk of pregnancy-induced hypertension. It is crucial to treat persistent resting hypertension and it appears reasonable to treat women normotensive at rest, but whose systolic blood pressure exceeds 200 mmHg at low levels of exercise on treadmill testing, especially in pregnancy. This is because pregnancy – with its increase in blood volume and cardiac output – can be regarded as a state of mild to moderate exercise [32, 33]. Women with unrecognised and untreated hypertension are at risk of developing superimposed preeclampsia with fetal growth restriction, placental abruption, congestive heart failure and acute renal failure [34], all of which may require preterm delivery. In every day clinical practice, blood pressure should be measured in both arms. If the left subclavian artery has been used as a part of the initial repair, then the left arm blood pressure may be falsely low. Blood pressure monitoring should be placed on the right arm [15]. Antihypertensive treatment in pregnancy generally consists of beta-blocker therapy while angiotensin-converting enzyme (ACE) inhibitors and angiotensin-receptor blockers are contraindicated [35].

13.3.2 Residual Coarctation and Re-coarctation

Residual coarctation and re-coarctation can be seen after all known surgical techniques (end-to-end anastomosis, prosthetic patch aortoplasty, subclavian flap aortoplasty) with the various incidence rates from 5 to 24 % [36–39]. In re-coarctation gradients are usually small and pregnancy is well tolerated. Sometimes it can be difficult to distinguish between restenosis and enhanced aortic stiffness. In this setting analysing diastolic flow patterns at the isthmus and verifying high flow during diastole, reflecting diastolic runoff, is the most important echocardiographic sign of restenosis. Further, women who have a residual coarctation or re-coarctation are at increased risk of developing systemic hypertension. On the other hand, if re-coarctation is significant, blood pressure in the lower part of the body can be reduced and endanger the fetus. Regular monitoring of mothers' blood pressure and fetal growth is mandatory. Depending on the severity, re-coarctation should be managed in the same as native coarctation [20, 32].

13.3.3 Aortic Aneurysm Formation

Late aneurysm formation has been reported after all types of CoA repair, but it occurs most frequently after Dacron patch repair [27, 40]. Dacron patch aortoplasty gained popularity in the mid-1960s because of its excellent haemodynamic result and because it avoided sacrifice of intercostal arteries and minimised restenosis. Due to the high incidence of late aneurysm formation, this technique has been abandoned. Nevertheless, we continue to see adult women of child-bearing age after these procedures highlighting the need to obtain information about previous operation techniques in other to evaluate potential risk factors before pregnancy [41, 42]. Furthermore, late aneurysm formation in the ascending aorta, proximal to the surgical repair site, has also been noted as a late complication [43]. Aneurysm formation can lead to aortic rupture and sudden death. Pregnancy appears to increase the risk of aneurysm rupture. This might be due to hemodynamic, hormonal and vascular changes [44]. The treatment decision depends on various factors, including the size of the aneurysm, gestational age and type of procedure. Current ESC Guidelines on the management of cardiovascular diseases during pregnancy state that depending of the aortic diameter, patients should be monitored by echocardiography every 4–12 weeks while maintaining strict blood pressure control. Prepregnancy surgical treatment is recommended when the ascending aorta is ≥45 mm. During pregnancy prophylactic surgery should be considered if the aortic diameter is ≥50 mm and increasing rapidly. When progressive dilatation occurs during pregnancy, before the fetus is viable, aortic repair with the fetus in utero can be considered. When the fetus is viable, caesarean delivery followed directly by aortic surgery is recommended [45]. Caesarean delivery should be considered when the aortic diameter exceeds 45 mm. A cardiac operation with cardiopulmonary bypass of a gravid patient still remains a high-risk procedure, especially for the fetus. Maternal mortality is similar to that of non-pregnant women but fetal mortality is 16–33% [46]. In the modern era, endovascular repair with stent graft could be a therapeutic alternative (minimally invasive approach) in pregnant patients with late thoracic aortic aneurysms after surgical repair of aortic coarctation [47–49]. However, to our knowledge, there are no literature reports of endovascular stent grafting for aneurysms in patients during pregnancy.

13.3.4 Timing and Mode of Delivery

Early discussion with the cardiologist, obstetrician and anaesthetist will facilitate optimal planning for the management of pregnancy and delivery. It appears that vaginal delivery with an effective epidural is the preferred method. It causes fewer and less dramatic changes in haemodynamic parameters and is associated with lower risk of maternal complications such as haemorrhage, infection and thrombosis. Vaginal delivery has also shown neonatal benefits in terms of a later delivery and greater birth weight [26]. During delivery, indication for antibiotic prophylaxis is controversial. We do not generally advocate antibiotic prophylaxis at the time of delivery. However, the only two cases of maternal death with coarctation and pregnancy in the UK mortality statistics from 1997 to 1999 were associated with endocarditis [22].

13.3.5 Postnatal Period

In the puerperium other antihypertensive drugs, contraindicated during pregnancy, can be considered. Caution is advised with beta-blocker therapy in mothers who are breastfeeding since they can cause neonatal bradycardia and the excretion of particular beta-blockers should be discussed with the obstetricians. In patients with severe aortic coarctation, repair should be planned early after delivery to avoid unnecessary complications.

13.4 The Effect of Pregnancy Adaptations

During normal pregnancy, women experience profound hemodynamic, hormonal and vascular changes. The first change is a profound fall in the peripheral vascular resistance [8], which results in a gradual increase in plasma volume of almost 50 % [6], heart rate by up to 20 % and cardiac output by 30–60 % [7]. During natural labour, there is a further increase in cardiac output due to increases in both stroke volume and heart rate and the phenomenon of autotransfusion during contractions, whereby blood is returned to the systemic circulation from the uterus during contractions [9]. The aorta itself also changes during normal human pregnancy, possibly induced by the marked changes in maternal hemodynamic parameters and the influence of local hormonal factors, particularly oestrogens, since the aortic wall contains oestrogen receptors [10]. Structurally, there is a reduction in mucopolysaccharides, multiplication and hypertrophy of smooth muscle cells and elastic fibre changes in the aortic wall [11]. The aortic diameter increases by approximately 5 % and the aorta becomes more compliant [12]. In pregnancy, these normal adaptive changes could increase the risk of aortic complications in patient with pre-existing arteriopathy [13, 14].

13.5 Preconception Counselling

Unrepaired, severe CoA is a high risk and considered to be World Health Organization class IV. This indicates that there is an extremely high risk of maternal mortality or morbidity and that pregnancy is generally contraindicated. Women found to have severe CoA during pregnancy should be seen by an experienced multidisciplinary team for counselling. If they decide to continue with the pregnancy, they should be intensively monitored throughout pregnancy, childbirth and the puerperium [45].

13.5.1 Risk of Recurrence of Congenital Heart Disease

An approximately 3 % incidence of congenital heart disease in the offspring has been reported, and fetal echocardiography at 20 weeks gestation should be considered in women with known CoA [50].

References

1. Baumgartner H et al (2010) ESC Guidelines for the management of grown-up congenital heart disease (new version 2010). Eur Heart J 31:2915–2957
2. Gatzoulis M, Webb G, Daubeney P (2011) Diagnosis and management of adult congenital heart disease. Diagn Manag Adult Congenit Heart Dis 261–270
3. Teo LLS, Cannell T, Babu-Narayan SV, Hughes M, Mohiaddin RH (2011) Prevalence of associated cardiovascular abnormalities in 500 patients with aortic coarctation referred for cardiovascular magnetic resonance imaging to a tertiary center. Pediatr Cardiol 32:1120–1127

4. Campbell M (1970) Natural history of coarctation of the aorta. Br Heart J 32:633–640
5. Kenny D, Hijazi ZM (2011) Coarctation of the aorta: from fetal life to adulthood. Cardiol J 18:487–495
6. Hytten F (1985) Blood volume changes in normal pregnancy. Clin Haematol 14:601–612
7. Robson SC, Hunter S, Boys RJ, Dunlop W (1989) Serial study of factors influencing changes in cardiac output during human pregnancy. Am J Physiol 256:H1060–H1065
8. Mashini IS et al (1987) Serial noninvasive evaluation of cardiovascular hemodynamics during pregnancy. Am J Obstet Gynecol 156:1208–1213
9. Robson SC, Dunlop W, Boys RJ, Hunter S (1987) Cardiac output during labour. Br Med J (Clin Res Ed) 295(1169–72)
10. Campisi D et al (1993) Evidence for soluble and nuclear site I binding of estrogens in human aorta. Atherosclerosis 103:267–277
11. Curry RA et al (2014) Marfan syndrome and pregnancy: maternal and neonatal outcomes. BJOG 121:610–617
12. Easterling TR, Benedetti TJ, Schmucker BC, Carlson K, Millard SP (1991) Maternal hemodynamics and aortic diameter in normal and hypertensive pregnancies. Obstet Gynecol 78:1073–1077
13. Steer PJ, Gatzoulis MA, Baker P (2006) Heart disease and pregnancy. At: https://books.google.de/books/about/Heart_Disease_and_Pregnancy.html?id=SHbUP_FW0EoC&pgis=1
14. Karas RH, Patterson BL, Mendelsohn ME (1994) Human vascular smooth muscle cells contain functional estrogen receptor. Circulation 89:1943–1950
15. Brickner ME, Hillis LD, Lange RA (2000) Congenital heart disease in adults. First of two parts. N Engl J Med 342:256–263
16. Prisant LM, Mawulawde K, Kapoor D, Joe C (2004) Coarctation of the aorta: a secondary cause of hypertension. J Clin Hypertens (Greenwich) 6:347–350, 352
17. Therrien J, Webb G (2003) Clinical update on adults with congenital heart disease. Lancet (London, England) 362:1305–1313
18. EAE textbook of echocardiography – Oxford Medicine. At: http://oxfordmedicine.com/view/10.1093/med/9780199599639.001.0001/med-9780199599639
19. Carvalho JS, Redington AN, Shinebourne EA, Rigby ML, Gibson D (1990) Continuous wave Doppler echocardiography and coarctation of the aorta: gradients and flow patterns in the assessment of severity. Br Heart J 64:133–137
20. Beauchesne LM, Connolly HM, Ammash NM, Warnes CA (2001) Coarctation of the aorta: outcome of pregnancy. J Am Coll Cardiol 38:1728–1733
21. Ural AV, Caglar IM, Caglar FNT, Ciftci S, Karakaya O (2014) Single therapeutic catheterization for treatment of late diagnosed native coarctation of aorta using a covered stent. J Clin Diagn Res 8:153–155
22. Venning S, Freeman LJ, Stanley K (2003) Two cases of pregnancy with coarctation of the aorta. J R Soc Med 96:234–236
23. Rodés-Cabau J et al (2007) Comparison of surgical and transcatheter treatment for native coarctation of the aorta in patients ≥1 year old. The Quebec Native Coarctation of the Aorta study. Am Heart J 154:186–192
24. Assaidi A, Sbragia P, Fraisse A (2013) Transcatheter therapy for aortic coarctation with severe systemic hypertension during pregnancy. Catheter Cardiovasc Interv 82:556–559
25. Drenthen W et al (2007) Outcome of pregnancy in women with congenital heart disease: a literature review. J Am Coll Cardiol 49:2303–2311
26. Ruys TPE et al (2015) Is a planned caesarean section in women with cardiac disease beneficial? Heart 101:530–536
27. Cohen M, Fuster V, Steele PM, Driscoll D, McGoon DC (1989) Coarctation of the aorta. Long-term follow-up and prediction of outcome after surgical correction. Circulation 80:840–845
28. Brown ML et al (2013) Coarctation of the aorta: lifelong surveillance is mandatory following surgical repair. J Am Coll Cardiol 62:1020–1025
29. Vriend JWJ et al (2005) Outcome of pregnancy in patients after repair of aortic coarctation. Eur Heart J 26:2173–2178

30. Celermajer DS, Greaves K (2002) Survivors of coarctation repair: fixed but not cured. Heart 88:113–114
31. Canniffe C, Ou P, Walsh K, Bonnet D, Celermajer D (2013) Hypertension after repair of aortic coarctation – a systematic review. Int J Cardiol 167:2456–2461
32. Gatzoulis, MA, MD, PhD, Webb, GD, MD, Broberg, C, MD, Uemura H (2010) Cases in adult congenital heart disease
33. Kaemmerer H et al (1998) Arterial hypertension in adults after surgical treatment of aortic coarctation. Thorac Cardiovasc Surg 46:121–125
34. Roberts JM, Pearson GD, Cutler JA, Lindheimer MD (2003) Summary of the NHLBI Working Group on research on hypertension during pregnancy. Hypertens Pregnancy 22:109–127
35. Drugs in pregnancy and lactation. At: http://www.lww.com/Product/9781451190823
36. Jahangiri M et al (2000) Subclavian flap angioplasty: does the arch look after itself? J Thorac Cardiovasc Surg 120:224–229
37. Rao PS, Thapar MK, Galal O, Wilson AD (1990) Follow-up results of balloon angioplasty of native coarctation in neonates and infants. Am Heart J 120:1310–1314
38. Walhout RJ et al (2003) Comparison of polytetrafluoroethylene patch aortoplasty and end-to-end anastomosis for coarctation of the aorta. J Thorac Cardiovasc Surg 126:521–528
39. Corno AF et al (2001) Surgery for aortic coarctation: a 30 years experience. Eur J Cardiothorac Surg 20:1202–1206
40. Dykukha SE, Naumova LP, Antoshchenko AA, Pavlov PV (1997) Late postoperative complications of coarctation of aorta. Klin Khir. pp. 78–80
41. Vossschulte K (1957) Plastic surgery of the isthmus in aortic isthmus stenosis. Thoraxchirurgie 4:443–450
42. Bergdahl L, Ljungqvist A (1980) Long-term results after repair of coarctation of the aorta by patch grafting. J Thorac Cardiovasc Surg 80:177–181
43. Heikkinen LO, Ala-Kulju KV, Salo JA (1991) Dilatation of ascending aorta in patients with repaired coarctation. Scand J Thorac Cardiovasc Surg 25:25–28
44. Parks WJ et al (1995) Incidence of aneurysm formation after Dacron patch aortoplasty repair for coarctation of the aorta: long-term results and assessment utilizing magnetic resonance angiography with three-dimensional surface rendering. J Am Coll Cardiol 26:266–271
45. Regitz-Zagrosek V et al (2011) ESC guidelines on the management of cardiovascular diseases during pregnancy: the Task Force on the Management of Cardiovascular Diseases during Pregnancy of the European Society of Cardiology (ESC). Eur Heart J 32:3147–3197
46. Sutton SW et al (2005) Cardiopulmonary bypass and mitral valve replacement during pregnancy. Perfusion 20:359–368
47. Erbel R et al (2014) 2014 ESC guidelines on the diagnosis and treatment of aortic diseases: document covering acute and chronic aortic diseases of the thoracic and abdominal aorta of the adult. The Task Force for the Diagnosis and Treatment of Aortic Diseases of the European. Eur Heart J 35:2873–2926
48. Juszkat R et al (2013) Endovascular treatment of late thoracic aortic aneurysms after surgical repair of congenital aortic coarctation in childhood. PLoS One 8:e83601
49. Botta L et al (2009) Role of endovascular repair in the management of late pseudo-aneurysms following open surgery for aortic coarctation. Eur J Cardiothorac Surg 36:670–674
50. Saidi AS, Bezold LI, Altman CA, Ayres NA, Bricker JT (1998) Outcome of pregnancy following intervention for coarctation of the aorta. Am J Cardiol 82:786–788

Ebstein Anomaly

14

Andrea Girnius, Gruschen Veldtman, Carri R. Warshak, and Markus Schwerzmann

Abbreviations

EA	Ebstein anomaly
NSAIDs	Nonsteroidal anti-inflammatory drugs
PPH	Postpartum hemorrhage
ESC	European Society of Cardiology
PPROM	Preterm premature rupture of membranes

A. Girnius, MD, PhD
Department of Anesthesiology, University of Cincinnati, Cincinnati, USA

G. Veldtman, MD, PhD
Department of Adolescent and Adult Congenital Heart Disease, Cincinnati Children's Hospital Medical Center, University of Cincinnati, Cincinnati, USA

C.R. Warshak, MD, PhD
Department of Matero-Fetal Medicine, University of Cincinnati, Cincinnati, USA

M. Schwerzmann, MD (✉)
University Hospital Inselspital, Center for Congenital Heart Disease, University of Bern, Bern, Switzerland
e-mail: Markus.Schwerzmann@insel.ch

© Springer International Publishing Switzerland 2017
J.W. Roos-Hesselink, M.R. Johnson (eds.), *Pregnancy and Congenital Heart Disease*, Congenital Heart Disease in Adolescents and Adults,
DOI 10.1007/978-3-319-38913-4_14

> **Key Facts**
> *Incidence*: 1–5/20,000 live births.
> *Inheritance*: 6%, but occurs sporadically, related to maternal age and maternal exposure to benzodiazepines or lithium therapy.
> *Medication*: Change antiarrhythmic drugs; a beta-blocker as an alternative is the first choice.
> *World Health Organization class*: Class II or III.
> *Risk of pregnancy*: Atrial arrhythmias, heart failure, thromboembolic events (possibly paradoxical in the presence of a shunt).
> *Life expectancy*: Reduced.

> **Key Management**
> *Preconception*: ECG, echo, exercise test; consider cMR.
> *Pregnancy*: Careful detection of arrhythmias and cardiac failure; consider thromboprophylaxis.
> *Labor*: Vaginal delivery.
> *Postpartum*: Consider thromboprophylaxis.

14.1 The Condition

Ebstein anomaly (EA) of the tricuspid valve was first described by Wilhelm Ebstein in 1866 [1]. It has important hemodynamic implications, which impacts not only symptoms and longevity but may also have important implications during pregnancy. An understanding of the EA-related cardiac abnormalities and their hemodynamic consequences is necessary for prepregnancy counseling and adequate perinatal care.

14.1.1 Anatomy and Physiology of Ebstein Anomaly

EA of the tricuspid valve is a rare (1–5/20,000 live births) congenital malformation [2] characterized by a spectrum of myocardial malformations including varying degrees of:

1. Failure of delamination of the tricuspid valve resulting in tricuspid valve regurgitation and leaflet abnormalities (muscularization, perforations, and/or tricuspid valve stenosis). The echocardiographic hallmark of this malformation is an excessive downward displacement of the hinge point of the septal and posterior tricuspid leaflets (>8 mm/m^2 of body surface area) below the mitral annular plane (see Fig. 14.1) [1].

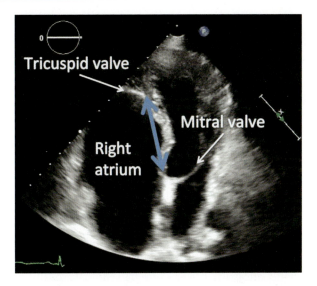

Fig. 14.1 Echo picture (four-chamber-view) of typical EA with apical displacement of the tricuspid valve

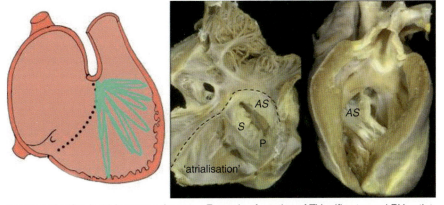

Rotation of orifice in 23 heart specimens   Example of rotation of TV orifice toward RV outlet

Fig. 14.2 Anatomical and schematic depiction of the tricuspid valve in EA. With the kind permission of Dr. Siew Yen Ho, Cardiac Morphologist, Royal Brompton and Harefield NHS Foundation Trust

2. Right atrial and functional right ventricular dilation increases as tricuspid regurgitation worsens. During childhood, already these chambers may be severely dilated giving rise to the term "wall-to-wall" heart.
3. Increasing degrees of anticlockwise rotation of the tricuspid valve (i.e., greater severity) annulus toward the right ventricular outflow with the fulcrum being the ventriculo-infundibular fold (see Fig. 14.2).
4. Right ventricular cardiomyopathy that includes myofibril loss and discontinuity and scarring of the right ventricular free wall, resulting in right ventricular dilation, thinning, and dysfunction.

5. Left ventricular cardiomyopathy, occurring in up to 18% [3]. This cardiomyopathy frequently resembles left ventricular non-compaction and occurs in combination with left heart structural abnormalities such as mitral valve prolapse and dysplasia, ventricular septal defect, and bicuspid aortic valve [4].
6. Atrial level shunt, ranging in size and degree as well as direction of shunt.
7. Bronchopulmonary segmental hypoplasia, particularly in more severe forms, and pulmonary vascular disease.
8. Altered and eventually diminished right atrial compliance, which dictates physiologic responses to tricuspid regurgitation and right ventricular dysfunction.

EA must be distinguished from other forms of congenital tricuspid regurgitation and/or right ventricular dilatation, such as an endocardial cushion defect, unguarded tricuspid valve, tricuspid valve prolapse, right ventricular dysplasia, or tricuspid valve dysplasia [5, 6].

The clinical presentation depends on the composite interaction of the above pathophysiologic perturbations. Up to half of all affected fetuses die in utero or shortly after birth because of right ventricular dysfunction, while other infants may need early surgery [7]. In milder forms, EA may not present until later life as symptoms may first occur in adult life, mainly due to arrhythmias [8]. Right bundle branch patterns due to infra-Hisian block are most often observed (up to 70%), and the extent of QRS duration correlates with the amount of right ventricular enlargement [9]. Other electrocardiographic and rhythm abnormalities include accessory atrioventricular or atriofascicular pathways (in 25%) of patients. These pathways are frequently right sided and multiple. Supraventricular tachyarrhythmias (atrioventricular reciprocating tachycardia, ectopic atrial tachycardia, and atrial fibrillation or flutter) are common and occur in 30–40% of adults with this anomaly [10].

14.1.1.1 Atrial Level Shunts in EA
Atrial shunting is present in up to 80–90% of EA patients [1]. The degree and nature of shunting depends on the relative compliances of the downstream respective ventricles. It plays various roles during the natural history of the disease. During early life, it may help to preserve cardiac output in the face of severe right heart disease. Eventually, it may become the mechanism for symptomatic cyanosis with exercise limitation and may be a vehicle for paradoxical embolism. As tricuspid regurgitation worsens, the right atrium enlarges, and the initial atrial septal defect or patent foramen ovale may be stretched providing a substrate for atrial level shunting. The decision to close the atrial shunt therefore needs to be taken with full appreciation of the potential hemodynamic impact [11, 12]. Atrial shunt closure can result in marked improvement in symptoms and volume unloading of the right ventricle especially in the presence of a predominant left-to-right shunt. In patients with right-to-left shunts, relief of cyanosis is very effective in improving symptoms.

14.1.1.2 Genetics
Most cases of EA occur sporadically [2]. Case-control studies have identified reproductive (e.g., maternal age) and environmental risk factors (e.g., maternal exposure

to benzodiazepines or lithium therapy) [1]. The genetic basis of isolated EA remains unknown. Studies show that EA is a genetically heterogeneous defect, with sporadic 1p36 and 8p23.1 chromosomal deletions being the most commonly associated imbalances in patients with syndromic EA [13]. Recent investigations have identified mutations in the gene MYH7, which encodes β-myosin heavy chain, in individuals with EA associated with left ventricular non-compaction [14].

14.1.1.3 Modified History

Medical therapy is used to relieve symptoms of right heart failure or to control arrhythmias, but a substantial proportion of patients will require tricuspid valve repair or replacement during their lifetime. The timing of surgical intervention depends on symptoms, exercise performance, heart size, the occurrence of arrhythmias, or the presence and consequences of interatrial shunting such as paradoxical embolism [15]. Usually, the exercise capacity of adults with EA is moderately impaired, comparable to the exercise capacity of adults with a systemic right ventricle. In a recent single-center study, the mean peak VO_2 in a cohort of >300 EA patients with a mean age of 28 years was 22 ml/kg/min or 60% of predicted [16].

14.2 Pregnancy Outcomes

The largest study investigating the outcome of pregnancies in mothers with EA included 44 women with 111 pregnancies, resulting in 85 live births (76%). The majority of women ($n=34$) had uncorrected EA. Sixteen women were cyanotic at the time of pregnancy due to interatrial shunting; five women had documented accessory conduction pathways. Twenty-three deliveries were premature, and there were 19 spontaneous miscarriages (17%), 7 therapeutic abortions, and 2 early neonatal deaths. There were no serious pregnancy-related maternal complications [17]. Patients with mild disease and little to no ventricular dysfunction tolerated pregnancy changes well. Patients with significant preexisting right or left heart dysfunction may experience more overt heart failure symptoms due to an inability to cope with the increased volume and cardiac output demands of pregnancy.

In the EA cohort from the ZAHARA study, 2 of 22 pregnancies were complicated by arrhythmias [18]. In case reports of pregnant women with EA, right heart failure or arrhythmias were the most commonly observed complications [19, 20]. In a recent literature review of pregnancy outcomes in CHD, including 127 completed pregnancies (>20 weeks gestation) in women with EA, arrhythmias complicated 4% and heart failure 3% of pregnancies [21]. No pregnancy-related death occurred. Overall, in the absence of maternal cyanosis or symptomatic arrhythmias prior to pregnancy, pregnancy was well tolerated.

Although there is scarce data for women with EA specifically, increased rates of adverse fetal outcomes have been observed in cohorts of women with diverse types of heart disease [21–23]. In a retrospective cohort of 331 women with both congenital and acquired heart disease, Gelson et al. found that low cardiac output and cyanosis are risk factors for adverse fetal outcomes [22]. In a large cohort, pregnancy completion rates in cyanotic women are <50% [21]. The use of cardiac medications and mechanical prosthetic valve has also been proposed as risk factors for adverse neonatal outcomes [18]. Cyanosis and the need of anticoagulation are not uncommon among EA patients. In the Mayo EA cohort, the mean birth weight of the infants born to cyanotic women was 2.5 kg, compared to 3.1 kg in acyanotic women [17]. There was no difference in late survival between children from mothers with cyanotic or non-cyanotic heart disease.

In a review by Drenthen et al., premature delivery was observed in 22% of EA pregnancies (vs. 10–12% expected occurrence), and 12% of babies were small for gestational age (vs. 10% of expected occurrence) [21]. None of the studies reported fetal mortality (intrauterine death >20 weeks gestation), but there was a 2% perinatal mortality (death within the first year of life). Overall, the risk of fetal or perinatal mortality seems to be low.

14.3 Pregnancy Management

14.3.1 Coordinated Care

During pregnancy, EA patients should be evaluated by an ACHD cardiologist, a maternal-fetal medicine specialist and an obstetric and/or cardiac anesthesiologist. Involvement of other consultants may be necessary based on patient's clinical presentation (i.e., critical care, cardiac surgery, hematology, etc.).

14.3.2 Frequency of Follow-Up

Frequency of follow-up is dictated by maternal cardiac status. Patients who are at low risk (WHO class II) can be seen by a cardiologist every trimester. For women in WHO class III, there is a higher risk of complications, and monthly or bimonthly cardiology follow-up is recommended to assess for changes in their cardiac status [24]. Arrhythmias, most commonly supraventricular tachycardia (SVT), may occur at any point in pregnancy. The patient should be counseled on vagal maneuvers that can potentially interrupt AV node-dependent arrhythmias. EA patients should also look for and report signs of heart failure. Although these are often difficult to distinguish from normal changes of pregnancy, concerning signs include peripheral edema, orthopnea, and rapidly progressive shortness of breath during exertion [24–26].

14.3.3 Fetal Echocardiography

Fetal echocardiography to screen for congenital heart disease is best done between 18 and 22 weeks gestation, when visualization of the heart and outflow tracts is optimal.

14.3.4 Management of Arrhythmias

For acute SVT, the initial recommended interventions in pregnancy are vagal maneuvers and IV adenosine. These are expected to have little effect on the fetus, as adenosine has an extremely short half-life and does not cross the placenta [27]. Additional interventions that may be considered include digoxin, beta-blockers, and verapamil. In the presence of an accessory pathway, SVTs (atrial flutter or atrial fibrillation) can lead to wide-complex tachycardias. In these circumstances, digoxin and calcium channel blockers are contraindicated, since they may increase the ventricular response rate by favoring conduction via the accessory pathway. For patients with an accessory pathway and symptomatic arrhythmias (reentry tachycardias and preexcited atrial fibrillation or atrial flutter), pharmacologic therapy to prevent further arrhythmias and/or slowing the ventricular response rate is necessary. Flecainide and propafenone possess favorable benefit/risk ratio. If the patient is hemodynamically unstable, synchronized cardioversion is recommended. There is no change in the recommended voltage in pregnancy, and the amount of electricity that reaches the fetus is extremely small [24, 27, 28]. Catheter ablation during pregnancy should only be considered for refractory and poorly tolerated cases of arrhythmia [27]. The presence of an atrial arrhythmia longer than 48 h can increase risk for atrial clot, so consideration should be given to anticoagulation in this situation [29].

14.3.5 Management of Progressive Heart Failure

Heart failure is one of the most common complications for women with heart disease during pregnancy [23, 25, 30, 31]. According to the available published information on EA in pregnancy, overt heart failure occurred in only 3 % of patients [21]. Ruys et al. looked retrospectively at heart failure during pregnancy in women with both congenital and acquired heart disease. They found an overall 13 % incidence of heart failure, the majority of which occurred at the end of the second trimester or in the peripartum period. Several parameters were associated with heart failure, including NYHA class ≥III, WHO pregnancy class ≥III, preexisting cardiomyopathy, preexisting pulmonary hypertension, and preexisting signs of heart failure [31]. Depressed subpulmonary ventricular function has been described as an additional risk factor for heart failure during pregnancy [32]. Measurement of natriuretic peptides (pro-BNP or BNP) can be useful to risk stratify patients. Normal levels of BNP (<100–128 pg/ml) at 20 weeks gestation have been found to have a 96–100 % negative predictive value for heart failure events associated with pregnancy. Patients with elevated BNP at 20 weeks gestation had a higher risk for heart failure [32, 33]. Most available treatment agents for heart failure are acceptable for the use during pregnancy, with the notable exception of ACE inhibitors and aldosterone antagonists. Admission to a tertiary care center may be necessary for careful management and titration of fluid status. In addition to bed rest and supplemental oxygen, furosemide can be used for diuresis, and nitrates or hydralazine can be used for afterload reduction. Inotropes can be considered if needed, although very little is known about the use of these agents during pregnancy [25, 26]. If the patient is placed on bed rest, consideration should be given to thromboembolic prophylaxis, particularly in an EA patient with an interatrial shunt.

14.3.6 Management of Progressive Cyanosis

Patients with cyanosis are at elevated risk for maternal and fetal complications during pregnancy. The management of progressive cyanosis and hypoxemia revolves around maintenance and improvement of oxygenation and oxygen-carrying capacity. Supplemental oxygen may be considered, but, in the presence of an atrial right-to-left shunt, it is unlikely to make a substantial difference [34]. Cardiac output should be maintained by avoiding dehydration, ambulation as tolerated, and compression stockings to optimize venous return. Hematocrit should be maintained in the physiologic range to maximize oxygen-carrying capacity. Low hematocrit may be due to iron deficiency and should be treated with iron supplementation. Elevated hematocrit (>65%) puts patients at risk of hyperviscosity syndrome, which can decrease oxygen delivery. If signs of hyperviscosity syndrome are seen, such as headache, lethargy, fatigue, dizziness, anorexia, or visual disturbances, hydration or exchange transfusion can be considered as indicated [34, 35]. In severe refractory cases, consideration can be given to percutaneous closure of the atrial septal defect. There are currently no reports in the literature regarding the effects of defect closure on pregnancy outcome in EA patients.

14.3.7 Mode and Timing of Delivery

In patients with EA, the largest available series show vaginal delivery to be safe [17, 20]. However, Caesarean delivery is still preferred for a select group of CHD patients, including cyanotic patients receiving warfarin anticoagulation within 2 weeks of delivery [34].

Timing of delivery should be discussed as a multidisciplinary group. Women with mild EA can be delivered at early term. In those with more significant complications, such as difficult to control arrhythmia, heart failure, or progressive cyanosis, the decision should be made on an individual basis, weighing the risks of prematurity vs. the risks to the mother of continuing the pregnancy.

14.3.8 Anesthesia Management During Delivery

Anesthetic management during labor and delivery is a vital component to the care of patients with EA. An obstetric anesthesiologist should be involved in the multidisciplinary planning prior to delivery in these patients. For vaginal delivery, early epidural analgesia is typically recommended for patients of all disease severity [24–26, 36]. Slow titration of local anesthetic and judicious fluid boluses before epidural placement can minimize rapid decreases in preload that are often seen with neuraxial anesthesia. For Caesarean section, epidural anesthesia can be slowly titrated to avoid hemodynamic disturbance while providing adequate anesthesia for the procedure. General anesthesia, with careful attention to hemodynamics and oxygenation, is also an option; however, it is generally not preferred in obstetrics [34].

14.3.9 Monitoring During Labor and Delivery

Patients with EA are at an increased risk for arrhythmia independent of symptoms or associated lesions. Therefore, they should be monitored on continuous telemetry during labor, delivery, and the immediate postpartum period. Hemodynamic monitoring during labor and delivery depends on the current status of each patient. Asymptomatic patients with minor disease and no associated lesions may not need additional hemodynamic monitoring. Patients with significant ventricular dysfunction, severe tricuspid regurgitation, heart failure, or cyanosis should have continuous pulse oximetry throughout labor and delivery. In rare cases, invasive hemodynamic monitoring may give useful additional information. Such monitoring may include invasive blood pressure monitoring, central venous pressure monitoring, minimally invasive cardiac output monitoring, and bioimpedance monitoring [26, 34, 37].

14.3.10 Specific Recommendations and Pitfalls

(i) *Paradoxical embolism*: Women with EA and an interatrial shunt are at risk for paradoxical embolus. To help prevent air entrainment into an IV causing a paradoxical embolus, air filters should be placed on all intravenous lines in patients with a known shunt.

(ii) *Preterm labor*: Medications used for premature contractions include tocolytics and drugs given to optimize neonatal outcome if premature labor progresses. The classes of tocolytics currently in use include nonsteroidal anti-inflammatory drugs (NSAIDs), calcium channel blockers, beta-agonists, and oxytocin antagonist atosiban (Europe only). Beta-agonists, such as terbutaline and hexoprenaline, have significant maternal side effects including tachycardia and an increased propensity for arrhythmias. These drugs should be avoided in EA patients. NSAIDs, such as indomethacin, have few maternal side effects. Commonly reported adverse effects include nausea, heartburn, and platelet inhibition. The platelet inhibition is rarely clinically significant unless there is another underlying bleeding disorder or therapeutic anticoagulation. They should not be used in the cyanotic EA patient. NSAIDs can have significant fetal side effects, including in utero constriction of the ductus arteriosus and oligohydramnios. These drugs are not used beyond 32 weeks of pregnancy and even before only under carefully monitoring of the ductus. Although calcium channel blockers can generally be used safely, they should be used with caution in patients with severe tricuspid regurgitation or other preload-dependent lesions, since the expected vasodilation will decrease preload [38]. Atosiban, an oxytocin receptor antagonist, is approved for use in Europe but not in the USA. It has been reported to cause pulmonary edema, hypotension, and tachycardia/dysrhythmia on rare occasions, but is generally considered safe [34]. Given its limited use, safety in the setting of maternal cardiac disease is unknown. Magnesium sulfate is commonly given in the setting of preterm labor for fetal neuroprotection. It has been shown to decrease the incidence and severity of cerebral palsy in premature infants [38]. At therapeutic levels, it can cause lethargy and hypotonia. Supratherapeutic Mg levels can cause pulmonary edema, cardiac arrhythmias, respiratory depression, and even cardiac arrest. It should be used with extreme caution in EA patients. Corticosteroids, given to improve fetal lung maturity when delivery is anticipated within 2 weeks at gestational ages of less than 34 weeks, can cause fluid retention. They should be used with care in patients with heart failure or depressed ventricular function. Potential fetal benefit of steroid administration should be weighed against maternal risk in individual circumstances.

(iii) *Induction of labor*: Cervical ripening is usually the first step in inducing labor. This is typically accomplished by vaginal application of a prostaglandin analogue, such as misoprostol (prostaglandin E1) and dinoprostone (prostaglandin E2). These agents can generally be used safely, although if there is excessive systemic absorption, they can cause vasodilation, which can lead to hypoxia in patients with a known shunt [34]. Pulse oximetry and blood pressure should be monitored during the use of these medications in these patients. Oxytocin is commonly given to augment uterine contraction strength during labor induction or during spontaneous labor. It is usually given as a continuous infusion at rates starting at 0.5–6 mU/min; a maximum dose has not been published [39]. For patients with heart failure and risk of fluid overload, the preparation can be concentrated to decrease fluid administered. When given with high volumes of fluids, oxytocin can cause fluid retention and hyponatremia due to its structural similarity to vasopressin [40]. Rapidly infused at rates of >2 units/min, oxytocin can cause systemic vasodilation and hypotension. For cyanotic patients with a right-to-left shunt, this may increase the degree of shunting. Although not well studied, oxytocin may increase pulmonary artery pressures [41, 42] and should therefore be used cautiously in patients with right heart dysfunction or existing pulmonary hypertension.

(iv) *Postpartum hemorrhage*: Uterine atony is the most common cause of postpartum hemorrhage (PPH). Therefore, the goal of pharmacological treatment of PPH is to increase uterine muscle tone. Oxytocin is the first-line treatment for PPH. It is more likely to be given rapidly this setting, so vigilance for the expected side effects of hypotension and reflex tachycardia is warranted. Misoprostol may also be administered for uterine atony. As with induction of labor, it can generally be used safely in this setting. Other agents used for the treatment of postpartum hemorrhage include methylergonovine (ergometrine in the UK) and carboprost (synthetic prostaglandin F2α); both are administered via intramuscular injection. Methylergonovine can cause arteriolar constriction and hypertension. It should be avoided in patients with heart disease. Carboprost can cause bronchoconstriction, especially in patients with a history of asthma. This can lead to increased pulmonary arterial pressures and increased hypoxemia, which would be especially detrimental to patients with an intracardiac shunt or right ventricular dysfunction and should be used under close observation.

(v) *Infective endocarditis prophylaxis*: EA patients with cyanosis or who have tricuspid valve replacement or repair using prosthetic material and residual valvular regurgitation should be considered at increased risk for infective endocarditis. Consideration of antibiotic prophylaxis is recommended in high-risk patients undergoing invasive dental procedures. However, vaginal delivery and Caesarean section are not considered high-risk procedures, and antibiotic prophylaxis is not recommended by the ESC or AHA/ACC unless the delivery is associated with an infection [43, 44]. However, other sources consider infective endocarditis prophylaxis reasonable for delivery in high-risk patients, including those with cyanosis [26, 34].

14.3.11 Postpartum Care

14.3.11.1 Monitoring
Where the patient will be recovered, postdelivery depends on the severity of her cardiac disease and consequently the level of required monitoring in the context of the logistics and capabilities of the institution. Patients who are NYHA class I throughout their pregnancy and are at elevated risk for arrhythmia should be monitored on cardiac telemetry. Patients with cyanosis or heart failure, or any other patients requiring invasive monitoring, may be best observed in an ICU for recovery. There is little evidence of the optimal duration of monitoring after delivery. Decisions regarding duration of monitoring should be made on a case-by-case basis. However, given the known increased cardiac demands for the first 24–48 h postpartum, monitoring for this length of time is reasonable, as this would be the time period at highest risk for cardiac complication. Patients with heart failure or cyanosis will likely require a longer duration of monitoring than patients with mild disease.

14.3.12 Specific Precautions in the Postpartum Period

(i) *Fluid management*: Ideally, EA patients should be euvolemic during the postpartum period. Patients with ventricular dysfunction, particularly left sided, and/or heart failure and cyanosis should be judiciously managed and excessive IV fluid replacement avoided. CVP monitoring may be a helpful adjunct guiding fluid replacement. Blood loss from delivery and the postpartum period is generally replaced with crystalloid, although colloid can also be used in patients at high risk for volume overload and pulmonary edema, and if needed, gentle diuresis can be undertaken.
(ii) *Antithrombotic regimen*: Patients continue to be at increased risk for thromboembolic events in the postpartum period. Patients who are known to be at high risk, including those with sustained atrial arrhythmia, severely depressed

ventricular function, or cyanosis, may already be receiving antithrombotic prophylaxis or treatment. Patients who received anticoagulation (therapeutic or prophylactic) are recommended to continue for at least 6 weeks postpartum [45]. Women with a high risk for venous thromboembolism are also recommended to wear graduated compression stockings in the postpartum period [45]. Patients who had a Caesarean delivery or are immobile after delivery should be considered for pharmacologic prophylaxis.

14.3.13 Discharge Plan

(i) *Duration of stay in hospital*: Postpartum hospital stay length varies by mode of delivery, underlying maternal condition, and complications encountered during delivery or in the postpartum period. For women with EA, a hospital stay of at least 48 h is recommended to monitor for arrhythmia and other complications. Women with heart failure or cyanosis will likely have a longer postpartum hospital stay, although the optimal length is unknown.
(ii) *Review of cardiac medication*: Before each patient's discharge, their current medications should be reviewed and updated as needed. Medications that were changed during pregnancy because of known fetal risk can be restarted in the postpartum period, but if the patient is breastfeeding, each medication should be reviewed for safety and risk of neonatal transmission.
(iii) *Follow-up plan*: Patients who tolerated labor and delivery well without cardiac complication should be seen for a routine postpartum visit after 6–8 weeks. If the patient has known valvular disease, right or left heart dysfunction or cyanosis, an echo can be performed at 6–8 weeks postpartum as well. Further follow-up should be based on the patient's clinical condition.

14.4 Impact of Physiological Changes of Pregnancy

The effect of pregnancy on EA circulatory function depends heavily on the preconception hemodynamic state of the EA patient. Tricuspid regurgitation may worsen as the circulatory volume augments and cardiac chamber dilation occurs. The clinical impact of this depends on preexisting right atrial compliance, which, if already diminished, is likely to provoke congestive heart failure. Worsened tricuspid regurgitation may also alter the degree of interatrial shunting. A greater degree of tricuspid regurgitation in the face of poor right atrial compliance may precipitate more right-to-left atrial shunting resulting in cyanosis [34]. Pregnancy physiology may also affect the relative compliances of the ventricles through a direct effect on the myocardium as well as through altered coupling of ventricle to the distal vascular beds. The systemic vascular resistance is likely to be reduced, in concert with greater stroke volume and cardiac output demands, altering the systolic and importantly the diastolic properties of the left ventricle. Similarly, the pulmonary vascular resistance may also diminish, albeit, to a lesser degree, altering coupling properties with the dysfunctional right ventricle. In a given pregnancy with EA, the effects of the altered pregnancy physiology may be difficult to predict on atrial shunting as so many factors play a potential role. In general, however, the decreased systemic vascular resistance and increased cardiac output seen in pregnancy tend to increase the degree of right-to-left shunt, worsening preexisting cyanosis.

Pregnancy is also a time of increased risk for arrhythmia [27]. Elevated adrenergic tone makes the myocardium more irritable and arrhythmogenic. In addition, the increased plasma volume in pregnancy causes dilation of heart chambers, resulting in unfavorable alteration in the refractoriness of the myocardium. This occurs through stimulation of stretch-activated ion channels. There is likely a synergistic effect through these pregnancy-induced phenomena and preexisting arrhythmia substrates that occur in EA. The net result is a greater degree of arrhythmia predisposition.

14.4.1 Interactions Between Pregnancy and EA Hemodynamics in Women with Common Underlying Comorbidities

The prevalence of obesity is increasing internationally [19] as are the associated cardiorespiratory problems such as obstructive sleep apnea (OSA). OSA is potentially devastating in EA as its adverse effects on pulmonary vascular physiology and autonomic tone may exacerbate EA circulatory dysfunction. Synergism may occur through the mass effect of pregnancy and the heightened CO_2 chemosensitivity to precipitate cardiorespiratory symptoms. Obese women are also at increased risk for hypertensive disorders of pregnancy (such as preeclampsia), diabetes, and thromboembolic disease [20, 21].

During pregnancy, smoking is associated with adverse events, including intrauterine growth restriction (IUGR) and abnormal placentation [22]. Although no direct interaction with cardiovascular physiology has been demonstrated, abnormal placentation, smoking, and EA pathophysiology are likely in severe cases to act synergistically in compromising fetal growth.

Preeclampsia complicates 2–8 % of pregnancies worldwide [23, 24]. Although it is fundamentally a microvascular disease of the placenta, it can have profound effects on the cardiovascular system. Preeclampsia increases systemic vascular resistance and potentially lowers cardiac output. Patients with severe forms of EA, especially those with left ventricular dysfunction, may already have a relatively low cardiac output. The further decrease seen in preeclampsia may trigger clinical heart failure [25]. Renal dysfunction and proteinuria, associated with cyanosis in EA, can complicate the diagnosis of preeclampsia. Thrombocytopenia and coagulation abnormalities seen in preeclampsia may also exacerbate preexisting coagulopathy of cyanotic heart disease, thereby increasing the bleeding risk [17].

Antepartum hemorrhage is most commonly secondary to placental disorders such as placenta previa and abruption. Postpartum hemorrhage, a common complication of pregnancy, can be caused by uterine atony, lacerations, surgical bleeding, and retained products of conception. The main physiologic concerns with obstetric hemorrhage are loss of intravascular volume and appropriate function of coagulation mechanisms. Patients with EA and cyanosis have a baseline increased bleeding risk secondary to cyanosis-related abnormalities in the coagulation system [26]. They are at higher risk for obstetrical hemorrhage, and it may be more difficult to control the bleeding if hemorrhage does occur.

Patients with congenital heart disease have a higher incidence of spontaneous preterm premature rupture of membranes (PPROM) and preterm labor [27–30]. The course after PPROM depends on the gestational age and clinical situation, as well as the risks and benefits to the patient. The patient may be managed expectantly or have labor induced with the goal of delivery. The most significant risks associated with expectant management in this population are the likelihood of prolonged immobility and concomitant increase risk of thromboembolic events and the progressive risk of infection.

14.5 Preconception Counseling

14.5.1 Fertility

Historically, many women with EA were counseled not to become pregnant, so their fertility status is unknown [17, 19, 20, 46, 47]. The fertility rate of EA women likely depends on the presence and degree of cyanosis. Canobbio et al. found that acyanotic women had similar menstrual patterns to control women [48]. On this basis, one would suspect that the fertility of acyanotic women is preserved. In contrast, women with cyanotic CHD are more likely to suffer from infertility. Indeed, in Canobbio et al.'s study, cyanotic women had significantly delayed onset of menstruation and a higher incidence of abnormal menstrual cycles, suggesting an abnormality in the hypothalamic-pituitary-ovarian axis [48]. It is reasonable to think that women with cyanotic heart disease, including EA patients with right-to-left shunts, have an increased rate of infertility. Women with more severe cyanosis (saturation <85% and hemoglobin >20 g/l) are also more likely to experience spontaneous early pregnancy losses [35].

14.5.2 Risk of Transmission

Although the literature on EA heritability is limited, transmission rates are reported to be 6% if the mother is affected and 1% if the father is affected. In a historical study of 26 families with EA, no case of inheritance of this anomaly was found in 93 first-degree relatives [49]. In a report from the Mayo Clinic, the overall incidence of CHD in 158 offspring of parents with EA was 4% (6 of 158), with one case of familial EA [17]. Consultation with a geneticist should be offered for a patient-specific discussion of risks and available testing options.

Table 14.1 WHO classification of risk for pregnancy in cardiovascular disease

WHO class	Description
I	Risk no higher than general population
II	Small increased risk of maternal morbidity and mortality
III	Significant expected increased risk of maternal morbidity and mortality. Expert cardiac and obstetric prepregnancy, antenatal and postnatal care required
IV	Pregnancy contraindicated; very high risk of maternal mortality or severe morbidity. Termination should be discussed. If pregnancy continues, care as for class III

Adapted from Thorne

14.5.3 EA Pregnancy Risk Scores

EA does not specifically appear in the WHO classification (see Table 14.1); however, patients can still be classified based on their individual manifestations of EA. Cyanotic heart disease and "other complex congenital heart disease," which would likely encompass many manifestations of EA, are considered WHO class III [50]. In their 2011 guidelines on the management of cardiovascular disease during pregnancy, the European Society of Cardiology (ESC) considered women with EA who did not have heart failure or cyanosis to be WHO class II, otherwise as class III [24].

14.5.4 Recommended Preconception Counseling Workup

Ideally, EA women should be seen while contemplating pregnancy. This should preferably be done by a maternal-fetal medicine specialist and an ACHD cardiologist. A thorough review of their cardiac and obstetric history should be obtained. A comprehensive, cardiac-focused physical exam should be conducted, honing in on signs and symptoms of chronic hypoxemia, congestive heart failure, arrhythmia, and any evidence of other systemic manifestations of EA. A baseline ECG and transthoracic echocardiogram should be obtained if they have not been done recently. Functional capacity and systemic saturation at rest and during exercise should be measured during cardiopulmonary exercise testing. Further testing, which may include a cardiac MRI, will depend on the severity of disease and the current cardiac status of each individual patient. Useful laboratory investigations include hemoglobin to assess for anemia or erythrocytosis secondary to a shunt-related cyanosis, platelet count and prothrombin time to assess coagulation status, and blood urea nitrogen and creatinine to assess renal function. In cyanotic patients, it may be useful to obtain a baseline urine protein measurement. A medication review should be undertaken, with particular attention to medications that should be avoided in pregnancy.

14.5.5 Review of Cardiac Medication

Patients with EA will have varied medications based on the severity of the lesion, associated conditions, and baseline cardiac status. Common considerations for EA patients are antiarrhythmic and heart failure medications. No antiarrhythmic drug has been shown completely safe during the first trimester, so continuation of maintenance antiarrhythmics during this time should be based on the frequency and tolerability of the underlying arrhythmia. If treatment is needed, the lowest effective dose should be used [24].

14.5.6 Effects of Pregnancy on Long-Term Outcome

Scant EA-specific data exist on the long-term cardiac effects of pregnancy. Several retrospective studies quantify long-term outcomes in women with CHD. A questionnaire-based study focused on functional status and ability to work and exercise in 267 women. Median follow-up time was 11 years. Sixty-seven percent of respondents were healthy and capable with a stable functional status. Thirty-three percent had pregnancies complicated by decrease in NYHA class. Sixty-six percent of those patients had recovered by the time of follow-up [51]. Others have studied the occurrence of adverse cardiac events (death, arrhythmia, stroke, heart failure/pulmonary edema) up to 5 years postpartum. Long-term cardiac event rates were 6.4–12 %. Patients with a cardiac event during pregnancy were significantly more likely to have a long-term cardiac incident [52, 53]. Risk factors for long-term cardiac events appear to be similar to those for peripartum cardiac events. The most common long-term complications seen in EA patients were arrhythmias [52, 53]. It is unknown if pregnancy altered the natural history of disease or if these arrhythmias would have been observed without pregnancy. Nonetheless, for EA patients with good prepregnancy functional status, there is a relatively low risk for long-term postpartum complication. Patients with cyanosis or heart failure are likely at higher risk for long-term complications, including worsening of functional status, given their higher risk for cardiac events during pregnancy.

References

1. Attenhofer Jost CH, Connolly HM, Dearani JA, Edwards WD, Danielson GK (2007) Ebstein's anomaly. Circulation 115:277–285
2. Lupo PJ, Langlois PH, Mitchell LE (2011) Epidemiology of Ebstein anomaly: prevalence and patterns in Texas, 1999–2005. Am J Med Genet A 155A:1007–1014
3. Attenhofer Jost CH, Connolly HM, O'Leary PW, Warnes CA, Tajik AJ, Seward JB (2005) Left heart lesions in patients with Ebstein anomaly. Mayo Clin Proc 80:361–368
4. Stähli BE, Gebhard C, Biaggi P et al (2013) Left ventricular non-compaction: prevalence in congenital heart disease. Int J Cardiol 167:2477–2481
5. Lang D, Oberhoffer R, Cook A et al (1991) Pathologic spectrum of malformations of the tricuspid valve in prenatal and neonatal life. J Am Coll Cardiol 17:1161–1167
6. Ammash NM, Warnes CA, Connolly HM, Danielson GK, Seward JB (1997) Mimics of Ebstein's anomaly. Am Heart J 134:508–513

7. Freud LR, Escobar-Diaz MC, Kalish BT et al (2015) Outcomes and predictors of perinatal mortality in fetuses with Ebstein anomaly or tricuspid valve dysplasia in the current era: a multicenter study. Circulation 132:481–489
8. Celermajer DS, Bull C, Till JA et al (1994) Ebstein's anomaly: presentation and outcome from fetus to adult. J Am Coll Cardiol 23:170–176
9. Egidy Assenza G, Valente AM, Geva T et al (2013) QRS duration and QRS fractionation on surface electrocardiogram are markers of right ventricular dysfunction and atrialization in patients with Ebstein anomaly. Eur Heart J 34:191–200
10. Khairy P, Marelli AJ (2007) Clinical use of electrocardiography in adults with congenital heart disease. Circulation 116:2734–2746
11. Atiq M, Lai L, Lee KJ, Benson LN (2005) Transcatheter closure of atrial septal defects in children with a hypoplastic right ventricle. Catheter Cardiovasc Interv 64:112–116
12. Agnoletti G, Boudjemline Y, Ou P, Bonnet D, Sidi D (2006) Right to left shunt through interatrial septal defects in patients with congenital heart disease: results of interventional closure. Heart 92:827–831
13. Digilio MC, Bernardini L, Lepri F et al (2011) Ebstein anomaly: genetic heterogeneity and association with microdeletions 1p36 and 8p23.1. Am J Med Genet A 155A:2196–2202
14. LaHaye S, Lincoln J, Garg V (2014) Genetics of valvular heart disease. Curr Cardiol Rep 16:487
15. Baumgartner H, Bonhoeffer P, De Groot NM et al (2010) ESC Guidelines for the management of grown-up congenital heart disease (new version 2010). Eur Heart J 31:2915–2957
16. Kempny A, Dimopoulos K, Uebing A et al (2012) Reference values for exercise limitations among adults with congenital heart disease. Relation to activities of daily life – single centre experience and review of published data. Eur Heart J 33:1386–1396
17. Connolly HM, Warnes CA (1994) Ebstein's anomaly: outcome of pregnancy. J Am Coll Cardiol 23:1194–1198
18. Drenthen W, Boersma E, Balci A et al (2010) Predictors of pregnancy complications in women with congenital heart disease. Eur Heart J 31:2124–2132
19. Chopra S, Suri V, Aggarwal N, Rohilla M, Vijayvergiya R, Keepanasseril A (2010) Ebstein's anomaly in pregnancy: maternal and neonatal outcomes. J Obstet Gynaecol Res 36:278–283
20. Donnelly JE, Brown JM, Radford DJ (1991) Pregnancy outcome and Ebstein's anomaly. Br Heart J 66:368–371
21. Drenthen W, Pieper PG, Roos-Hesselink JW et al (2007) Outcome of pregnancy in women with congenital heart disease. J Am Coll Cardiol 49:2303–2311
22. Gelson E, Curry R, Gatzoulis MA et al (2011) Effect of maternal heart disease on fetal growth. Obstet Gynecol 117:886–891
23. Siu SC, Sermer M, Colman JM et al (2001) Prospective multicenter study of pregnancy outcomes in women with heart disease. Circulation 104:515–521
24. European Society of G, Association for European Paediatric C, German Society for Gender M et al (2011) ESC guidelines on the management of cardiovascular diseases during pregnancy: the Task Force on the Management of Cardiovascular Diseases during Pregnancy of the European Society of Cardiology (ESC). Eur Heart J 32:3147–3197
25. Greutmann M, Pieper PG (2015) Pregnancy in women with congenital heart disease. Eur Heart J 36:2491–2499
26. Rao S, Ginns JN (2014) Adult congenital heart disease and pregnancy. Semin Perinatol 38:260–272
27. Knotts RJ, Garan H (2014) Cardiac arrhythmias in pregnancy. Semin Perinatol 38:285–288
28. Adamson DL, Nelson-Piercy C (2008) Managing palpitations and arrhythmias during pregnancy. Postgrad Med J 84:66–72
29. Khairy P, Van Hare GF, Balaji S et al (2014) PACES/HRS expert consensus statement on the recognition and management of arrhythmias in adult congenital heart disease. Heart Rhythm 11:e102–e165
30. Khairy P, Ouyang DW, Fernandes SM, Lee-Parritz A, Economy KE, Landzberg MJ (2006) Pregnancy outcomes in women with congenital heart disease. Circulation 113:517–524

31. Ruys TPE, Roos-Hesselink JW, Hall R et al (2014) Heart failure in pregnant women with cardiac disease: data from the ROPAC. Heart 100:231–238
32. Kampman MM, Balci A, van Veldhuisen DJ et al (2014) N-terminal pro-B-type natriuretic peptide predicts cardiovascular complications in pregnant women with congenital heart disease. Eur Heart J 35:708–715
33. Tanous D, Siu SC, Mason J et al (2010) B-type natriuretic peptide in pregnant women with heart disease. J Am Coll Cardiol 56:1247–1253
34. Koos BJ (2004) Management of uncorrected, palliated, and repaired cyanotic congenital heart disease in pregnancy. Prog Pediatr Cardiol 19:25–45
35. Presbitero P, Somerville J, Stone S, Aruta E, Spiegelhalter D, Rabajoli F (1994) Pregnancy in cyanotic congenital heart disease. Outcome of mother and fetus. Circulation 89:2673–2676
36. Goldszmidt E, Macarthur A, Silversides C, Colman J, Sermer M, Siu S (2010) Anesthetic management of a consecutive cohort of women with heart disease for labor and delivery. Int J Obstet Anesth 19:266–272
37. Levin H, LaSala A (2014) Intrapartum obstetric management. Semin Perinatol 38:245–251
38. American College of Obstetricians and G. P R AC T I C E (2012) Management of preterm labor. Obstet Gynecol 119:1308–1317
39. American Congress of O, Gynecologists (2009) Practice bulletin clinical management guidelines for obstetrician-gynecologists induction of labor. Obstet Gynecol 114:386–397
40. Bergum D, Lonnée H, Hakli TF (2009) Oxytocin infusion: acute hyponatraemia, seizures and coma. Acta Anaesthesiol Scand 53:826–827
41. Roberts NV, Keast PJ, Brodeky V, Oates A, Ritchie BC (1992) The effects of oxytocin on the pulmonary and systemic circulation in pregnant ewes. Anaesth Intensive Care 20:199–202
42. Secher NJ, Arnsbo P, Wallin L (1978) Haemodynamic effects of oxytocin (syntocinon) and methyl ergometrine (methergin) on the systemic and pulmonary circulations of pregnant anaesthetized women. Acta Obstet Gynecol Scand 57:97–103
43. Habib G, Lancellotti P, Antunes M et al (2015) ESC Guidelines for the management of infective endocarditis. Eur Heart J 2015:ehv319-ehv319
44. Nishimura RA, Otto CM, Bonow RO et al (2014) 2014 AHA/ACC guideline for the management of patients with valvular heart disease. J Thorac Cardiovasc Surg 148:e1–e132
45. Marik PE, Plante L (2008) Venous thromboembolic disease and pregnancy. N Engl J Med 359:2025–2033
46. Katsuragi S, Kamiya C, Yamanaka K et al (2013) Risk factors for maternal and fetal outcome in pregnancy complicated by Ebstein anomaly. Am J Obstet Gynecol 209:452 e1–6
47. Zhao W, Liu H, Feng R, Lin J (2012) Pregnancy outcomes in women with Ebstein's anomaly. Arch Gynecol Obstet 286:881–888
48. Canobbio MM, Rapkin AJ, Perloff JK, Lin A, Child JS (1995) Menstrual patterns in women with congenital heart disease. Pediatr Cardiol 16:12–15
49. Emanuel R, O'Brien K, Ng R (1976) Ebstein's anomaly. Genetic study of 26 families. Br Heart J 38:5–7
50. Thorne S, MacGregor A, Nelson-Piercy C (2006) Risks of contraception and pregnancy in heart disease. Heart 92:1520–1525
51. Wacker-Gussmann A, Thriemer M, Yigitbasi M, Berger F, Nagdyman N (2013) Women with congenital heart disease: long-term outcomes after pregnancy. Clin Res Cardiol: Off J Ger Card Soc 102:215–222
52. Balint OH, Siu SC, Mason J et al (2010) Cardiac outcomes after pregnancy in women with congenital heart disease. Heart (Br Card Soc) 96:1656–1661
53. Kampman MAM, Balci A, Groen H et al (2015) Cardiac function and cardiac events 1-year postpartum in women with congenital heart disease. Am Heart J 169:298–304

Fontan

15

Margherita Ministeri and Michael A. Gatzoulis

Abbreviations

ACC	American College of Cardiology
AHA	American Heart Association
BP	Blood pressure
CHD	Congenital heart disease
CO	Cardiac output
CPET	Cardiopulmonary exercise test
CT	Computed tomography
ECG	Electrocardiogram
EF	Ejection fraction
FC	Fontan circulation
LMWH	Low molecular weight heparin
MR	Magnetic resonance
NYHA	New York Heart Association
SVT	Supraventricular tachycardia
TCPC	Total cavopulmonary conversion

M. Ministeri, MD (✉)
Adult Congenital Heart Centre and Centre for Pulmonary Hypertension,
Royal Brompton Hospital, London, UK

National Heart & Lung Institute, Imperial College, London, UK

Division of Cardiology, Ferrarotto Hospital, University of Catania, Catania, Italy
e-mail: M.Ministeri@rbht.nhs.uk; margheritaministeri@yahoo.it

M.A. Gatzoulis, MD, PhD, FACC, FESC
Adult Congenital Heart Centre and Centre for Pulmonary Hypertension,
Royal Brompton Hospital, London, UK

National Heart & Lung Institute, Imperial College, London, UK
e-mail: m.gatzoulis@rbht.nhs.uk

> **Key Facts**
>
> *Incidence:* The Fontan operation is a palliative procedure for patients with tricuspid atresia, double-inlet ventricle, double-outlet ventricle, pulmonary atresia with intact septum and hypoplastic left heart syndrome, all rare congenital lesions. About 5% of all patients with congenital heart disease need a Fontan operation.
>
> *Inheritance:* Between 3 and 10% of offspring.
>
> *Medication:* Oral anticoagulation should be replaced by LMWH for at least the first trimester.
>
> *World Health Organization class:* III–IV.
>
> *Risk of pregnancy:* 40% risk of miscarriage. Risk of deterioration in ventricular function and increasing atrioventricular valve regurgitation. Elevation in the right atrial pressure increases tachyarrhythmias.
>
> *Life expectancy:* Clearly decreased. After successful surgery, 70–76% are alive at 25 years.

> **Key Management**
>
> *Preconception:* Physical examination, ECG, echo, BNP and CMR. Exercise testing to assess increase cardiac output and oxygen saturation. Consider the left/right heart catheterisation or CT scan. Arrhythmias, haemodynamic lesions, anaemia and infection diagnosed and treated.
>
> *Pregnancy:* Intensive monitoring in a tertiary, multidisciplinary environment. Key to detect early signs of heart failure, arrhythmia, thromboembolic complications and worsening cyanosis. Serial echocardiograms are needed. Limit exercise and take adequate rest.
>
> *Labour:* Vaginal delivery is preferable.
>
> *Postpartum:* Infuse oxytocin at lowest effective dose. In-hospital observation for at least 48 h longer (1 week) where the risk of cardiac decompensation is high.

15.1 The Condition

The Fontan operation was originally introduced, in 1971, as a palliative procedure for patients with tricuspid atresia [1]. It has since been used extensively to provide palliation for patients with several forms of congenital heart disease unsuitable for biventricular circulation including double-inlet ventricle, double-outlet ventricle, pulmonary atresia with intact septum and hypoplastic left heart syndrome. The vena cava flow is directed to the pulmonary arteries bypassing the ventricle. Since the first description, the Fontan procedure has evolved over the years, most notably with the substitution of the right atrial to pulmonary artery anastomosis with cavopulmonary

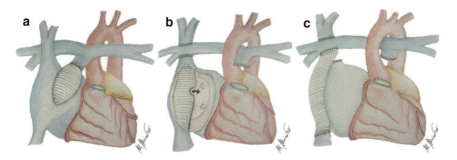

Fig. 15.1 Variations of Fontan operation. (**a**) The modified classic Fontan procedure: direct communication between the right atrium and the pulmonary artery. (**b**) The total cavopulmonary connection (TCPC) with an intra-atrial lateral tunnel: the blood from the inferior vena cava is directed to the inferior portion of the right pulmonary artery, and the superior vena is directly connected to the pulmonary artery via a Glenn shunt. There is a fenestration in the lateral tunnel allowing shunting from the Fontan to common atrium. (**c**) Total cavopulmonary connection (TCPC) with an extracardiac conduit: the right atrium is excluded, the synthetic conduit is placed from the inferior vena cava to the right pulmonary artery, and the superior vena cava is connected to the right pulmonary artery via a Glenn shunt. This is the most widely used Fontan procedure

connections [2]. Whether achieved by direct atriopulmonary anastomoses or via intra- or extracardiac total cavopulmonary connections, the objective of Fontan surgery is to separate systemic from pulmonary circulations and reduce or abolish cyanosis (Fig. 15.1). In short, Fontan physiology consists of one functional ventricle that generates systemic blood flow, with systemic venous return directed into the pulmonary arteries. The pulmonary circulation is driven by the remaining kinetic energy from the single ventricle output, the transpulmonary gradient (the difference between mean central venous pressure and systemic ventricle end-diastolic pressure) and the negative intrathoracic pressure created by inspiration. Therefore, the Fontan circulation is volume dependent that requires an adequate preload and normal to low afterload to maintain cardiac output.

The surgical progress resulted in significantly improved long-term survival (90 % at 10 years, 83 % at 20 years, and 70–76 % at 25 years), and an increasing number of women who have undergone the Fontan surgery in childhood are surviving into adulthood; some of them become pregnant [3, 4]. While the growing body of literature is improving efforts to predict risk and provide evidence-based counselling, data remain scarce for certain subtypes of congenital heart disease, including complex congenital heart defects with Fontan palliation. In general, patients with Fontan circulation can be hampered by various late complications that can perturb the delicate physiologic balance that allows venous propulsion of blood flow through the pulmonary circulation. Common long-term sequel includes severe right atrium dilatation, atrial bradyarrhythmias and tachyarrhythmias, thromboemboli, hepatic dysfunction, progressive ventricular dysfunction, atrioventricular valve regurgitation, protein-losing enteropathy and worsening cyanosis from systemic venous collateralisation, pulmonary arteriovenous malformations and pulmonary vein compression. Based on the complexity of this patient population, historically women who

Table 15.1 Most common maternal and neonatal complications in pregnant women with the Fontan circulation

Maternal complications
Cardiac
Arrhythmias, SVT
Heart failure
Thromboembolic episodes
Obstetric
Miscarriages
Premature rupture of membrane
Premature labour and delivery
Postpartum haemorrhage
Neonatal complications
Intrauterine growth retardation
Prematurity
Small for gestational age birthweight

SVT supraventricular tachycardia

had a Fontan operation were advised to refrain from pregnancy. Currently Fontan circulation is not an absolute contraindication to pregnancy; however, risks must be thoughtfully considered. In this setting, a multidisciplinary approach is clearly necessary, including high-risk obstetric care, specialised cardiology assessment and follow-up, genetic counselling and anaesthetic and neonatal care.

15.2 Pregnancy Outcome

15.2.1 Fetal Outcomes

In women with Fontan circulation, there is a higher risk of fetal and neonatal adverse events (Tables 15.1 and 15.2). The fetus is at risk of miscarriage, intrauterine growth retardation and prematurity. If the mother is cyanotic, this risk is even higher [5]. In addition, maternal drug therapy may adversely affect the fetus; the most common of these are oral anticoagulants [6] and beta-blockers [7]. The high incidence of miscarriage could be also the effect of ovarian dysfunction and pelvic venous hypertension. The most common neonatal complications are prematurity and small for gestational age birthweight [8–10]. Different causes may account for this: (a) obstetric complications such as premature rupture of membranes and preterm labour, (b) the limited ability of the heart after a Fontan operation to increase cardiac output and cope with the increased demands of pregnancy and delivery, and (c) the decreased placental oxygen delivery and poor neonatal outcome in a cyanotic patient. In any case, premature delivery is a leading cause of infant morbidity and mortality. Growth of the fetus should be monitored frequently throughout pregnancy.

Despite the severe complexity of mother's heart condition, the overall incidence of congenital heart disease (CHD) in the children is not high (5.6% and 6.9%, respectively, in the French and Mayo Clinic series). Furthermore, when CHD recurs, it does not need to be severe (overall one case with the single ventricle, one with the left superior vena cava, one with the patent ductus arteriosus and one with

Table 15.2 Key points in the management of pregnant women with the Fontan circulation

Preconception counselling
Offer a timely pre-pregnancy counselling in a joint clinic
Discuss reproductive health to prevent false perceptions and reveal reproductive disorders
Asses carefully maternal cardiac status (using clinical examination and full investigations)
Give information on fetal risk
Address and treat all reversible causes of failing FC and precipitating factors
Discuss about effective contraceptive methods in high-risk patients
Gestation period
Offer a close cardiovascular monitoring in a tertiary, multidisciplinary environment
Use medications with the lowest-risk profile for the fetus
Limit strenuous exercise and advise against lying flat to avoid aortocaval compression
Consider some form of antithrombotic therapy:
Full anticoagulation with LMWH in higher thrombotic risk patients
Prophylactic weight-adjusted LMWH or aspirin in the lower thrombotic risk patients
Offer a detailed fetal echocardiogram at 16–23 weeks' gestation
Monitor growth of the fetus frequently throughout pregnancy
Offer early termination in cases of unintended/high-risk pregnancy
Delivery/postpartum period
Reserve Caesarean section for obstetric indications and for patients in severe heart failure
Prefer spinal-epidural anaesthesia with spontaneous ventilation to general anaesthesia
Maintain left lateral decubitus position to assure a good preload
Ensure good control of pain and anxiety during delivery using regional techniques, intravenous pain medications and other non-pharmacological techniques
Assure maternal monitoring during labour and delivery including continuous ECG/BP monitoring and pulse oximetry and occasionally invasive BP recording
Consider antibiotic prophylaxis at the time of delivery
If necessary to support systemic CO, use milrinone instead of ephedrine and phenylephrine
Assure adequate hydration and use of compression stockings to reduce the risk of thrombotic events
Infuse oxytocin at the slowest effective dose to avoid significant vasodilation and hypotension

FC Fontan circulation, *LMWH* low molecular weight heparin, *ECG* electrocardiogram, *BP* blood pressure, *CO* cardiac output

the membranous ventricular septal defect) [9, 10]. However, all pregnant patients with Fontan circulation should be offered a detailed fetal echocardiogram at 16–23 weeks of gestation.

15.2.2 Maternal Outcomes

Maternal complications are low in a well-functioning Fontan patient. In the largest series of pregnant women with Fontan operation published to date (59 pregnancies in 37 patients from a multicentre French study [9]; 70 pregnancies in 19 patients from the Mayo Clinic's experience [10]), there have been no reported maternal deaths; medical issues with earlier pregnancies were not always predictive of difficulties with later pregnancies in the multiparous women. Although there is a risk of maternal morbidity, most complications are treatable (Table 15.1).

15.2.3 Arrhythmias

The most common cardiac complication reported is a supraventricular arrhythmia. Past medical history of arrhythmia was significantly predictive of atrial arrhythmia during pregnancy, while no association was found with the type of palliation, although review of the literature indicates that the type of Fontan palliation may play a role in arrhythmia genesis during pregnancy [8]. The mechanism behind this complication involves scar tissue formation in the right atrium, damage to the sinoatrial node during previous atriotomy and exposure of the right atrium tissue to elevated pressures. In addition, pregnancy increases plasma volumes, and elevated levels of oestrogen and progesterone cause augmentation of adrenergic receptor activity. Atrial arrhythmias are considered to be a medical emergency and are notoriously resistant to pharmacological therapy. Hence, electrical cardioversion is often required. In this case, the fetal heart rate should be checked before and after for the risk of fetal bradycardias. However, energies of up to 300 W/s have been used without affecting the fetus or inducing premature labour. Recurrent arrhythmias may be managed with catheter ablation using CARTO navigation system without fluoroscopy in tertiary ACHD centres [11].

15.2.4 Heart Failure

Physiological changes related to pregnancy may worsen the mother's functional capacity and symptoms of heart failure [12], particularly those with morphological right ventricles [13], who, when compared to patients with a left ventricle, are more prone to failure. As a result, there is a high incidence of miscarriage, prematurity and intrauterine fetal growth retardation. Depending on the woman's clinical status, in-patient bed rest, oxygen supplementation and medical treatment of arrhythmia (diuretic, etc.) should be considered, especially during the third trimester.

15.2.5 Thromboembolism

Thromboembolic complications are possible in patients with the Fontan circulation. However, in the largest series, the incidence was low, three cases in 59 pregnancies, two during the antepartum period and one during the peripartum, and there were no thromboembolic complications amongst 70 pregnancies from the French and American experience [9, 10]. One can speculate, if these lower complication rates may be at least in part due to the anticoagulation/antiplatelet therapy and the lower thrombotic profile of TCPC, present in the majority of the younger pregnant women with the Fontan circulation.

15.2.6 Obstetric Complications

Obstetric complications appear to be a major problem of pregnancy in the context of Fontan palliation: miscarriages with higher rates observed in cyanotic patients, preterm rupture of membranes, premature labour and delivery between 26 and 33 weeks and postpartum haemorrhage are the most common complications. Although these complications do not lead to maternal mortality, they pose a major morbidity and mortality risk to the fetus.

15.3 Management

Patients with the Fontan circulation should be cared for in a tertiary, multidisciplinary environment where a 24 h service of experienced obstetricians, anaesthetists, cardiologists, cardiac surgeons and neonatologists is available. Careful planning for antenatal care and delivery is needed. According to cardiovascular changes occurring in pregnancy, it is appropriate to consider three periods, each with its own risks.

15.3.1 Pregnancy

The duration of gestation period is often reduced in women with a Fontan circulation (between 26 and 36 weeks) due to preterm rupture of membranes, premature labour and delivery [8–10]. Monitoring should focus on early signs of heart failure, arrhythmia, thromboembolic complications and worsening cyanosis. Serial echocardiograms are needed to assess overall ventricular size and function and valve gradients and determine any changes, which may influence delivery plans. In this phase, Fontan patients should limit strenuous exercise, obtain adequate rest and be advised against lying flat during pregnancy to avoid aortocaval compression (rolling from the supine to the left lateral position increases the stroke volume and cardiac output). Depending on the individual's clinical status, in-patient bed rest and oxygen supplementation may be considered during the third trimester.

15.3.2 Labour and Delivery

The cardiovascular system is affected by pain, uterine contractions, medications, maternal position and type of delivery. The timing and mode of delivery and anaesthesia may be selected according to the specific clinical scenario; in general it should be agreed after a multidisciplinary case discussion including the patient. Vaginal delivery is preferable because it is associated with less blood loss, less risk of infection and fewer thromboembolic events [14]. However, it should be undertaken at institutions where there is considerable experience in neuraxial blockade and assisted vaginal deliveries. It is important to ensure good control of pain and anxiety to minimise any further increase in cardiac output. This is achieved using regional techniques, intravenous pain medications and other non-pharmacological techniques [15]. From a haemodynamic point of view, the uterine contractions result in a further increase in cardiac output by up to 60%, and after immediately delivery, stroke volume increases due to autotransfusion of uterine blood and enhanced venous return following relief of vena cava obstruction [7, 16].

There is no consensus regarding absolute contraindications to vaginal delivery, but Caesarean section is reserved for obstetric indications and for patients in severe heart failure [15]. Delivery by Caesarean section does provide the benefits of minimising the deleterious cardiovascular effects caused by repeated Valsalva manoeuvres and the increases in positive intrathoracic pressure required to achieve a vaginal delivery. Furthermore, a delivery should be scheduled at the time when maximum clinical support is available, which is more difficult to arrange in the case of an attempted vaginal delivery. Maternal monitoring during labour and delivery is obviously necessary and usually includes continuous electrocardiographic, blood pressure monitoring and pulse oximetry and occasionally invasive blood pressure recording. It is important to avoid dehydration, which may reduce central venous pressure and blood flow through the cavopulmonary connection to the lungs. With adequate hydration in combination with the use of compression stockings, it is also possible to minimise the risk of thrombotic events during labour and delivery.

15.3.3 Postpartum

The immediate postpartum period is the third phase and also a potentially high-risk period. It is characterised by further 30 % increase in cardiac output. Despite an estimated 500–1,000 mL of blood lost during delivery, blood volume expands as a consequence of the loss of the placental circulatory bed and the contracting uterus. Hence, there is a risk of cardiac decompensation up to 1 week postpartum. Oxytocin should be infused at the slowest effective dose in such patients because it can produce significant vasodilation and hypotension, which may result in devastating cardiovascular consequences in single ventricle patients [17].

15.3.4 Medical Therapy

Patients with good function of the Fontan circulation usually do not need regular/chronic medications, with the exception of anticoagulation/antiplatelet therapy. However, if the patient with single ventricle physiology is optimised with cardiac drugs, these medications should be continued throughout pregnancy, but the lowest possible effective dose should be applied. The use of various cardiovascular drugs during pregnancy has been recently and comprehensively reviewed [18–20]. With the exception of heparin, almost all cardiovascular medications can be expected to cross the placental barrier. Whenever possible, medications with the lowest-risk profile should be used for the management of cardiac disease during pregnancy. Commonly used cardiac medications that can have detrimental effects on the fetus or neonate include warfarin, angiotensin-converting enzyme inhibitors and angiotensin receptor blockers. Timing of exposure may be important, and risks and benefits of the medications for the mother need to be considered.

15.3.5 Infectious Endocarditis Prophylaxis

Due to lack of evidence that infective endocarditis is related to vaginal or Caesarean section, antibiotic prophylaxis is not generally recommended by the American Heart Association (AHA)/American College of Cardiology (ACC) or European guidelines [20, 21]. Nevertheless, antibiotic prophylaxis is helpful at the time of delivery for repaired single ventricle patients. These patients are considered to be at risk because of the prosthetic material used in the procedure; further the presence of a shunt increases the risk of a paradoxical septic embolism [17].

15.3.6 Anticoagulation

Patients with the Fontan operation are at increased risk of intracardiac thrombus formation with a reported incidence ranging from 17 to 33 % [22, 23]. This risk is due to a combination of factors, including the existence of prosthetic material, increased risk of atrial arrhythmia and low cardiac output resulting in a low-flow prothrombotic state [24]. In addition, there is evidence that single ventricle physiology is associated with a baseline deficiency in anticoagulant factors, such as antithrombin III and proteins C and S. However, this finding may be balanced by an equivalent deficiency in procoagulant factors [25]. Overall, there remains controversy regarding the need for routine anticoagulation in all patients following Fontan surgery. Some groups, such as patients with a history of thrombosis, low cardiac output, arrhythmias, atrial dilation and original right atrium-pulmonary artery connection, are more routinely anticoagulated. A randomised trial suggested that aspirin is as effective as coumadin in preventing thrombotic events. However, despite full anticoagulation, thromboembolic events may still occur in these patients [26]. As showed by Tomkiewicz-Pajak et al. patients with a Fontan circulation, despite having significantly reduced platelet numbers, have increased basal platelet activity, increased thrombogenesis, endothelial dysfunction and evidence of systemic inflammation. Although these data support the use of anti-platelet therapy in the same study, a significant proportion of aspirin-treated adults with a Fontan circulation were resistant to aspirin, which may account for the inability of aspirin to prevent thrombotic complications in these patients [27]. Pregnancy itself intensifies the risk of venous thromboembolic complications, with an estimated eightfold increase, which rises to 11-fold during the peripartum period [28]. Therefore, despite the lack of solid evidence, pregnant women with Fontan circulation should be considered for some form of antithrombotic therapy, either full anticoagulation with low molecular weight heparin in higher thrombotic risk patients, prophylactic weight-adjusted low molecular weight heparin (owing to the teratogenic effects of coumadin) or aspirin. The last can be used either in isolation or combined with anticoagulant agents but should be stopped at 35 weeks of gestation.

15.3.7 Anaesthetic Management

The goal of any anaesthetic should be to balance the pulmonary and systemic blood flow by preserving ventricular systolic function, minimising the cardiac depressant effects of anaesthetic agents, keeping pulmonary vascular resistance low and maintaining sinus rhythm, all of which are crucial in maintaining an adequate cardiac output. Spontaneous ventilation is beneficial in that the negative intrathoracic pressure created during inspiration augments blood flow to the lungs and thus improves oxygenation [29]. The use of low-dose epidural analgesia or sequential low-dose combined spinal-epidural anaesthesia may therefore be preferred to general anaesthesia since positive pressure ventilation may result in decreased preload and thus a decreased cardiac output. A decrease in pulmonary vascular resistance is facilitated by providing supplemental oxygen, keeping the PCO_2 level normal to low normal, and preventing and treating respiratory acidosis. Regional anaesthesia also provides the theoretical benefit of avoiding the negative inotropic effects of most anaesthetic agents. If general anaesthesia is necessary, in addition to the standard pregnancy precautions, the left lateral decubitus position is crucial in maintaining preload in patients with single ventricle physiology. Ventilatory parameters should keep peak airway pressures low in order to decrease pulmonary vascular resistance and maintain oxygenation; spontaneous ventilation should be resumed as soon as possible. Haemodynamically stable induction agents such as ketamine and etomidate also should be considered. When it is necessary to support systemic cardiac output, milrinone, an inotrope and vasodilator acting through increases in contractility and decreases in pulmonary vascular resistance, may be the drug of choice in patients with single ventricle physiology, significant baseline cyanosis, and a low cardiac output state [30]. The commonly used vasopressors (ephedrine and phenylephrine) have disadvantages for patients with single ventricle physiology, causing excessive tachycardia (which can cause decreased preload and cardiac output) and increasing in pulmonary vascular resistance and systemic vascular resistance, both of which may negatively affect cardiac output.

For either vaginal delivery or Caesarean section, it is advisable to monitor the patients with a continuous ECG, have large-bore intravenous access and place an arterial catheter for constant BP evaluation. For patients with decreased cardiac function, reliable central access for vasoactive medications should be achieved with a central catheter [31]. An echocardiogram assessing structure and ventricular function helps guide decisions and optimisation of cardiac function. It is important to avoid hypovolaemia during the labour and postpartum period because it may reduce central venous pressure and blood flow through the cavopulmonary connection to the lungs. Sinus rhythm should be maintained with medications such as beta-blockers, channel blockers or DC cardioversion, if necessary, in a haemodynamically unstable parturient.

15.4 Impact of Physiological Changes of Pregnancy

The first trimester of gestation is characterised by several changes in haemodynamic parameters: (a) increase in total blood volume, plasma volume and red blood cell volume; (b) increase in cardiac output, stroke volume and heart rate; and (c) decrease in systemic and pulmonary vascular resistance a consequence of hormonal influences and the later development of the high-flow, low-resistance maternal-placental circulation [7, 16]. At the end of gestation, i.e. third trimester, rapid growth of the fetus and enlargement of the uterus result in haemodynamically significant compression of the inferior vena cava and a resultant drop in venous return to the heart and in cardiac output especially in supine position [32]. These changes pose particular challenges to Fontan patients who are very sensitive to preload and thus at risk for oedema, ascites and arrhythmias. Hence, frequent cardiac assessment should be in place throughout pregnancy.

15.5 Preconception Counselling

The different biopsychological periods in a woman's life, including menarche, sexuality, pregnancies, and menopause, are all interactively associated with the cardiovascular system [33]. The causal biologic pathway between the cardiac anomaly and ovarian function has never been studied in depth and no prospective data are available. Drenthen et al. reported on a series of 38 female patients with Fontan palliation, whereas age at menarche was on average 14.6 years, which is significantly higher than the 13.0–13.2 years found in the general population in the Netherlands and Belgium. The incidence of primary amenorrhoea furthermore was particularly high [8]. It has been hypothesised that in Fontan patients, abnormal menstrual patterns represent recurrent anovulatory cycles, dysfunction of the hypopituitary-ovarian axis or disturbed uterine homeostasis due to chronic hypoxemia before the palliation, chronic venous congestion or hyperviscosity [34]. In addition to the cardiac defect itself, repeat surgical interventions during childhood might have interfered with the complex physiologic processes involved in the ovarian cycle. Recent data derived from a multicentre French study revealed that the infertility rate is high in Fontan population compared to healthy women of the same age (6%) [9]. These data are consistent with the Mayo Clinic's experience regarding 138 women with available contraception/pregnancy data; there were 35 women with known pregnancies amongst them but only 49/138 (36%) patients with previous counselling against pregnancy [10]. This may suggest possible difficulty of Fontan female patients in becoming pregnant, independent of cardiac concerns, due to an underling infertility problem.

Vigl et al. showed that women with complex or cyanotic cardiac anomalies experienced reproductive and sexuality disorders: amongst 536 adult female patients with CHD, menarche was significantly delayed with increased risk of menstrual irregularities and menstrual discomfort and increased or altered cardiac symptoms during sexual activity [35]. It is difficult to ascertain how much of these reports relate to biological-organic dysfunction or to psychosocial issues in the context of chronic illness. Scars and cyanosis in adult patients with CHD as well as the fear of physical overexertion increase self-consciousness and decrease body image, which could account for the decreased levels of sexual activity in these patients [36, 37]. Although patients with CHD are physically limited by their condition, anxiety about possible complications could also play a role. Reid et al. reported that women with complex CHD, like Fontan patients, have the highest levels of concern regarding their fertility and risk of genetic transmission of CHD, as well as concerns about adverse effects of pregnancy on their own health [38].

These data emphasise the need to be particularly attentive to the discussion on sexual health with female patients to prevent false perceptions. In addition, it is important for the medical point of view to consider the clinical implications of chronic anovulation, deciding whether they represent an underactivity of the hypothalamic pituitary ovarian axis, and so cause a hypo-oestrogenic state with risks of bone under-mineralisation or a polycystic ovarian situation, where high baseline levels of oestrogen promote unopposed endometrial growth resulting in an increased risk of endometrial hyperplasia, the formation of polyps, fibroids and histologic atypia. In fact, menorrhagia after anovulatory cycles is a relevant cause of iron-deficiency anaemia. Furthermore, menorrhagia has been named a possible prothrombotic condition in itself, increasing the risk of thrombotic events [39].

All Fontan women of reproductive age should undergo thorough evaluation prior to becoming pregnant. This should be provided in a joint clinic by an obstetrician with expertise in high-risk pregnancy and a cardiologist with special training in adult congenital heart disease. This evaluation should focus first on identifying and quantifying the risk to the mother. Second, it should address potential risks to the fetus, including the risk of recurrence of congenital heart disease. Parental life expectancy should be discussed, as also premature death, disability, or the need for major surgery will obviously affect a couple's ability to care for their child. This consultation allows women to make an informed decision. Furthermore, the evaluation prior to counselling may uncover an anatomical or functional problem that should be addressed before pregnancy. These may include arrhythmias, decreased systolic function of the systemic ventricle, cyanosis, heart failure, venous pathway obstruction or leak, protein-losing enteropathy, etc. Hence, a preconception evaluation should involve at a minimum a physical examination, electrocardiogram, echocardiogram and blood tests. Cardiac magnetic resonance imaging should also be part of this evaluation because transthoracic echocardiography may provide only limited information on ventricular function. Cardiopulmonary exercise testing may be helpful to assess the woman's ability to increase cardiac output and preserve oxygen saturation during exercise. Further investigations should be considered on a case-by-case basis, but may include left/right heart catheterisation or CT scan. All reversible causes of failing Fontan circulation (arrhythmias, haemodynamic lesions) and precipitating factors such as anaemia should be sought and treated, Fig. 15.2.

Pregnancy, with the increased blood volume and tendency for thrombosis, is a risk for patients with Fontan circulation. This can result in deterioration in ventricular function and increasing atrioventricular valve regurgitation. The inevitable elevation in the right atrial pressure predisposes to tachyarrhythmias and worsening of cyanosis if a right-to-left shunt is present [40, 41]. There is no standardised risk stratification system, which is able to distinguish between high-risk and low-risk Fontan women during pregnancy. According to the risk assessment analysis of pregnant women with congenital and acquired heart disease proposed by Siu et al. it is

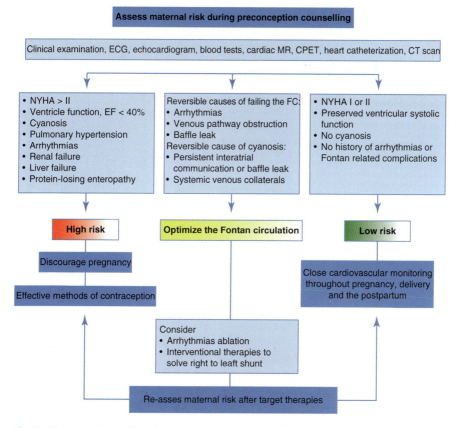

Fig. 15.2 Proposed algorithm for maternal risk assessment during pregnancy in women with the Fontan circulation (FC). *ECG* electrocardiogram, *MR* magnetic resonance, *CPET* cardiopulmonary exercise test, *CT* computed tomography. *EF* ejection fraction

possible to recognise specific clinical situations that significantly increase the risk of cardiac events during pregnancy [42, 43]:

- Fontan women with poor functional class before pregnancy (New York Heart Association functional classification > II)
- Cyanosis
- Impaired systemic ventricular function (ejection fraction <40%)
- Pulmonary hypertension
- Preconception history of adverse cardiac events such as symptomatic arrhythmia, stroke, transient ischaemic attack and pulmonary oedema
- Other major complications related to Fontan physiology

In presence of one or more of these clinical circumstances, a woman should be discouraged from becoming pregnant as there is a high risk of significant morbidity or mortality. Effective methods of contraception should be discussed, and, in the case of an unintended pregnancy, early termination should be offered. Combined oral contraceptives should be avoided because of the prothrombotic effects of oestrogen. Depot injections of progestogen, or an intrauterine device impregnated with progestogen, are highly effective and safe. Sterilisation should be considered for women in whom pregnancy would carry a prohibitively high risk or when a couple decide that they never want to have children. However, it is important to consider the surgical risks associated with the procedure.

Women with Fontan palliation can have a much lower pregnancy-related risk if they are functional class (NYHA) I or II, have preserved ventricular function, have no cyanosis at rest or during exercise and have no history of arrhythmia. Although in this scenario maternal mortality risk appears low, arrhythmias, heart failure and thromboembolic events may still occur. All women should be aware, therefore, that they will need close cardiovascular monitoring in a tertiary, multidisciplinary environment throughout pregnancy, delivery and the postpartum.

15.5.1 Preconception Interventions to Reduce Cyanosis

In the absence of an atrial fenestration, patients with a Fontan circulation have systemic arterial O_2 saturation over 94 % and normal haemoglobin level [44]. Common causes of worsening hypoxemia include shunting through a persistent interatrial communication or a baffle leak [45], systemic venous collaterals, pulmonary arteriovenous malformations, progressive ventricular dysfunction with or without atrioventricular valve regurgitation, pulmonary venous compression [46] and pulmonary restrictive pathology. If a patient is cyanotic, she has a greater chance of complications during pregnancy [47]. In their literature review of 2,491 pregnancies in women with congenital heart disease, Drenthen et al. reported that cyanotic patients (the single ventricle with cyanosis was not a separate category) had a 40 % spontaneous abortion rate, 3 % developed arrhythmias, 14 % developed heart failure, and 3 % developed endocarditis. In contrast, patients with cyanosis in the setting of Fontan had rates of spontaneous abortion and dysrhythmias equal to 40 % and 16 %, respectively, but no episodes of heart failure or endocarditis. Perinatal mortality was 3 % in the overall cyanotic group and less than 1 % in the Fontan group [5]. Such findings reinforce the need to prevent or minimise cyanosis. If cyanosis is the major concern in a woman with good function of the Fontan circuit, closure of the right-to-left shunt secondary to atrial fenestration or baffle leak before pregnancy should be undertaken to improve the outcome of the pregnancy. Usually, the procedure can be performed percutaneously with transcatheter umbrella devices or covered stents [45]. Obliteration of systemic venous collaterals or pulmonary arteriovenous malformations by detachable coils may also be considered, albeit often complicated by high rates of recurrence [48].

15.5.2 Total Cavopulmonary Conversion (TCPC)

Despite a higher incidence of arrhythmias and thromboembolic complications with classical Fontan circuits, the desire to pursue pregnancy cannot currently be considered a sufficient indication for TCPC, given the associated surgical risks and residual poorly defined maternal and fetal complication rates.

15.5.3 Fertility Treatment

Therapeutic interventions to overcome infertility may carry risks, in particular thromboembolic complications and fluid overload. During in vitro fertilisation, controlled ovarian stimulation leads to multiple oocytes and supraphysiological levels of oestrogens [49, 50]. The consequence is an increase in the procoagulant state during pregnancy and the possibility of multiple pregnancies. Both of these conditions can worsen the outcome of pregnancy in these women.

15.5.4 Termination of Pregnancy

Unplanned pregnancies in women with high risk of morbidity/mortality may require termination as a therapeutic intervention. It should be performed as soon as the decision has been made because the risk of termination of pregnancy increases with increasing gestational age. Ideally, in the first trimester, suction curettage under local anaesthesia is the preferred method. Medical abortion with oral antiprogesterones and vaginally administered prostaglandins is probably contraindicated because of the haemodynamic and other adverse effects (systemic vasodilation with hypotension, increasing cyanosis, heavy bleeding and retention of products with infection) are unpredictable.

References

1. Fontan F, Baudet E (1971) Surgical repair of tricuspid atresia. Thorax 26:240–248
2. Reul GJ, Gregoric ID (1992) Recent modifications of the Fontan procedure for complex congenital heart disease. Tex Heart Inst J 19:223–242
3. Khairy P, Fernandes SM, Mayer JE Jr et al (2008) Long-term survival, modes of death, and predictors of mortality in patients with Fontan surgery. Circulation 117(1):85–92
4. d'Udekem Y, Iyengar AJ, Galati JC et al (2014) Redefining expectations of long-term survival after the Fontan procedure: twenty-five years of follow-up from the entire population of Australia and New Zealand. Circulation 130(11 Suppl 1):S32–S38
5. Drenthen W, Pieper PG, Roos-Hesselink JW, ZAHARA Investigators et al (2007) Outcome of pregnancy in women with congenital heart disease: a literature review. J Am Coll Cardiol 49:2303–2311
6. Mehndiratta S, Suneja A, Gupta B et al (2010) Fetotoxicity of warfarin anticoagulation. Arch Gynecol Obstet 282:335–337

7. Gelson E, Curry R, Gatzoulis MA et al (2011) Effect of maternal heart disease on fetal growth. Obstet Gynecol 118:364. [29] Fujitani S, Baldisseri MR (2005) Hemodynamic assessment in a pregnant and peripartum patient. Crit Care Med 33(10 Suppl):S354–S361
8. Drenthen W, Pieper PG, Roos-Hesselink JW et al (2006) Pregnancy and delivery in women after Fontan palliation. Heart 92:1290–1294
9. Gouton M, Nizard J, Patel M et al (2015) Maternal and fetal outcomes of pregnancy with Fontan circulation: a multicentric observational study. Int J Cardiol 187:84–89
10. Pundi NK, Pundi K, Johnson JN et al (2015) Contraception practices and pregnancy outcome in patients after Fontan operation. Congenit Heart Dis
11. Kozluk E, Gawrysiak M, Piatkwoska A et al (2013) Radiofrequency ablation without the use of fluoroscopy: in what kind of patients is it feasible? Arch Med Sci 9(5):821–825
12. Fernandes SM, McElhinney DB, Khairy P et al (2010) Serial cardiopulmonary exercise testing in patients with previous Fontan surgery. Pediatr Cardiol 31(2):175–180
13. Jain VD, Moghbeli N, Webb G et al (2011) Pregnancy in women with congenital heart disease: the impact of a systemic right ventricle. Congenit Heart Dis 6(2):147–156
14. Bonanno C, Gaddipati S (2008) Mechanisms of hemostasis at caesarean delivery. Clin Perinatol 35:531–547
15. European Society of Gynecology (ESG), Association for European Paediatric Cardiology (AEPC), German Society for Gender Medicine (DGesGM), Regitz-Zagrosek V, Blomstrom Lundqvist C, Borghi et al (2011) ESC Guidelines on the management of cardiovascular diseases during pregnancy: the Task force on the Management of Cardiovascular Diseases during Pregnancy of the European Society of Cardiology (ESC). Eur Heart J 32:3147–3197
16. Hunter S, Robson SC (1992) Adaptation of the maternal heart in pregnancy. Br Heart J 68(6):540–543
17. Uebing A, Steer PJ, Yentis SM, Gatzoulis MA (2006) Pregnancy and congenital heart disease. BMJ 332(7538):401–406
18. Bonow RO, Carabello BA, Kanu C et al (2006) ACC/AHA 2006 guidelines for the management of patients with valvular heart disease: a report of the American College of Cardiology/American Heart Association Task Force on Practice Guidelines (writing committee to revise the 1998 Guidelines for the Management of Patients With Valvular Heart Disease): developed in collaboration with the Society of Cardiovascular Anesthesiologists: endorsed by the Society for Cardiovascular Angiography and Interventions and the Society of Thoracic Surgeons. Circulation 114:e84–e231
19. Khalil A, O'Brien P (2006) Cardiac drugs in pregnancy. In: Steer P, Gatzoulis M, Baker P (eds) Heart disease and pregnancy. RCOG Press, London, pp 79–95
20. Regitz-Zagrosek V, Blomstrom Lundqvist C, Borghi C et al (2011) ESC Guidelines on the management of cardiovascular diseases during pregnancy: the Task Force on the Management of Cardiovascular Diseases during Pregnancy of the European Society of Cardiology (ESC). Eur Heart J 32:3147–3197
21. Warnes CA, Williams RG, Bashore TM et al (2008) ACC/AHA 2008 guidelines for the management of adults with congenital heart disease a report of the American College of Cardiology/American Heart Association Task Force on Practice Guidelines (Writing Committee to Develop Guidelines on the Management of Adults With Congenital Heart Disease): Developed in Collaboration With the American Society of Echocardiography, Heart Rhythm Society, International Society for Adult Congenital Heart Disease, Society for Cardiovascular Angiography and Interventions, and Society of Thoracic Surgeons. Circulation 118:e714–e833
22. Gewillig M, Goldberg DJ (2014) Failure of the Fontan circulation. Heart Fail Clin 10:105–116
23. Tomkiewicz-Pajak L, Hoffman P, Trojnarska O et al (2013) Long term follow-up in adult patients after Fontan operations. Pol J Cardiothorac Surg 10:357–363
24. Aboul Hosn JA, Shavelle DM, Castellon Y et al (2007) Fontan operation and the single ventricle. Congenit Heart Dis 2:2–11
25. Walker HA, Gatzoulis MA (2005) Prophylactic anticoagulation following the Fontan operation. Heart 91:854–856

26. Monagle P, Cochrane A, Roberts R, Fontan Anticoagulation StudyGroup et al (2011) A multicenter, randomized trial comparing heparin/warfarin and acetylsalicylic acid as primary thromboprophylaxis for 2 years after the Fontan procedure in children. J Am Coll Cardiol 58:645–651
27. Tomkiewicz-Pajak L, Wojcik T, Chłopicki S (2015) Aspirin resistance in adult patients after Fontan surgery. Int J Cardiol 181:19–26
28. Heit JA, Kobbervig CE, James AH et al (2005) Trends in the incidence of venous thromboembolism during pregnancy or postpartum: a 30-year population-based study. Ann Intern Med 143(10):697–706
29. Naguib MA, Dob DP, Gatzoulis MA (2010) A functional understanding of moderate to complex congenital heart disease and the impact of pregnancy. Part II: tetralogy of Fallot, Eisenmenger's syndrome and the Fontan operation. Int J Obstet Anesth 19:306–312
30. Bailey PD Jr, Jobes DR (2009) The Fontan patient. Anesthesiol Clin 27:285–300
31. Jooste EH, Haft WA, Ames WA et al (2013) Anesthetic care of parturients with single ventricle physiology. J Clin Anesth 25:417–423
32. Clark SL, Cotton DB, Pivarnik JM et al (1991) Position change and central hemodynamic profile during normal third-trimester pregnancy and post partum. Am J Obstet Gynecol 164:883–887
33. Somerville J (1989) Congenital heart disease in the adolescent. Arch Dis Child 64:771–773
34. Canobbio MM, Mair DD, Rapkin AJ et al (1990) Menstrual patterns in females after the Fontan repair. Am J Cardiol 66:238–240
35. Vigl M, Kaemmerer M, Niggemeyer E et al (2010) Sexuality and reproductive health in women with congenital heart disease. Am J Cardiol 105:538–541
36. Kovacs AH, Sears SF, Saidi AS (2005) Biopsychosocial experiences of adults with congenital heart disease: review of the literature. Am Heart J 150:193–201
37. Karsdorp PA, Kindt M, Rietveld S, Everaerd W, Mulder BJ (2008) Interpretation bias for heart sensations in congenital heart disease and its relation to quality of life. Int J Behav Med 15:232–240
38. Reid G, Siu S, McCrindle B et al (2008) Sexual behavior and reproductive concerns among adolescents and young adults with congenital heart disease. Int J Cardiol 125:332–338
39. Sundström A, Seaman H, Kieler H, Alfredsson L (2009) The risk of venous thromboembolism associated with the use of tranexamic acid and other drugs used to treat menorrhagia: a case-control study using the general practice research database. Br J Obstet Gynaecol 116:91–97
40. Gewillig M (2005) The Fontan circulation. Heart 91:839–846, 4
41. Walker F (2007) Pregnancy and the various forms of the Fontan circulation. Heart 93:152–154
42. Siu SC, Sermer M, Harrison DA, Grigoriadis E, Liu G, Sorensen S et al (1997) Risk and predictors for pregnancy-related complications in women with heart disease. Circulation 96:2789–2794
43. Siu SC, Sermer M, Colman JM, Alvarez AN, Mercier LA, Morton BC et al (2001) Prospective multicenter study of pregnancy outcomes in women with heart disease. Circulation 104:515–521
44. Magee AG, McCrindle BW, Mawson J et al (1998) Systemic venous collateral development after the bidirectional cavopulmonary anastomosis. Prevalence and predictors. J Am Coll Cardiol 32(2):502–508
45. Gamillscheg A, Beitzke A, Stein JI et al (1998) Transcatheter coil occlusion of residual interatrial communications after Fontan procedure. Heart 80(1):49–53
46. O'Donnell CP, Lock JE, Powell AJ, Perry SB (2003) Compression of pulmonary veins between the left atrium and the descending aorta. Am J Cardiol 91(2):248–251
47. Presbitero P, Somerville J, Stone S et al (1994) Pregnancy in cyanotic congenital heart disease. Outcome of mother and fetus. Circulation 89(6):2673–2676
48. Hsu HS, Nykanen DG, Williams WG et al (1995) Right to left interatrial communications after the modified Fontan procedure: identification and management with transcatheter occlusion. Br Heart J 74(5):548–552
49. Szecsi PB, Jorgensen M, Klajnbard A, Andersen MR, Colov NP, Stender S (2010) Haemostatic reference intervals in pregnancy. Thromb Haemost 103:718–727
50. Hansen AT, Kesmodel US, Juul S et al (2014) Increased venous thrombosis incidence in pregnancies after in vitro fertilization. Hum Reprod 29(3):611–617

Cyanotic Lesions

16

Matthias Greutmann and Daniel Tobler

Abbreviation

SpO_2 Transcutaneous oxygen saturation

> **Key Facts**
> *Incidence*: The number of women with cyanotic heart defects in childbearing age become increasingly rare. These women are however at high risk during pregnancy
> *Inheritance*: 3–5 %, In the case of associaten with 22q11-microdeletion syndrome (autosomal dominant inheritance) the risk is much higher.
> *Medication*: Angiotensin-converting enzyme inhibitors, angiotensin and aldosterone antagonists are contraindicated.
> *World Health Organization class*: III, but with pulmonary hypertension, IV.
> *Risk of pregnancy*: Spontaneous abortion (50 %), maternal complications (heart failure (18.9 %), arrhythmias (4.8 %), endocarditis (4.1 %) and thromboembolic complications (3.6 %).
> *Life expectancy*: Markedly reduced.

M. Greutmann, MD (✉)
University Heart Center, Department of Cardiology, University Hospital Zurich,
Zurich, Switzerland
e-mail: matthias.greutmann@usz.ch

D. Tobler, MD
Department of Cardiology, University Hospital Basel,
Basel, Switzerland
e-mail: daniel.tobler@usb.ch

> **Key Management**
> *Preconception*: Detailed review of diagnostic procedures, interventions and previous complications. Echocardiography: valve and ventricular function, estimate pulmonary artery pressure (if uncertain then cardiac catheterisation). If complex anatomy: CMR or CT. Exercise testing. Blood: BNP, full blood count and iron stores.
> *Pregnancy*: Intensive follow-up minimum of four weekly, resting oxygen saturations, blood tests and echocardiography (at least twice). Iron deficiency must be avoided
> *Labour*: There are no data on mode of delivery. Careful multidisciplinary delivery planning is important
> *Postpartum*: At least 48 h. Meticulous thromboembolic prophylaxis and use of air bubble filters for intravenous lines are mandatory.

16.1 The Condition

Cyanotic heart defects are a heterogeneous group of congenital heart defects with an estimated incidence at birth of about 1.3/1,000 live births [1]. The natural history of cyanotic congenital heart defects is bleak, and without intervention, childhood mortality is high [2]. With the advent of surgical palliation and intracardiac repair operations, the fate of patients born with cyanotic congenital heart defects has changed dramatically. Currently almost all such patients undergo timely intracardiac repair in childhood, alleviating cyanosis and allowing survival to adulthood in the large majority. Survival with non-cyanotic unrepaired shunt lesions is better, but if left unrepaired, many patients with large shunts develop irreversible pulmonary vascular disease and eventually Eisenmenger syndrome associated with shunt reversal and right-to-left shunting leading to progressive cyanosis. In developed countries, most shunt lesions are repaired in a timely manner, and the number of patients who develop Eisenmenger syndrome is now exceedingly small. Given these trends of early repair of shunt lesions and timely repair of complex cyanotic defects, the number of adult survivors with cyanotic lesions is decreasing in developed countries, particularly the number of young adults with cyanotic lesions and hence the number of affected women of childbearing age (Fig. 16.1) [3]. This decreasing number of adults with cyanotic defects is in sharp contrast to the rapidly expanding cohorts of adult survivors with repaired defects [4]. Adults with unrepaired cyanotic heart defects are a vulnerable patient group with a high risk of morbidity and a markedly increased risk of premature death as young adults [3].

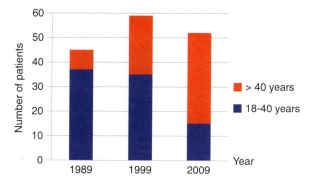

Fig. 16.1 Evolution of numbers of adults with unrepaired cyanotic heart defects stratified for age 18–40 years and >40 years followed at the Toronto Congenital Cardiac Centre for Adults between 1980 and 2009 (Modified from Ref. [3] with permission)

Table 16.1 Types of cyanotic congenital heart defects in adults

Group 1: unrepaired cyanotic defects with obligatory right-to-left shunting
Pulmonary atresia with multicentric pulmonary perfusion
Unrepaired tetralogy of Fallot (in rare cases with only mild right ventricular outflow tract obstruction at rest, the patient may not be cyanotic at rest)
Single ventricle physiology with obstructed pulmonary blood flow
Cyanotic defects after palliative shunt operations without intracardiac repair
Group 2: shunt lesions with resulting irreversible pulmonary hypertension
Eisenmenger syndrome caused by pre-tricuspid shunt lesions (e.g. atrial septal defects)
Eisenmenger syndrome caused by post-tricuspid shunt lesions (e.g. ventricular septal defects)
Eisenmenger syndrome caused by complex congenital heart defects (e.g. single ventricle physiology with unobstructed lung perfusion)
Group 3: congenital cardiac lesions with facultative right-to-left shunting
Ebstein anomaly with interatrial communication
Congenitally corrected transposition of the great arteries associated with ventricular septal defect and pulmonary stenosis (the degree of pulmonary stenosis determines shunt direction)
Group 4: repaired defects with residual lesions leading to right-to-left shunting
Fontan palliation for single ventricle physiology and residual fenestrations or veno-venous collaterals
Patients after atrial switch repair for transposition of the great arteries and residual baffle leaks
Lesions associated with right ventricular diastolic dysfunction (restrictive right ventricular physiology) and residual interatrial shunts

16.1.1 Types of Defects and Pathophysiology of Cyanotic Heart Disease

Cyanotic congenital heart defects that may be encountered in women of childbearing age are summarised in Table 16.1. In this chapter, specific problems pertinent to all congenital cardiac conditions with cyanosis are discussed, but the focus will be on women with unrepaired cyanotic defects with obligatory right-to-left shunting (see Table 16.1 group 1 and Fig. 16.2). More detailed discussion of other lesions potentially associated with cyanosis is found in other chapters (Chaps. 14, 15 and 17).

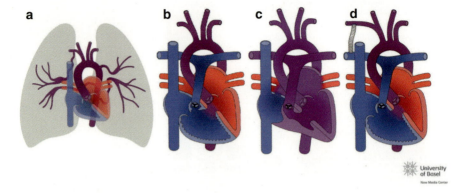

Fig. 16.2 Unrepaired cyanotic defects with obligatory right-to-left shunting (Copyright © 2014 New Media Center, University of Basel. All Rights Reserved). (**a**) Pulmonary atresia with multicentric pulmonary perfusion. (**b**) Unrepaired tetralogy of Fallot. (**c**) Tricuspid atresia with atrial septal defect. (**d**) Tetralogy of Fallot, palliated with right-sided modified Blalock-Taussig shunt

16.1.2 General Aspects and Pathophysiology of Cyanotic Congenital Heart Defects

All cyanotic congenital cardiac defects have in common that deoxygenated systemic venous blood returning to the heart mixes with oxygenated pulmonary venous blood before being ejected into the systemic circulation. Cyanosis is a manifestation of arterial hypoxemia, which can be estimated by transcutaneous oxygen saturation (SpO_2). The degree of hypoxemia depends on the magnitude of right-to-left shunting, which is determined by the size of the shunt lesion (i.e. restrictive or nonrestrictive ventricular septal defect), the amount of pulmonary blood flow and cardiac output. While the size of the shunt lesion is typically fixed, cardiac output and pulmonary blood flow are variable and depend on heart rate, stroke volumes of the ventricles and the ratio of vascular resistance between systemic and pulmonary circulations.

16.2 Pregnancy Outcomes

Risk assessment in women with cyanotic heart defects is a multidisciplinary and multistep endeavour that has to take into account all cardiac and noncardiac aspects impacting the individual [5]. Given the decreasing number of women with unrepaired cyanotic heart defects in childbearing age, this patient group is underrepresented in studies that investigated the outcome of women with congenital heart disease in pregnancy [6–8]. Apart from case reports, only few studies have systematically addressed pregnancy outcomes in women with cyanotic heart defects. The largest study, published in 1994, reported the outcome of 96 pregnancies in 44 women with cyanotic heart defects identified from two European centres [9].

16.2.1 Maternal Outcome

The risk of cardiovascular complications during pregnancy in women with cyanotic congenital heart defects is high, affecting about one third of such women [9, 10]. The most common complication is heart failure, affecting 18.9 % of pregnancies, as reported in the meta-analysis by Drenthen et al. [10]. Other common complications are arrhythmias (4.8 %), endocarditis (4.1 %) and thromboembolic complications (3.6 %). In contrast to cardiovascular complications, obstetric complications seem not to be particularly increased, apart from postpartum haemorrhage, which may be related to coagulation abnormalities and thrombocytopenia, frequently observed in patients with long-standing cyanosis. Nonetheless, the occurrence of obstetric complications, such as hypertensive disorders of pregnancy, pre-eclampsia or multiple pregnancies, increases the haemodynamic load of pregnancy and thus increases the risk of maladaptation and subsequently increases the risk of cardiovascular complications in vulnerable patients [6, 7, 11, 12]. The increased risk of multiple pregnancies may be of particular importance in women seeking assisted fertilisation and underscores the need for optimal multidisciplinary pre-pregnancy communication, counselling and planning.

The occurrence of cardiovascular complications, such as tachyarrhythmias during pregnancy and peripartum may further impair the adaptive capacity of the cardiovascular system and precipitate decompensation. The impact of pregnancy on long-term outcomes in women with cyanotic heart defects is not well defined. Pregnancy may, however, lead to worsening of functional capacity [9].

16.2.2 Fetal Outcomes

Based on data from lesion-specific outcome series and multicentre studies, the risk of adverse fetal events is extremely high in women with unrepaired cyanotic defects [6, 7, 9]. About half of pregnancies end in spontaneous abortion [9]. In on-going pregnancies beyond 20 weeks of gestation the risk of premature delivery is more than 40 % and two thirds of babies are born small for gestational age

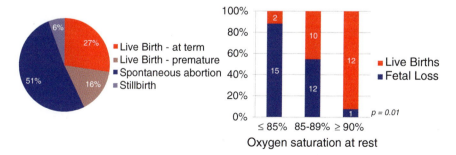

Fig. 16.3 Fetal outcomes. (Panel **a**) Proportion of live births, spontaneous abortion and stillbirths among 96 pregnancies. (Panel **b**) Proportion of live births in relation to resting oxygen saturations (Modified from Ref. [9])

[10]. Prematurity can result from spontaneous premature labour but also from early, induced delivery for maternal (cardiac) reasons. For women with cyanotic congenital heart defects, the risk of having a stillbirth is among the highest in all congenital cardiac defects. The high rate of offspring outcomes is illustrated in Fig. 16.3a, adapted from the study of Presbitero et al. [9]. As illustrated in Fig. 16.3b, the risk of fetal complications is strongly predicted by the severity of cyanosis. The fact that women with resting oxygen saturations below 85 % have a very low chance of delivering a viable offspring may have an important bearing on pregnancy counselling and pre-pregnancy optimisation of the underlying cardiac condition.

Apart from the maternal cardiac condition, the risk for offspring events is also determined by obstetric risk factors, such as maternal age, multiple gestations, history of premature delivery or rupture of membranes, incompetent cervix or antepartum bleeding and placental abnormalities [13]. This underscores the need for a multidisciplinary team approach not only during pregnancy but for pre-pregnancy risk assessment and counselling as well.

The recurrence risk of isolated congenital heart defects in the offspring ranges on average between 3 and 5 % [14]. There is however substantial variability in recurrence risk, depending on familial occurrence and type of defect [15, 16]. Some congenital heart defects that may be encountered in women with unrepaired cyanotic defects (i.e. pulmonary atresia or tetralogy of Fallot) are associated with the 22q11 microdeletion syndrome. The inheritance of the 22q11 microdeletion syndrome is autosomal dominant, and recurrence risk is thus 50%, with a high risk of congenital cardiac defects (particularly conotruncal defects) in the affected offspring.

16.3 Management of Pregnancy

Pregnancies in women with cyanotic congenital heart defects are considered high-risk pregnancies and thus should be managed by a dedicated experienced multidisciplinary team at a tertiary care centre. For each pregnancy, a clear management and follow-up plan must be developed. The frequency of cardiologic and obstetric follow-up visits during pregnancy must be individualised, but most women require close follow-up including frequent assessment of adequate fetal growth. Fetal outcome is associated with uteroplacental blood flow characteristics, and recent evidence suggests that uteroplacental blood flow is associated with maternal haemodynamics in women with congenital heart disease [17]. The impact of changes in uteroplacental blood flow on management decisions needs to be further investigated but may provide an elegant option for additional monitoring maternal haemodynamics [18]. In addition, all pregnant women with CHD should be offered fetal echocardiography between 18 and 21 weeks of gestation.

Assessment at the time of cardiology visits usually includes thorough clinical examination with serial measurements of resting oxygen saturations, blood work to ensure adequate secondary erythrocytosis and adequate iron stores, as well as transthoracic echocardiography at least at baseline and between 28 and 30 weeks of gestation at the haemodynamic peak of pregnancy. Depending on the clinical course, symptoms and findings on clinical examination, echocardiography may be needed more often.

The importance of patient education at each clinic visit cannot be overemphasised. Every woman who experiences novel or worsening symptoms during pregnancy (i.e. palpitations or increasing shortness of breath) should be encouraged to seek prompt assessment by her specialised multidisciplinary team.

As women with unrepaired cyanotic heart defects have a high risk of paradoxical systemic embolism, meticulous thromboembolic prophylaxis is mandatory at times of increased risk, particularly in women requiring bed rest.

16.3.1 Management of Heart Failure in Pregnancy and Peripartum

Women with unrepaired cyanotic heart defects may be prone to develop heart failure, as many have diastolic ventricular dysfunction and may not tolerate the increasing volume load of pregnancy. Serial measurements of natriuretic peptides (Pro-BNP or BNP) may help in diagnosis and risk stratification of heart failure during pregnancy [19, 20].

In women with unrepaired cyanotic heart defects, heart failure may present with worsening cyanosis, as shifts in the balance between systemic and pulmonary vascular resistance may precipitate increased right-to-left shunting. For these women, the mainstay of therapy is bed rest to reduce further exacerbation of cyanosis triggered by physical activity.

If overt heart failure occurs, patients should be admitted to a specialised centre, and precipitating factors, such as infection or arrhythmias, should be actively sought and excluded. Bed rest, supplemental oxygen and careful fluid balance with daily weight measurements should be initiated. Careful administration of diuretics may be used but with caution to avoid overdiuresis which can reduce uteroplacental blood flow.

In the case of refractory heart failure, delivery should be contemplated as soon as the fetus is viable, or, in the case of persistent haemodynamic instability, irrespective of the duration of gestation. Antenatal steroids to improve fetal lung maturity may lead to maternal fluid retention and worsening of heart failure.

16.3.2 Multidisciplinary Delivery Plan

There are no data on whether vaginal delivery or Caesarean section is superior in women with cyanotic heart defects. Depending on the type of defect, myocardial function and residual haemodynamic lesions, women with cyanotic heart defects may have limited cardiovascular reserves to cope with the haemodynamic needs of labour and delivery. Effective analgesia and assisted second stage of delivery can effectively decrease the additional haemodynamic load of labour. Assisted delivery may however be associated with a higher risk of postpartum haemorrhage and high-degree lacerations [21]. The average blood loss during vaginal delivery of 500 ml counteracts the impact of autotransfusion from the contracting uterus at stage 3 of delivery. Blood loss with Caesarean section is usually higher (on average 1,000 ml) which may be a disadvantage in women for whom (relative) anaemia may be deleterious.

A multidisciplinary delivery plan, based on local experience, logistics and infrastructure (e.g. possibilities for monitoring on labour ward), should be developed early in all women with cyanotic heart defects. Given the high rate of premature delivery, this detailed delivery plan must be available and easily accessible as soon as the fetus is viable. Early involvement of experienced obstetric anaesthetists and, if required, the input of cardiac anaesthetists are vital. Important aspects that need to be covered by the delivery plan are summarised in Table 16.2. A schematic drawing of the patient's cardiac anatomy is always helpful and may be of critical importance if emergency central venous line or temporary pacemaker insertion is required in women with unusual systemic venous anatomy. It is wise to ensure that air bubble filters are easily available on the labour ward.

The issue regarding endocarditis prophylaxis remains controversial. Although antibiotic prophylaxis for uncomplicated deliveries is not routinely recommended in currently available guidelines, in the largest series assessing the outcome of cyanotic defects in pregnancy, two women experienced endocarditis peripartum. Thus, some experts advocate routine antibiotic prophylaxis for delivery in all women with cyanotic heart defects [9, 22].

16.4 Impact of the Physiological Changes of Pregnancy

Depending on the type of cyanotic heart defect, the impact of pregnancy on oxygen saturations may vary considerably. For example, in patients with large shunts at the ventricular level and limited pulmonary blood flow, the pregnancy-associated decrease in systemic vascular resistance may unfavourably impact the balance between systemic and pulmonary vascular resistance enhancing right-to-left shunting and aggravating cyanosis. In contrast, in a woman after Fontan palliation with a residual restrictive fenestration between the Fontan pathway and the systemic circulation, the increase in cardiac output during pregnancy may decrease the proportion of right-to-left shunting, and hence, oxygen saturations may even increase during pregnancy.

An important compensatory mechanism to maintain oxygen carrying capacity in patients with chronically decreased systemic arterial oxygen saturation is secondary erythrocytosis. Many cyanotic patients have haemoglobin levels well above 200 g/l (12.4 mmol/l). Hyperviscosity symptoms such as headaches, blurry vision and dizziness are rare and usually respond well to hydration. Iron deficiency impedes this important compensatory mechanism, actually increases blood viscosity at lower levels of haemoglobin and must be avoided.

Patients with cyanotic heart defects are especially vulnerable to the complications of respiratory tract infection, and thus, its prevention by annual vaccination

Table 16.2 Requirements for a comprehensive multidisciplinary delivery plan

Content of a comprehensive multidisciplinary delivery plan			
1. Information on the underlying heart defect and current haemodynamics			
☑ Exact cardiac diagnosis, previous surgical and interventional procedures			
☑ Schematic drawing of the woman's heart is mandatory as most have complex anatomy			
☑ Previous cardiovascular complications			
☑ Current cardiovascular findings and important residual lesions			
2. Specific recommendations and pitfalls			
☑ Use of air bubble filters for intravenous lines to reduce the risk of paradoxical embolism			
☑ (if the delivery of large volumes or radiopaque contrast is required, administration without bubble filters is required – on these occasions, meticulous de-bubbling of IV lines is important)			
☑ Recommendations on type and dosage of thromboembolic prophylaxis			
☑ Site of blood pressure measurements in women with occlusion of arm arteries (i.e. after previous classical Blalock-Taussig shunts)			
3. Anticipated complications			
☑ Type and expected timing of the occurrence			
☑ Suggested management in the case of complications (e.g. arrhythmias, heart failure)			
☑ Contact details of involved cardiologists in case of complications			
☑ List of specific drugs that need to be immediately available on the labour ward. In the case of drugs that are not commonly used on the labour ward (e.g. amiodarone), clear instructions on how to prepare and use such drugs should be provided			
4. Caution about obstetric drugs if adverse effects are expected			
☑ Beta-mimetics (e.g. hexoprenaline)	☐ No restriction	☐ Caution	☐ Do not use
☑ Atosiban (oxytocin antagonist)	☐ No restriction	☐ Caution	☐ Do not use
☑ Misoprostol	☐ No restriction	☐ Caution	☐ Do not use
☑ Oxytocin	☐ No restriction	☐ Caution	☐ Do not use
☑ Prostaglandin F analogues	☐ No restriction	☐ Caution	☐ Do not use
5. Detailed list of medications			
6. Allergies			
7. Information on important obstetric issues			
☑ Previous obstetric history and complications			
☑ Estimated date of delivery			
8. Recommendation for delivery			
☑ Mode and timing of delivery (i.e. spontaneous delivery or induction at pre-specified date)			
☑ Recommendation for anaesthesia during delivery			
☑ Recommendation for rhythm monitoring during labour and delivery			
☑ Recommendation for type and duration of haemodynamic monitoring during labour and delivery			
9. Detailed plan for postpartum care			
☑ Place of postpartum care (intensive care unit, cardiology ward, obstetric ward)			
☑ Necessity and duration of rhythm monitoring postpartum			
☑ Recommendation for type and duration of haemodynamic monitoring postpartum			
☑ Recommendation for duration of postpartum stay in hospital (usually >72 h)			
☑ Specific precautions and treatment recommendations (e.g. careful fluid balance)			
☑ Recommendation for investigations postpartum (e.g. predischarge echocardiography)			
10. Follow-up plan after discharge from hospital			

Modified from Ref. [5] with permission

against seasonal influenza and vaccination against pneumococcal disease is very important in this patient group.

16.4.1 Haemodynamic Challenges of Pregnancy in Women with Cyanotic Congenital Heart Defects

Pregnancy is associated with profound changes of the cardiovascular system starting early in the course of pregnancy and plateauing at their peak around 30 weeks of gestation. Systemic vascular resistance decreases by more than 30%; heart rate and stroke volume increase resulting in an increase of cardiac output by about 50%. The ability to adapt to these cardiovascular demands of pregnancy may be markedly impaired in women with cyanotic congenital heart defects. A greater decrease of systemic compared to pulmonary vascular resistance may lead to a decrease in pulmonary blood flow and worsening cyanosis during pregnancy. Many patients with long-standing cyanotic heart defects suffer from myocardial dysfunction; in particular diastolic ventricular dysfunction is very common [23]. The volume load of pregnancy may thus lead to exaggerated rises in ventricular filling pressure and precipitate heart failure.

Apart from the haemodynamic challenges of pregnancy, women with cyanotic congenital heart defects also have an increased risk of paradoxical systemic thromboembolism, which may be further heightened by the pro-thrombotic state of pregnancy. Other complications not reserved to the time of pregnancy are an increased risk of endocarditis, brain abscesses and, particularly in patients with pulmonary hypertension, pulmonary haemorrhage.

16.5 Preconception Assessment and Counselling

16.5.1 Pre-pregnancy Assessment

Careful and comprehensive pre-pregnancy assessment not only allows estimation of maternal and fetal risks, it is also an important opportunity to identify residual lesions that can be improved or optimised to increasing the chance of a successful pregnancy [5]. Conversely, it is an opportunity to define situations in which maternal risk is very high and the likelihood of a live born fetus very low, such that pregnancy should not be further considered.

Pre-pregnancy assessment starts with a detailed chart review. Every effort should be made to obtain previous notes from diagnostic procedures (i.e. cardiac catheterisation reports) and previous interventions. Careful history taking may reveal previous complications (i.e. arrhythmias or heart failure) and allows the estimation of exercise capacity. History taking is followed by a thorough clinical examination, importantly with measurement of resting oxygen saturation.

Detailed cardiac imaging is key for risk assessment and usually starts with a comprehensive transthoracic echocardiography to assess valvular and ventricular function and to estimate pulmonary artery pressures. In patients with complex anatomy, cardiac magnetic resonance imaging or cardiac computed tomography may be helpful for delineation of the exact cardiac anatomy, particularly to visualise extra-cardiac structures, such as aortopulmonary collateral arteries or branch pulmonary arteries. If pulmonary artery pressures cannot be adequately estimated by non-invasive imaging, cardiac catheterisation should be performed, as increased pulmonary artery pressures may importantly increase maternal risks during a pregnancy [24].

Formal exercise testing (with measurement of transcutaneous oxygen saturation) provides information about the woman's exercise tolerance, heart rate and blood pressure response and the extent of desaturation during exercise. Although no formal study has assessed the impact of exercise parameters on pregnancy risks in women with cyanotic congenital cardiac defects, this information is clearly useful during individual risk assessment.

Blood work, including at least a full blood count and assessment of iron stores, is mandatory to assure adequate secondary erythrocytosis. Iron deficiency with (relative) anaemia may be deleterious in patients with cyanotic congenital cardiac conditions. The correction of any iron deficiency is mandatory in all women before embarking on pregnancy.

Cyanotic congenital heart defects with long-standing chronic cyanosis should be considered to be a systemic disease, involving not only the cardiovascular but also many different organ systems. Systemic afflictions may include renal failure, gout, gallstones and coagulation disorders. Directed by history taking, chart review and physical examination, more extensive blood work or additional testing may be required.

One of the key questions of pre-pregnancy assessment in women with unrepaired cyanotic defects is whether the patient's physiology can be improved. This is particularly important in those women with oxygen saturations below 85 % in room air. In such patients creation of surgical aortopulmonary shunts or dilatation/stenting of existing shunts may improve pulmonary blood flow and hence oxygen saturation and consequently may improve the chances of a successful pregnancy. We should, however, be aware that such procedures are deemed to be high-risk procedures in adults with cyanotic heart disease and the price paid for increasing pulmonary blood flow in such patients is additional volume loading to the ventricles which may precipitate heart failure in patients with diastolic dysfunction. These aspects have to be carefully discussed with the woman seeking advice regarding pregnancy.

Occasionally careful assessment may identify adult patients with cyanotic heart defects that may still be amenable to intracardiac repair (i.e. patients with tetralogy of Fallot, in whom the pulmonary circulation is protected by right ventricular outflow tract obstruction). This may be particularly important in women who have immigrated from developing countries where programmes for paediatric heart surgery may not have been available. If repair with alleviation of cyanosis is an option, pregnancy should be delayed until surgical repair has been undertaken.

An important part of pre-pregnancy assessment and counselling is the education of patients regarding potential cardiovascular complications (e.g. arrhythmias, endocarditis), and appropriate behaviour should symptoms of such complications occur. Regular dental care with the use of endocarditis prophylaxis should be reinforced.

Pre-pregnancy assessment requires a review of the patient's medication, as some may be contraindicated in pregnancy (i.e. angiotensin-converting enzyme inhibitors, angiotensin or aldosterone antagonists). In patients requiring anticoagulation, careful consideration of the most appropriate type(s) of drugs and management regimen is required, depending on the individual risk of thromboembolic complications.

16.5.2 Preconception Counselling

Pre-pregnancy counselling is important, as only detailed discussions of all aspects of maternal and fetal risks will allow the affected woman to make an informed decision. Importantly, in women with unrepaired cyanotic heart defects, pre-pregnancy counselling is a multidisciplinary task that should be provided by dedicated cardiologists and obstetricians of a dedicated high-risk pregnancy programme and may involve other specialists. Although detailed information on pregnancy risks is usually provided at the time when a patient wishes to become pregnant, it is important to emphasise that general information on contraception and pregnancy risks should be part of every routine clinic visit, starting in early adolescence.

Apart from detailed discussions about maternal and fetal risks of pregnancy, an important aspect of comprehensive pre-pregnancy counselling includes discussions about the potential impact of pregnancy on long-term outcomes of the underlying heart defects. As the prognosis of the woman with cyanotic congenital heart defects may interfere with the ability to raise children, discussions about the prognosis and potential long-term complications should be offered to women seeking advice about risks of pregnancy [25, 26]. Such discussions are difficult as the prognosis may be uncertain and a number of barriers impair these discussions [26]. The discussion about pregnancy risks may however be a good setting to explore the women's wishes to discuss these issues. It is well known that patient knowledge about long-term risks of the underlying heart defects is often inappropriate [27]. To abstain from discussions about long-term prognosis of the underlying congenital heart defect may impede informed decision making about family planning in affected women. It should also be emphasised that it is important to offer these discussions not only to our female patients but also to our male patients with cyanotic congenital heart defects when they contemplate starting a family.

In all patients with congenital heart defects, including male patients, recurrence risk should be discussed and counselling by a clinical geneticist should be offered.

Once a woman has made a decision whether or not to accept the risks of a pregnancy, it is important to plan future management. For women not wishing to become pregnant, safe and effective contraception should be provided [28, 29]. When there is no current but possible future pregnancy wish, the woman should be instructed to use safe and effective contraception and, when she desires to embark on a pregnancy, to visit her cardiologist for an up-to-date assessment of pregnancy risk and construction of a pregnancy management plan before discontinuing her contraceptive.

For women, who wish to become pregnant, it is important to clearly define management during pregnancy and to provide obstetric assessment to ascertain up-to-date vaccination and initiation of appropriate prophylactic measures, such as folic acid supplementation as well as recommendations for smoking cessation and abstinence from alcohol.

Acknowledgements We wish to thank Prof. Jack M. Colman for the thorough review of the manuscript.

References

1. Hoffman JI, Kaplan S (2002) The incidence of congenital heart disease. J Am Coll Cardiol 39(12):1890–1900
2. Warnes CA, Liberthson R, Danielson GK, Dore A, Harris L, Hoffman JI, Somerville J, Williams RG, Webb GD (2001) Task force 1: the changing profile of congenital heart disease in adult life. J Am Coll Cardiol 37(5):1170–1175
3. Greutmann M, Tobler D, Kovacs AH, Greutmann-Yantiri M, Haile SR, Held L, Ivanov J, Williams WG, Oechslin EN, Silversides CK, Colman JM (2015) Increasing mortality burden among adults with complex congenital heart disease. Congenit Heart Dis 10(2):117–127
4. Marelli AJ, Ionescu-Ittu R, Mackie AS, Guo L, Dendukuri N, Kaouache M (2014) Lifetime prevalence of congenital heart disease in the general population from 2000 to 2010. Circulation 130(9):749–756
5. Greutmann M, Pieper PG (2015) Pregnancy in women with congenital heart disease. Eur Heart J 36(37):2491–2499
6. Drenthen W, Boersma E, Balci A, Moons P, Roos-Hesselink JW, Mulder BJ, Vliegen HW, van Dijk AP, Voors AA, Yap SC, van Veldhuisen DJ, Pieper PG, Investigators Z (2010) Predictors of pregnancy complications in women with congenital heart disease. Eur Heart J 31(17):2124–2132
7. Siu SC, Sermer M, Colman JM, Alvarez AN, Mercier LA, Morton BC, Kells CM, Bergin ML, Kiess MC, Marcotte F, Taylor DA, Gordon EP, Spears JC, Tam JW, Amankwah KS, Smallhorn JF, Farine D, Sorensen S (2001) Cardiac disease in pregnancy I. Prospective multicenter study of pregnancy outcomes in women with heart disease. Circulation 104(5):515–521
8. Roos-Hesselink JW, Ruys TP, Stein JI, Thilen U, Webb GD, Niwa K, Kaemmerer H, Baumgartner H, Budts W, Maggioni AP, Tavazzi L, Taha N, Johnson MR, Hall R, Investigators R (2013) Outcome of pregnancy in patients with structural or ischaemic heart disease: results of a registry of the European Society of Cardiology. Eur Heart J 34(9):657–665
9. Presbitero P, Somerville J, Stone S, Aruta E, Spiegelhalter D, Rabajoli F (1994) Pregnancy in cyanotic congenital heart disease. Outcome of mother and fetus. Circulation 89(6):2673–2676
10. Drenthen W, Pieper PG, Roos-Hesselink JW, van Lottum WA, Voors AA, Mulder BJ, van Dijk AP, Vliegen HW, Yap SC, Moons P, Ebels T, van Veldhuisen DJ, Investigators Z (2007) Outcome of pregnancy in women with congenital heart disease: a literature review. J Am Coll Cardiol 49(24):2303–2311
11. Robson SC, Hunter S, Boys RJ, Dunlop W (1989) Hemodynamic changes during twin pregnancy. A Doppler and M-mode echocardiographic study. Am J Obstet Gynecol 161(5):1273–1278
12. Greutmann M, Von Klemperer K, Brooks R, Peebles D, O'Brien P, Walker F (2010) Pregnancy outcome in women with congenital heart disease and residual haemodynamic lesions of the right ventricular outflow tract. Eur Heart J 31(14):1764–1770
13. Siu SC, Colman JM, Sorensen S, Smallhorn JF, Farine D, Amankwah KS, Spears JC, Sermer M (2002) Adverse neonatal and cardiac outcomes are more common in pregnant women with cardiac disease. Circulation 105(18):2179–2184
14. Burn J, Brennan P, Little J, Holloway S, Coffey R, Somerville J, Dennis NR, Allan L, Arnold R, Deanfield JE, Godman M, Houston A, Keeton B, Oakley C, Scott O, Silove E, Wilkinson J, Pembrey M, Hunter AS (1998) Recurrence risks in offspring of adults with major heart defects: results from first cohort of British collaborative study. Lancet 351(9099):311–316

15. Fesslova V, Brankovic J, Lalatta F, Villa L, Meli V, Piazza L, Ricci C (2011) Recurrence of congenital heart disease in cases with familial risk screened prenatally by echocardiography. J Pregnancy 2011:368067
16. Gill HK, Splitt M, Sharland GK, Simpson JM (2003) Patterns of recurrence of congenital heart disease: an analysis of 6,640 consecutive pregnancies evaluated by detailed fetal echocardiography. J Am Coll Cardiol 42(5):923–929
17. Pieper PG, Balci A, Aarnoudse JG, Kampman MA, Sollie KM, Groen H, Mulder BJ, Oudijk MA, Roos-Hesselink JW, Cornette J, van Dijk AP, Spaanderman ME, Drenthen W, van Veldhuisen DJ, investigators ZI (2013) Uteroplacental blood flow, cardiac function, and pregnancy outcome in women with congenital heart disease. Circulation 128(23):2478–2487
18. Wald RM, Silversides CK, Kingdom J, Toi A, Lau CS, Mason J, Colman JM, Sermer M, Siu SC (2015) Maternal cardiac output and fetal doppler predict adverse neonatal outcomes in pregnant women with heart disease. J Am Heart Assoc 4(11)
19. Tanous D, Siu SC, Mason J, Greutmann M, Wald RM, Parker JD, Sermer M, Colman JM, Silversides CK (2010) B-type natriuretic peptide in pregnant women with heart disease. J Am Coll Cardiol 56(15):1247–1253
20. Kampman MA, Balci A, van Veldhuisen DJ, van Dijk AP, Roos-Hesselink JW, Sollie-Szarynska KM, Ludwig-Ruitenberg M, van Melle JP, Mulder BJ, Pieper PG, investigators ZI (2014) N-terminal pro-B-type natriuretic peptide predicts cardiovascular complications in pregnant women with congenital heart disease. Eur Heart J 35(11):708–715
21. Ouyang DW, Khairy P, Fernandes SM, Landzberg MJ, Economy KE (2010) Obstetric outcomes in pregnant women with congenital heart disease. Int J Cardiol 144(2):195–199
22. European Society of G, Association for European Paediatric C, German Society for Gender M, Regitz-Zagrosek V, Blomstrom Lundqvist C, Borghi C, Cifkova R, Ferreira R, Foidart JM, Gibbs JS, Gohlke-Baerwolf C, Gorenek B, Iung B, Kirby M, Maas AH, Morais J, Nihoyannopoulos P, Pieper PG, Presbitero P, Roos-Hesselink JW, Schaufelberger M, Seeland U, Torracca L, Guidelines ESCCfP (2011) ESC Guidelines on the management of cardiovascular diseases during pregnancy: the Task Force on the Management of Cardiovascular Diseases during Pregnancy of the European Society of Cardiology (ESC). Eur Heart J 32(24):3147–3197
23. Saab FG, Aboulhosn JA (2013) Hemodynamic characteristics of cyanotic adults with single-ventricle physiology without Fontan completion. Congenit Heart Dis 8(2):124–130
24. Bedard E, Dimopoulos K, Gatzoulis MA (2009) Has there been any progress made on pregnancy outcomes among women with pulmonary arterial hypertension? Eur Heart J 30(3):256–265
25. Tobler D, Greutmann M, Colman JM, Greutmann-Yantiri M, Librach LS, Kovacs AH (2012) End-of-life in adults with congenital heart disease: a call for early communication. Int J Cardiol 155(3):383–387
26. Greutmann M, Tobler D, Colman JM, Greutmann-Yantiri M, Librach SL, Kovacs AH (2013) Facilitators of and barriers to advance care planning in adult congenital heart disease. Congenit Heart Dis 8(4):281–288
27. Reid GJ, Webb GD, Barzel M, McCrindle BW, Irvine MJ, Siu SC (2006) Estimates of life expectancy by adolescents and young adults with congenital heart disease. J Am Coll Cardiol 48(2):349–355
28. Thorne S, Nelson-Piercy C, MacGregor A, Gibbs S, Crowhurst J, Panay N, Rosenthal E, Walker F, Williams D, de Swiet M, Guillebaud J (2006) Pregnancy and contraception in heart disease and pulmonary arterial hypertension. J Fam Plann Reprod Health Care 32(2):75–81
29. Silversides CK, Sermer M, Siu SC (2009) Choosing the best contraceptive method for the adult with congenital heart disease. Curr Cardiol Rep 11(4):298–305

Pulmonary Hypertension

17

Werner Budts

Abbreviations

BMPR2	Bone morphogenetic protein receptor type 2
CS	Caesarean section
EIF2AK4	Eukaryotic translation initiation factor 2 alpha kinase 4
HIV	Human immunodeficiency virus
LVEF	Left ventricle ejection fraction
NYHA	New York Heart Association
PAH	Pulmonary arterial hypertension
PH	Pulmonary hypertension
WHO	World Health Organization

Key Facts

Incidence: 5–10 % of congenital heart disease patients.
Inheritance: Variable.
Medication: Advanced therapies (prostacyclin analogues, phosphodiesterase inhibitors, and endothelin-receptor antagonists) are contraindicated during pregnancy. However, sildenafil has been taken safely in severe PH.
World Health Organization class: IV.
Risk of pregnancy: High risk of severe right ventricular failure, cardiac arrest, pulmonary embolism, endocarditis, and uncontrollable bleeding. High risk of death in pregnancy and puerperium.
Life expectancy: Markedly shortened.

W. Budts, MD, PhD
Congenital and Structural Cardiology, University Hospitals Leuven,
Department of Cardiovascular Sciences, Catholic University Leuven, Leuven, Belgium
e-mail: werner.budts@uzleuven.be

> **Key Management**
> *Preconception*: Discourage pregnancy.
> *Pregnancy*: If the pregnancy is unplanned, termination should be discussed and performed in an experienced tertiary care center. Frequent visits are required throughout pregnancy. Hospitalization during the third trimester may facilitate management and a safer delivery.
> *Labor*: Planned Caesarean delivery and vaginal delivery are favored over emergency Caesarean delivery. During labor, delivery, and in the postpartum period intensive monitoring is recommended (arterial and central venous lines).
> *Postpartum*: In-hospital monitoring for at least 2 weeks after delivery.

17.1 The Condition

Pulmonary hypertension (PH) is defined as an increase in mean pulmonary artery pressure ≥25 mmHg at rest as assessed by right heart catheterization [1]. Pulmonary *arterial* hypertension (PAH) is characterized by the presence of precapillary PH, defined as a pulmonary artery wedge pressure of ≤15 mmHg and a pulmonary vascular resistance of >3 Wood units. Congenital heart disease is mostly associated with PAH, although other types of PH occur in the adult population. Table 17.1 summarizes the recently updated clinical classification of PH [1, 2]. PAH associated with congenital heart disease is a very heterogeneous group requiring the development of an additional clinical classification. (1) *Eisenmenger's syndrome* is characterized by a large intra- and/or extracardiac congenital heart defect that starts with a systemic-to-pulmonary shunt. After a certain period of time, the pulmonary vascular resistance starts to increase, pressures in the right heart and pulmonary circulation elevate, and the shunt reverses to pulmonary-to-systemic or becomes bidirectional. As a consequence, central cyanosis and secondary erythrocytosis occur and lead finally to multi-organ involvement. (2) PAH might also occur with a *prevalent systemic-to-pulmonary shunt*. This occurs in the context of moderate to large defects and a mildly to moderately increased pulmonary vascular resistance. Cyanosis is not present at rest. Some of these defects are considered to be correctable while others are not [3]. (3) PAH may be present in patients who also have small, and therefore probably incidental, defects. The pulmonary vascular resistance in these patients is disproportionately elevated given the size of the defect and these patients are considered to suffer from idiopathic pulmonary hypertension. (4) Finally, PAH might persist or even (re)-occur after shunt closure [4].

Epidemiological data about PAH in congenital heart disease are scarce. However, a European survey reported a PAH prevalence between 5% and 10% among

Table 17.1 Clinical classification of pulmonary hypertension

1. Pulmonary arterial hypertension
   1.1 Idiopathic
   1.2 Heritable
      1.2.1 BMPR2 mutation
      1.2.2 Other mutations
   1.3 Drugs and toxins induced
   1.4 Associated with:
      1.4.1 Connective tissue disease
      1.4.3 Portal hypertension
            1.4.4 Congenital heart disease
      1.4.5 Schistosomiasis
1'. Pulmonary veno-occlusive disease and/or pulmonary capillary hemangiomatosis
   1'.1 Idiopathic
   1'.2 Heritable
      1'.2.1 EIF2AK4 mutation
      1'.2.2 Other mutations
   1'.3 Drugs, toxins, and radiation induced
   1'.4 Associated with:
      1'.4.1 Connective tissue disease
      1'.4.2 HIV infection
1''. Persistent pulmonary hypertension of the newborn
2. Pulmonary hypertension due to left heart disease
      2.1 Left ventricular systolic dysfunction
      2.2 Left ventricular diastolic dysfunction
   2.3 Valvular disease obstruction and congenital cardiomyopathies
   2.4 Congenital/acquired left heart inflow/outflow tract
   2.5 Congenital/acquired pulmonary veins stenosis
3. Pulmonary hypertension due to lung diseases and/or hypoxia
   3.1 Chronic obstructive pulmonary disease
   3.2 Interstitial lung disease
   3.3 Other pulmonary diseases with mixed restrictive and obstructive pattern
   3.4 Sleep-disordered breathing
   3.5 Alveolar hypoventilation disorders
   3.6 Chronic exposure to high altitude
   3.7 Developmental lung diseases
4. Chronic thromboembolic pulmonary hypertension and other pulmonary artery obstructions
   4.1 Chronic thromboembolic pulmonary hypertension
   4.2 Other pulmonary artery obstructions
      4.2.1 Angiosarcoma
      4.2.2 Other intravascular tumors
      4.2.3 Arteritis
      4.2.4 Congenital pulmonary arteries stenosis
      4.2.5 Parasites (hydatidosis)
5. Pulmonary hypertension with unclear and/or multifactorial mechanisms
   5.1 Hematological disorders: chronic hemolytic anemia, myeloproliferative disorders, splenectomy

(continued)

Table 17.1 (continued)

5.2 Systemic disorders: sarcoidosis, pulmonary histiocytosis, lymphangioleiomyomatosis, neurofibromatosis
5.3 Metabolic disorders: glycogen storage disease, Gaucher disease, thyroid disorders
5.4 Others: pulmonary tumor thrombotic microangiopathy, fibrosing mediastinitis, chronic renal failure (with/without dialysis), segmental pulmonary hypertension

BMPR2 bone morphogenetic protein receptor, type 2, *EIF2AK4* eukaryotic translation initiation factor 2 alpha kinase 4, *HIV* human immunodeficiency virus

congenital heart disease patients [5]. In the Dutch CONCOR registry, a PAH prevalence of 3.2% in congenital heart disease patients and of 100 per million in the general population was found [6]. PAH prevalence increases with age, from 2.5% in those less than 30 years to 35% in older people. However, it is unclear whether the elevated pulmonary artery pressures diagnosed at older age can still be categorized as precapillary. It is possible that in an aging population postcapillary PH might play a more important role [4].

17.2 Pregnancy Outcome

Pregnancy in women with PAH is associated with *high maternal morbidity and mortality*. In one of the oldest series of 44 well-documented cases with Eisenmenger's syndrome and 70 pregnancies, Gleicher et al. found a maternal mortality of 52% in 1979 [7]. Twenty years later perinatal mortality decreased to 36% [8], but has since declined little as reported by Bédard et al. in 2009 who found that the maternal mortality was still 28% [9]. Remarkably, in this study none of the patients died during the pregnancy, but all of them within the first months after the delivery [8, 9]. Causes of death were severe right ventricular failure, cardiac arrest, pulmonary embolism, endocarditis, and uncontrollable bleeding (Fig. 17.1).

Pregnancy induces systemic vasodilation and increases cardiac output. In patients with a persistent defect, the pulmonary-to-systemic shunt worsens and more hypoxia occurs. This leads to further vasoconstriction and higher pulmonary vascular resistance. Hemodynamic stress during labor and delivery induces more CO_2 retention and acidosis, which, in turn, acutely increases the pulmonary artery pressures and precipitates refractory heart failure [9, 10]. The effect of pregnancy on the cardiovascular system may persist for several months after delivery [11], and it fits with the hypothesis that most severe complications occur shortly of delivery. However, the prepregnancy severity of PH might be associated with outcome. A more recent study from Katsuragi et al. suggested that women with mild pulmonary arterial hypertension, who were more often NYHA class I or II in early pregnancy, had a less marked increase in pulmonary artery pressures during pregnancy. Only a few people with mild PAH deteriorated from NYHA class II to class

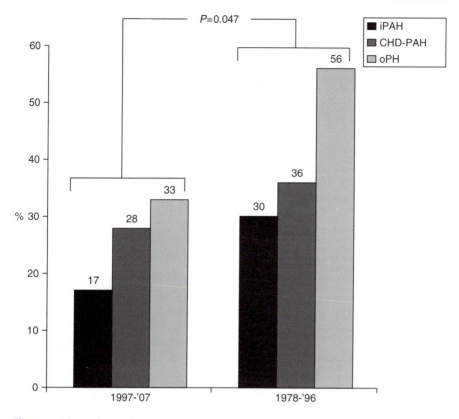

Fig. 17.1 Maternal mortality among pregnant women with pulmonary arterial hypertension: comparison between 1997 and 2007 and previous era (1978–1996) [9]

III/IV. Women with severe pulmonary hypertension delivered earlier than women with mild pulmonary hypertension and no patients died in the mild form of pulmonary arterial hypertension [12].

The neonatal outcome in PAH-congenital heart disease pregnancies is also compromised. Bedard et al. found a neonatal or fetal death of 7 % and a rate of fetal growth restriction of 24 %. Premature delivery, defined as delivery before 37 weeks of gestation, occurred in 86 % [9]. Earlier series report an even higher perinatal mortality of 28.3 %, which was significantly associated with prematurity [7].

17.3 Pregnancy Management

The best management of a PAH patient with congenital heart disease is to discourage pregnancy. Remarkably, in 27 % of the PAH cases in pregnant women with congenital heart disease, the diagnosis of PAH was first made during the pregnancy [9]. There are currently no guidelines or recommendations relating to the management of PAH in pregnant women. In the review from Bédard et al., the current status of management is discussed [9]. In general, patients are hospitalized earlier (median 32 weeks of gestation, range 17–40), probably related to complications occurring during pregnancy, the awareness of premature delivery, and the choice for elective delivery by Caesarean section. Caesarean section is electively planned in 31 % of the pregnant general heart disease population, but seems not to have any advantage over planned vaginal delivery [13]. However, one might suggest that Caesarean section is preferred in more complex heart diseases [9]. Indeed, 72 % of cases were delivered by CS in the report of Bédard et al. [9]. However, the hemodynamic impact of a vaginal delivery is held to be lower than that of a Caesarean section. Less blood loss causes smaller volume shifts, less clotting and bleeding disorders; moreover, a vaginal delivery is associated with a lower risk of infection [14]. During delivery, the Valsalva manoeuvre increases both heart rate and vascular resistance, both of which might increase the workload on the right heart [15].

The anesthetic management is closely related to the mode of the delivery. Bédard et al. found that in 31 % of cases, the Caesarean section was performed under general anesthesia in PAH patients with congenital heart disease. This was associated with a higher maternal mortality [9]. Although it is possible that more severe cases had a general anesthetic accounting for the greater maternal mortality, an alternative explanation would be that general anesthesia is not the best option since it might disturb the balance between the pulmonary and systemic circulations by differentially influencing the vascular resistance [16]. Pulmonary vascular resistance is increased by hypoxia, hypercarbia, high hematocrit levels, positive pressure ventilation, cold, metabolic acidosis, and alpha-adrenergic stimulation. The systemic vascular resistance decreases by the use of vasodilators, spinal and epidural anesthesia, deep general anesthesia, and hyperthermia. In case of a persistent shunt defect, the pulmonary-to-systemic shunt might increase and lead to more pronounced systemic desaturation. In the presence of PAH without a shunt defect, the increase of pulmonary vascular resistance will aggravate the pressure load on the subpulmonary ventricle and might induce acute heart failure. Moreover, all anesthetic agents depress myocardial contractility [17]. The choice between epidural and general anesthesia has to be left to an experienced anesthetist with sufficient expertise in the management of complex congenital heart disease to find the best compromise in this highly challenging situation [14].

Intensive monitoring is recommended for patients with PAH during labor, delivery, and in the postpartum period. An arterial line to measure blood pressure and oxygen saturation and a central venous line to control right atrial pressures seem to be useful in the peripartum period [18]. Acid–base status should be checked frequently, since undetected acidosis can exacerbate pulmonary hypertension [18]. Bédard et al. noted the use of radial artery and/or central venous pressure catheter in 38 % and the use of a pulmonary artery catheter in 31 % of the cases [9]. However, invasive pulmonary arterial pressure monitoring remains controversial and does not seem to influence outcome in a positive or negative way [9]. Nevertheless, more invasive monitoring is related to a higher risk for potential complications [19]. In-hospital monitoring is suggested for at least 2 weeks after delivery [18]. Indeed, the effect of pregnancy on the cardiovascular system may persist for several months after delivery [11].

The occurrence of thrombosis and/or pulmonary embolism raises the question about the usefulness of thrombosis prophylaxis in PAH patients. Although oral anticoagulation is the standard of care for patients with idiopathic PAH [1], thromboprophylaxis in idiopathic PAH was used in 52 % and 41 % during pregnancy and after delivery, respectively [9]. These numbers were even lower in PAH patients with congenital heart disease, 24 % received thromboprophylaxis during pregnancy and 31 % after delivery [9]. This is probably explained by the controversy that exists about the use of oral anticoagulants in PAH-congenital heart disease patients [20]. This is especially so in patients with the Eisenmenger's syndrome, where the balance between thrombosis and bleeding is very delicate and explaining why severe bleeding is in the list of peripartum complications [21]. However, anti-thromboembolic stockings or compression pumps can be used to help prevent peripheral venous thrombosis with no adverse effects [18]. The ESC guidelines on pregnancy suggest that in PAH associated with congenital cardiac shunts and in the absence of significant hemoptysis, anticoagulant treatment should be considered in the presence of pulmonary artery thrombosis or signs of heart failure [22].

At least 50 % of pregnant women with PAH and congenital heart disease patients receive advanced therapy for PAH [9]. Prostacyclin analogues, phosphodiesterase inhibitors, and endothelin-receptor antagonists are proven to have a beneficial effect on exercise performance and functional capacity [23–25], whereas inhaled NO decreases pulmonary vascular resistance [26]. However, the number of case reports and the series, in which advanced therapy was used, is too small to draw conclusions on safety and efficiency for pregnant women and the fetus [27–32]. However, there tended to be a beneficial effect of advanced therapy on outcome, but there may be a publication bias toward positive results. The guanylate cyclase stimulator, riociguat [33], might cause fetal harm and was shown to have teratogenic effects. Calcium channel blockers are mainly used in idiopathic pulmonary arterial hypertension, but are relatively contraindicated in congenital heart disease patients with PAH and a persistent shunt, as they might increase pulmonary-to-systemic shunt by a decrease of systemic vascular resistance [20]. Although the use of oxygen is controversial in adult patients with the Eisenmenger syndrome, increased oxygen might lower pulmonary vascular resistance during labor and delivery [34].

If an unplanned pregnancy occurs in a PAH-congenital heart disease patient, termination should be discussed and performed in an experienced tertiary center [22]. However, even when the pregnancy is stopped at this stage, maternal mortality rates of up to 7 % are reported [7]. Dilatation and curettage in the first trimester is probably the procedure of choice, preferably with general anesthesia [18].

Women who opt to continue the pregnancy need to be referred to a tertiary center urgently for follow-up and delivery by a multidisciplinary team with experienced congenital cardiologists, experts in pulmonary hypertension, obstetricians, anesthetists, neonatologists, and experts in intensive care. Moreover, the psychological stress of such a high-risk pregnancy should not be underestimated and support by a psychological team beneficial. Frequent visits throughout pregnancy are recommended, and hospitalization during the third trimester may facilitate management and safer delivery [9].

17.4 The Effect of Pregnancy Adaptations

During pregnancy the plasma volume increases and peaks at about 50 % above baseline early in the third trimester. The red blood cell mass increases by 20–30 % too [35]. The extra volume might compromise the function of the right ventricle and precipitate right heart failure since the higher pulmonary vascular resistance increases right ventricular pressure and work. In addition, systemic vascular resistance decreases in normal pregnancy, and in patients with a persistent shunt defect, this will result in a more pronounced pulmonary-to-systemic flow, which will exacerbate the preexisting hypoxia and result in greater pulmonary vasoconstriction. Once set in train, this sequence of events will lead to a self-perpetuating deterioration in the patient's clinical state.

The physiological changes in labor may also challenge the circulation of those women with PAH and persisting shunt. Midwall et al. demonstrated that uterine contractions are associated with a substantial decrease in the ratio of pulmonary-to-systemic blood flow [34]. Normally, uterine contractions cause an increase in cardiac output and right ventricular pressures [36]; however, if this occurs when the pulmonary vascular resistance does not decrease or remains fixed, more pulmonary-to-systemic flow will occur. Also, when traction forceps were used during a uterine contraction, the pulmonary flow decreased further [34]. Moreover, in late pregnancy and during labor, the gravid uterus might compromise cardiac output by compression of the inferior vena cava in supine position. Some recommend delivery in the lateral position to avoid compression of the inferior vena cava and maintain sufficient systemic venous return [18]. Furthermore, at the time of labor and delivery, acidosis and hypercarbia may further increase pulmonary vascular resistance. Any hypovolemia resulting from blood loss or hypotension from a vasovagal response to pain may result in insufficient cardiac output and sudden death [18]. On the other hand, a temporary increase in venous return may occur immediately following delivery due to relief of inferior vena cava pressure which at times results in a substantial rise in ventricular filling pressures, which might unbalance the shunt flow [15]. Therefore, postpartum patients should continue to be monitored hemodynamically for 24–48 h to detect any deterioration due to the postpartum increase in venous return to the heart [15].

17.5 Preconception Counseling

Because of the high maternal and fetal mortality in women with PAH in the context of congenital heart disease, pregnancy should be discouraged. The risks of severe complications are unacceptably high. Unfortunately, this is not clear from all risk score models. Currently, three predictive scoring models are used to estimate the maternal risk for a pregnancy. In the model of the *CARPREG study*, cyanosis was related to cardiac events, neonatal complications, and postpartum hemorrhage [37]. However, no Eisenmenger patients were included in the study so that cyanosis was related to congenital heart defects with pulmonary-to-systemic shunts and normal pulmonary artery pressures. Moreover, no relationship between PH and an adverse pregnancy outcome was found. This does not mean that PH is not important in determining outcome, but that the study sample size was too small to show any significant association between PH and outcome. Consequently, the risk model based on the CARPREG study cannot be used in the context of PAH. Similarly, the risk model, based on the ZAHARA study [38], has the same problem. Only four patients suffered from PH or Eisenmenger's syndrome. In this study, cyanotic heart disease was significantly associated with cardiac and neonatal complications, but several of these patients underwent corrective surgery, or had a pulmonary-to-systemic shunt with presumably normal pulmonary artery pressures. Consequently, as for the CARPREG study, the risk model based on the ZAHARA study cannot be used in the context of PAH. In contrast, the modified World Health Organization (WHO) risk classification includes contraindications for pregnancy that are not present in the CARPREG and ZAHARA risk scores/predictors, including PAH [39]. PAH is listed in WHO risk class IV: extremely high risk of maternal mortality or severe morbidity and pregnancy contraindicated (Table 17.2) [22]. Importantly, following this risk classification, the risk of maternal death is also to be considered high even in the presence of mild pulmonary hypertension [39]. The risk probably increases as pulmonary pressures rise. However, even moderate forms of pulmonary vascular disease can worsen during pregnancy as a result of the decrease in systemic vascular resistance and overload of the right ventricle, and there is no safe cutoff value prompting the ESC guidelines to conclude: "Whether the risk is also high for congenital patients after successful shunt closure with mildly elevated pulmonary pressures is not well known, but these risks are probably lower and pregnancy can be considered after a careful risk assessment" [22]. Therefore, it is the safest to rely on the WHO risk classification when counseling a PAH patient for pregnancy. Balci et al. concluded in their comparative study between risk scores that the WHO classification was the best available risk assessment model for estimating cardiovascular risk in pregnant women with CHD [40]. However, no offspring prediction models seem to perform adequately [40] nor include PAH to predict neonatal events (Table 17.3) [22]. Although cyanosis is also here used as predictor, it refers mainly to the situation of congenital heart defects with pulmonary-to-systemic shunts and normal pulmonary artery pressures [37].

Table 17.2 Conditions in which pregnancy risk is WHO IV (pregnancy contraindicated)

1. Pulmonary arterial hypertension of any cause
2. Severe systemic ventricular dysfunction (LVEF <30%, NYHA III-IV)
3. Previous peripartum cardiomyopathy with any residual impairment of left ventricular function
4. Severe mitral stenosis, severe symptomatic aortic stenosis
5. Marfan syndrome with aorta dilated >45 mm
6. Aortic dilatation >50 mm in aortic disease associated with bicuspid aortic valve
7. Native severe coarctation

WHO World Health Organization, *LVEF* left ventricle ejection fraction, *NYHA* New York Heart Association

Table 17.3 Maternal predictors of neonatal events in women with heart disease

1. Baseline NYHA class > II or cyanosis
2. Maternal left heart obstruction
3. Smoking during pregnancy
4. Multiple gestation
5. Use of oral anticoagulants during pregnancy
6. Mechanical valve prosthesis

17.5.1 Contraception in Pulmonary Arterial Hypertension and Congenital Heart Disease

Barrier methods such as condoms, diaphragms, and cervical caps give protection against sexual transmittable diseases and do not have health risks, but their high failure rate with typical use (15–30%) makes them an inappropriate contraceptive for women with PH [35].

Sterilization seems to be the best choice for women who should not become pregnant and is rated WHO II for contraceptive method [41]. WHO risk for contraceptive method by medical condition is summarized in Table 17.4. The safest surgical technique to sterilize patients with pulmonary vascular disease is probably the mini-laparatomy or minimal laparascopy (with <200 ml CO_2 and minimal increase in intra-abdominal pressure) [41]. Indeed, during laparoscopic sterilization under general anesthesia, the combination with positive pressure ventilation, abdominal inflation with CO_2, and intermittent head down tilt might decrease venous return and negatively affects the circulation. Vagal reaction under local anesthesia must be avoided because of the decrease in systemic vascular resistance, aggravating a pulmonary-to-systemic shunt. Finally, patients with a persistent shunt might have an increased risk for paradoxical air embolism, not only from venous catheters but also from the soluble CO_2 used for inflation [41].

The use of *contraceptive hormonal treatment* and its WHO classification are summarized in Table 17.5 [41]. Combined oral contraceptives (progestogen and estrogen) are safe and very effective as contraception. However, the estrogen component is responsible for an increased risk of arterial and venous thromboembolism and is therefore unsuitable for patients with pulmonary-to-systemic shunts who are

Table 17.4 WHO risk classifications by medical condition for contraceptive methods [41]

WHO Class	Risk for contraceptive method by medical condition	
I	Condition with no restriction for the use of the contraceptive method	Always usable
II	Condition where the advantages of the method generally outweigh the risks	Broadly usable
III	Condition where the risks of the method usually outweigh the advantages: alternatives are usually preferable. Exceptions if: (i) Patient accepts risks and rejects alternatives (ii) The risk of pregnancy is very high and the only acceptable alternative methods are less effective	Caution in use
IV	Condition where the method represents an unacceptable health risk	Do not use

WHO World Health Organization

Table 17.5 World Health Organization class for contraceptive methods in pulmonary arterial hypertension and Eisenmenger's syndrome [41]

Contraception	WHO classification
Combined contraceptives	I
Standard-dose progestogen-only pill	I[a] (IV[b])
High-dose progestogen-only pill	I (III[b])
Injectable progestogen	I
Implantable progestogen	I (IV[b])
Hormone-releasing intrauterine device	III–IV

[a]Although safe, the limited efficacy of the progestogen-only pill limits its use in women in whom pregnancy carries a particular risk (PAH and Eisenmenger's syndrome)
[b]For patients treated with bosentan

at risk for paradoxical embolism and stroke (WHO IV). Combined non-oral contraceptives (skin patch or vaginal ring) have the same potential side effects as the combined oral contraceptives. Therefore, WHO IV is also recommended for the non-oral forms in PAH patients with a persistent shunt. Progestogen-only methods are not associated with increased risk for arterial or venous thrombosis [42]. Unfortunately, although the standard progestogen-only pills are very safe, contraception is not always reliable; consequently, standard progestogen-only pills are not recommended for patient with PAH or the Eisenmenger's syndrome. In addition standard progestogen-only pills are contraindicated for patients treated with bosentan. Bosentan might reduce the efficacy of progestogen-only contraceptives. However, high-dose progestogen-only pills are a more reliable form of contraception [41]. After systematic use of the injectable and implantable form, many women become amenorrheic, which might be an advantage in cyanotic patients who suffer from menorrhagia [41]. The hormone-releasing intrauterine device does not have the risk of increased vaginal bleeding and pain, as seen in the copper devices. However, implantation of this device is still categorized in the risk classification WHO III-IV as 5% of patients experience a vasovagal response that might lead to cardiovascular collapse in patients with PAH and/or the Eisenmenger's syndrome. A skilled operator is recommended for this choice of contraceptive. There are no data regarding the use of emergency contraception.

References

1. Galiè N, Humbert M, Vachiery JL, Gibbs S, Lang I, Torbicki A, Simonneau G, Peacock A, Vonk Noordegraaf A, Beghetti M, Ghofrani A, Gomez Sanchez MA, Hansmann G, Klepetko W, Lancellotti P, Matucci M, McDonagh T, Pierard LA, Trindade PT, Zompatori M, Hoeper M, Members: ATF, Members ATF (2015) 2015 esc/ers guidelines for the diagnosis and treatment of pulmonary hypertension: The joint task force for the diagnosis and treatment of pulmonary hypertension of the european society of cardiology (esc) and the european respiratory society (ers)endorsed by: Association for european paediatric and congenital cardiology (aepc), international society for heart and lung transplantation (ishlt). Eur Heart J. 2016;37(1):67–119
2. Simonneau G, Galiè N, Rubin LJ, Langleben D, Seeger W, Domenighetti G, Gibbs S, Lebrec D, Speich R, Beghetti M, Rich S, Fishman A (2004) Clinical classification of pulmonary hypertension. J Am Coll Cardiol 43:5S–12S
3. Baumgartner H, Bonhoeffer P, De Groot NM, de Haan F, Deanfield JE, Galie N, Gatzoulis MA, Gohlke-Baerwolf C, Kaemmerer H, Kilner P, Meijboom F, Mulder BJ, Oechslin E, Oliver JM, Serraf A, Szatmari A, Thaulow E, Vouhe PR, Walma E, (ESC) TFotMoG-uCHDotESoC, (AEPC) AfEPC, (CPG) ECfPG (2010) Esc guidelines for the management of grown-up congenital heart disease (new version 2010. Eur Heart J 31:2915–2957
4. Gabriels C, De Meester P, Pasquet A, De Backer J, Paelinck BP, Morissens M, Van De Bruaene A, Delcroix M, Budts W (2014) A different view on predictors of pulmonary hypertension in secundum atrial septal defect. Int J Cardiol 176:833–840
5. Engelfriet PM, Duffels MG, Möller T, Boersma E, Tijssen JG, Thaulow E, Gatzoulis MA, Mulder BJ (2007) Pulmonary arterial hypertension in adults born with a heart septal defect: the euro heart survey on adult congenital heart disease. Heart 93:682–687
6. van Riel AC, Schuuring MJ, van Hessen ID, Zwinderman AH, Cozijnsen L, Reichert CL, Hoorntje JC, Wagenaar LJ, Post MC, van Dijk AP, Hoendermis ES, Mulder BJ, Bouma BJ (2014) Contemporary prevalence of pulmonary arterial hypertension in adult congenital heart disease following the updated clinical classification. Int J Cardiol 174:299–305
7. Gleicher N, Midwall J, Hochberger D, Jaffin H (1979) Eisenmenger's syndrome and pregnancy. Obstet Gynecol Surv 34:721–741
8. Weiss BM, Zemp L, Seifert B, Hess OM (1998) Outcome of pulmonary vascular disease in pregnancy: a systematic overview from 1978 through 1996. J Am Coll Cardiol 31:1650–1657
9. Bédard E, Dimopoulos K, Gatzoulis MA (2009) Has there been any progress made on pregnancy outcomes among women with pulmonary arterial hypertension? Eur Heart J 30:256–265
10. Metcalfe J, Ueland K (1974) Maternal cardiovascular adjustments to pregnancy. Prog Cardiovasc Dis 16:363–374
11. Clapp JF, Capeless E (1997) Cardiovascular function before, during, and after the first and subsequent pregnancies. Am J Cardiol 80:1469–1473
12. Katsuragi S, Yamanaka K, Neki R, Kamiya C, Sasaki Y, Osato K, Miyoshi T, Kawasaki K, Horiuchi C, Kobayashi Y, Ueda K, Yoshimatsu J, Niwa K, Takagi Y, Ogo T, Nakanishi N, Ikeda T (2012) Maternal outcome in pregnancy complicated with pulmonary arterial hypertension. Circ J 76:2249–2254
13. Ruys TP, Roos-Hesselink JW, Pijuan-Domènech A, Vasario E, Gaisin IR, Iung B, Freeman LJ, Gordon EP, Pieper PG, Hall R, Boersma E, Johnson MR, investigators R (2015) Is a planned caesarean section in women with cardiac disease beneficial? Heart 101:530–536
14. Uebing A, Steer PJ, Yentis SM, Gatzoulis MA (2006) Pregnancy and congenital heart disease. BMJ 332:401–406
15. Sahni S, Palkar AV, Rochelson BL, Kępa W, Talwar A (2015) Pregnancy and pulmonary arterial hypertension: a clinical conundrum. Pregnancy Hypertens 5:157–164
16. Cannesson M, Earing MG, Collange V, Kersten JR (2009) Anesthesia for noncardiac surgery in adults with congenital heart disease. Anesthesiology 111:432–440
17. Williams GD, Philip BM, Chu LF, Boltz MG, Kamra K, Terwey H, Hammer GB, Perry SB, Feinstein JA, Ramamoorthy C (2007) Ketamine does not increase pulmonary vascular

resistance in children with pulmonary hypertension undergoing sevoflurane anesthesia and spontaneous ventilation. Anesth Analg 105:1578–1584, table of contents
18. Warnes CA (2004) Pregnancy and pulmonary hypertension. Int J Cardiol 97(Suppl 1):11–13
19. Barash PG, Nardi D, Hammond G, Walker-Smith G, Capuano D, Laks H, Kopriva CJ, Baue AE, Geha AS (1981) Catheter-induced pulmonary artery perforation. Mechanisms, management, and modifications. J Thorac Cardiovasc Surg 82:5–12
20. Budts W (2005) Eisenmenger syndrome: medical prevention and management strategies. Expert Opin Pharmacother 6:2047–2060
21. Pitts JA, Crosby WM, Basta LL (1977) Eisenmenger's syndrome in pregnancy: does heparin prophylaxis improve the maternal mortality rate? Am Heart J 93:321–326
22. Regitz-Zagrosek V, Blomstrom Lundqvist C, Borghi C, Cifkova R, Ferreira R, Foidart JM, Gibbs JS, Gohlke-Baerwolf C, Gorenek B, Iung B, Kirby M, Maas AH, Morais J, Nihoyannopoulos P, Pieper PG, Presbitero P, Roos-Hesselink JW, Schaufelberger M, Seeland U, Torracca L, (ESG) ESoG, (AEPC) AfEPC, (DGesGM) GSfGM, Guidelines ECfP (2011) ESC guidelines on the management of cardiovascular diseases during pregnancy: the task force on the management of cardiovascular diseases during pregnancy of the european society of cardiology (esc). Eur Heart J 32:3147–3197
23. Bharani A, Patel A, Saraf J, Jain A, Mehrotra S, Lunia B (2007) Efficacy and safety of pde-5 inhibitor tadalafil in pulmonary arterial hypertension. Indian Heart J 59:323–328
24. Galiè N, Beghetti M, Gatzoulis MA, Granton J, Berger RM, Lauer A, Chiossi E, Landzberg M, Investigators BRToEAT-B (2006) Bosentan therapy in patients with eisenmenger syndrome: a multicenter, double-blind, randomized, placebo-controlled study. Circulation 114:48–54
25. Thomas IC, Glassner-Kolmin C, Gomberg-Maitland M (2013) Long-term effects of continuous prostacyclin therapy in adults with pulmonary hypertension associated with congenital heart disease. Int J Cardiol 168:4117–4121
26. Budts W, Van Pelt N, Gillyns H, Gewillig M, Van De Werf F, Janssens S (2001) Residual pulmonary vasoreactivity to inhaled nitric oxide in patients with severe obstructive pulmonary hypertension and eisenmenger syndrome. Heart 86:553–558
27. Molelekwa V, Akhter P, McKenna P, Bowen M, Walsh K (2005) Eisenmenger's syndrome in a 27 week pregnancy – management with bosentan and sildenafil. Ir Med J 98:87–88
28. Goodwin TM, Gherman RB, Hameed A, Elkayam U (1999) Favorable response of eisenmenger syndrome to inhaled nitric oxide during pregnancy. Am J Obstet Gynecol 180:64–67
29. Lacassie HJ, Germain AM, Valdés G, Fernández MS, Allamand F, López H (2004) Management of eisenmenger syndrome in pregnancy with sildenafil and l-arginine. Obstet Gynecol 103:1118–1120
30. Lust KM, Boots RJ, Dooris M, Wilson J (1999) Management of labor in eisenmenger syndrome with inhaled nitric oxide. Am J Obstet Gynecol 181:419–423
31. Rosenthal E, Nelson-Piercy C (2000) Value of inhaled nitric oxide in eisenmenger syndrome during pregnancy. Am J Obstet Gynecol 183:781–782
32. Geohas C, McLaughlin VV (2003) Successful management of pregnancy in a patient with eisenmenger syndrome with epoprostenol. Chest 124:1170–1173
33. Ghofrani HA, Galiè N, Grimminger F, Grünig E, Humbert M, Jing ZC, Keogh AM, Langleben D, Kilama MO, Fritsch A, Neuser D, Rubin LJ, Group P-S (2013) Riociguat for the treatment of pulmonary arterial hypertension. N Engl J Med 369:330–340
34. Midwall J, Jaffin H, Herman MV, Kupersmith J (1978) Shunt flow and pulmonary hemodynamics during labor and delivery in the eisenmenger syndrome. Am J Cardiol 42:299–303
35. Pieper PG, Lameijer H, Hoendermis ES (2014) Pregnancy and pulmonary hypertension. Best Pract Res Clin Obstet Gynaecol 28:579–591
36. Lees MM, Scott DB, Kerr MG (1970) Haemodynamic changes associated with labour. J Obstet Gynaecol Br Commonw 77:29–36
37. Siu SC, Sermer M, Colman JM, Alvarez AN, Mercier LA, Morton BC, Kells CM, Bergin ML, Kiess MC, Marcotte F, Taylor DA, Gordon EP, Spears JC, Tam JW, Amankwah KS, Smallhorn JF, Farine D, Sorensen S, Investigators CDiPC (2001) Prospective multicenter study of pregnancy outcomes in women with heart disease. Circulation 104:515–521

38. Drenthen W, Boersma E, Balci A, Moons P, Roos-Hesselink JW, Mulder BJ, Vliegen HW, van Dijk AP, Voors AA, Yap SC, van Veldhuisen DJ, Pieper PG, Investigators Z. (2010) Predictors of pregnancy complications in women with congenital heart disease. Eur Heart J 31:2124–2132
39. Thorne S, MacGregor A, Nelson-Piercy C (2006) Risks of contraception and pregnancy in heart disease. Heart 92:1520–1525
40. Balci A, Sollie-Szarynska KM, van der Bijl AG, Ruys TP, Mulder BJ, Roos-Hesselink JW, van Dijk AP, Wajon EM, Vliegen HW, Drenthen W, Hillege HL, Aarnoudse JG, van Veldhuisen DJ, Pieper PG, investigators Z-I (2014) Prospective validation and assessment of cardiovascular and offspring risk models for pregnant women with congenital heart disease. Heart 100:1373–1381
41. Thorne S, Nelson-Piercy C, MacGregor A, Gibbs S, Crowhurst J, Panay N, Rosenthal E, Walker F, Williams D, de Swiet M, Guillebaud J (2006) Pregnancy and contraception in heart disease and pulmonary arterial hypertension. J Fam Plann Reprod Health Care 32:75–81
42. Heinemann LA, Assmann A, DoMinh T, Garbe E (1999) Oral progestogen-only contraceptives and cardiovascular risk: results from the transnational study on oral contraceptives and the health of young women. Eur J Contracept Reprod Health Care 4:67–73

Pulmonary Stenosis

18

Marianna Stamatelatou and Lorna Swann

Abbreviations

PS	Pulmonary stenosis
DCRV	Double-chambered RV
RVOT	Right ventricular outflow tract
MPA	Main pulmonary artery

> **Key Facts**
> *Incidence*: 0.5 per 1,000 births.
> *Inheritance*: 3–5 %.
> *Medication*: None
> *World Health Organization class*: I–II.
> *Risk of pregnancy*: low risk. Arrhythmias and heart failure may occur. Poor RV function, severe pulmonary regurgitation, cyanosis or a history of prior arrhythmia increase the risk.
> *Life expectancy*: normal or nearly normal.

M. Stamatelatou, MD, MSc • L. Swann, MB, ChB, MD, FRCP (✉)
Department of Adult Congenital Heart Disease, Royal Brompton Hospital, London, UK
e-mail: lornaswan@yahoo.com

> **Key Management**
> *Preconception*: If stenosis is at valve level and minor then ECG and echo are usually sufficient. Otherwise a full assessment with MRI and exercise testing is required.
> *Pregnancy*: In simple mild valve stenosis review in early pregnancy and again in the early third trimester.
> *Labour*: vaginal delivery.
> *Post-partum*: Routine unless complicated by cyanosis, arrhythmia or RV dysfunction.

18.1 The Condition

Pulmonary stenosis (PS) is part of the spectrum of right heart obstructive lesions and is usually defined as an obstructive lesion at the level of, or just above or below, the pulmonary valve. Pulmonary stenosis demonstrates a wide spectrum of disease severity, and therefore its clinical presentation varies from critical PS in the neonate to the finding of mild PS in the older patient evaluated for an asymptomatic murmur. Pulmonary stenosis is one of the more common forms of congenital heart disease, and its prevalence does show some geographic variation with an increased incidence in Asian populations [1].

There are many subtypes of pulmonary stenosis, but the classic PS valve is a mobile, dome-shaped valve with a small opening orifice [2, 3]. Ten to 20 % of PS is due to a dysplastic valve. In this setting the valve is trileaflet and thickened with myxomatous change in the leaflets [4]. These dysplastic valves are more frequently associated with inherited genetic syndromes such as Noonan syndrome [5]. Unicuspid and bicuspid pulmonary valves are also uncommon and are often associated with more complex lesions, such as tetralogy of Fallot which is described in Chap. 6 [6].

18.1.1 Other Forms of Pulmonary Stenosis

Subvalvular pulmonary stenosis includes infundibular PS and double-chambered RV (DCRV). Infundibular stenosis can be primarily caused by discrete fibromuscular obstruction or hypertrophic myocardium. In the setting of severe valvular pulmonary stenosis, reactive ventricular hypertrophy can cause a secondary infundibular stenosis and a further dynamic right ventricular outflow tract (RVOT) obstruction.

In double-chambered RV, the RV cavity is divided into a high-pressure inlet part and a low-pressure outlet part by anomalous muscle bundles. This is often associated with a ventricular septal defect, and the obstruction is usually progressive [7, 8].

Supravalvar PS occurs above the valve in the main pulmonary artery (MPA), bifurcation or pulmonary artery branches. It is described as part of several syndromes including Williams syndrome and Alagille syndrome [9]. It is also a common finding in congenital rubella syndrome. Congenital supravalvar stenosis can be caused by a discrete ridge or by a diffusely hypoplastic segment of the main pulmonary artery. Pulmonary atresia is a different entity and will be discussed in relation to tetralogy of Fallot.

Pulmonary stenosis is also commonly seen in relation to previous surgical intervention. Previously "repaired" or replaced valves may become stenotic over time. This includes any form of valved conduit between the heart and the pulmonary arteries. On average a replaced pulmonary valve, which is almost always a tissue valve, will be significantly dysfunctioning by 15 years post implantation. The principles of assessing native and post-surgical pulmonary stenosis are essentially the same.

Post-repair supravalvar PS is also relatively common. Examples of this are stenosis at the site of previous pulmonary artery banding or post arterial switch operation at the level of the distal anastomosis between the neo-pulmonary "root" and the MPA.

18.1.2 Pathophysiology

The clinical consequences of pulmonary stenosis are directly related to the degree of stenosis. Severe PS increases right ventricular afterload causing ventricular hypertrophy and a reduced end systolic deformation of the RV [10]. Significant elevation of RV systolic and diastolic pressures also leads to an increase in right atrial pressure, right atrial stretch and a propensity towards atrial arrhythmia. Increased right atrial pressures can also cause right to left shunting across an atrial communication (such as a patent foramen ovale) and secondary tricuspid regurgitation. In more complex lesions, the same is also true for shunts at ventricular level. However this chapter will focus, in the main, on isolated PS.

Right ventricular dysfunction and overt right heart failure are a late finding in the pathophysiology of PS. Even lifelong PS may not ever progress to cause frank heart failure.

Overall the long-term outlook for patients with PS is excellent. Those with gradients less than 20 mmHg rarely progress. In contrast those with gradients over 50 mmHg are likely to require intervention in later years [11]. Intervention, whether catheter-based or surgical, is relatively straightforward and is expected to return the patient to full health with no symptoms.

18.1.3 Clinical Presentation

A wide range of pulmonary stenosis may be present in women of childbearing age. Many of these patients will have had little, or no, previous intervention.

The usual clinical findings in these patients include:

- An ejection click that decreases with inspiration (if valve mobile).
- An ejection systolic murmur at the upper left sternal border radiation through to the back. During pregnancy the intensity of the murmur may increase as pulmonary blood flow increases.
- A split-second sound.
- Occasionally a diastolic pulmonary regurgitation murmur (especially if previous intervention).
- A fourth heart sound if severe stenosis is present.
- There may be signs of secondary tricuspid regurgitation or cyanosis if there are associated complications. Cyanosis may only manifest itself on exercise and should be actively looked for especially if there is the finding of unexplained erythrocytosis.

The majority of patients with pulmonary stenosis are asymptomatic. Symptoms usually only occur when there is loss of sinus rhythm or RV pressure exceeds 50 % of LV pressure. When symptoms do occur, they tend to be a slow progressive onset of effort intolerance, breathlessness and fatigue. Palpitation is common. Cardiogenic ankle oedema is a rare but concerning symptom that requires further assessment. Chest pain, syncope and even sudden death are rarely seen but if present are thought to be driven by RV ischaemia and ventricular arrhythmia.

18.1.4 Diagnostic Tools

The electrocardiogram is often normal, and ECG changes only occur when the RV pressure is significantly elevated. Important stenosis is associated with evidence of right atrial enlargement, right axis deviation and RV hypertrophy. In severe stenosis there may be a pure R or Rs, or QR is the usual pattern in the right precordial leads, and the R wave is usually greater than 20 mm (Fig. 18.1).

18.1.5 Echocardiography

Echocardiography is the diagnostic tool of choice (Fig. 18.2). It morphologically classifies the different types and locations of PS, evaluates the hemodynamic implications and delineates coexisting lesions. Doppler echocardiography provides the gradient across the obstruction, the presence and severity of pulmonary and tricuspid regurgitation and an estimate of the RV systolic pressure. Pressure gradients depend on the amount of flow across PV, the RV function and the pulmonary artery pressure. Care therefore needs to be taken in assessing the degree of stenosis. During

18 Pulmonary Stenosis

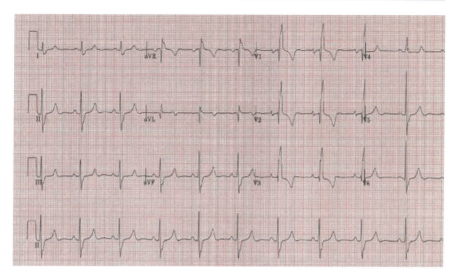

Fig. 18.1 12-lead ECG of a patient with significant pulmonary stenosis. There is a right bundle branch block, evidence of RV hypertrophy and a slightly peaked P wave

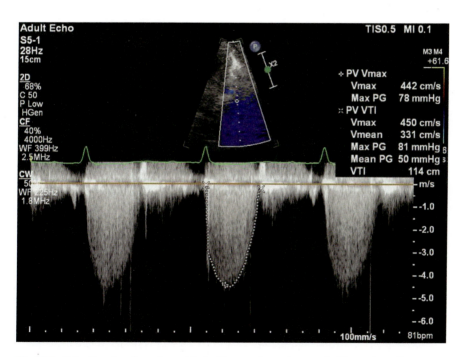

Fig. 18.2 Echo Doppler of a patient with significant pulmonary stenosis. The peak gradient across the valve is 78 mmHg with a mean gradient of 50 mmHg

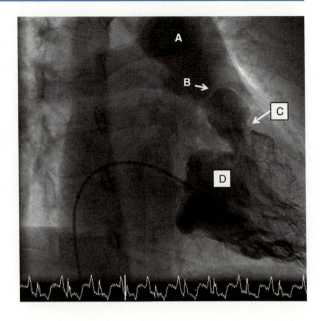

Fig. 18.3 Angiogram of a patient with severe pulmonary stenosis pre-balloon angioplasty. (**a**) Dilated main pulmonary artery. (**b**) Stenosis at the valve level. (**c**) Secondary infundibular stenosis. (**d**) Hypertrophied and trabeculated right ventricle

pregnancy one would expect the pressure gradient to increase as flow increases. PS is considered mild when the peak gradient across the obstruction is <36 mmHg (peak velocity <3 m/s), moderate from 36 to 64 mmHg (peak velocity 3–4 m/s) and severe when the gradient is >64 mmHg (peak velocity>4 m/s). These gradients are often a little higher than invasive gradients but correlate well with catheter-based measurements (Fig. 18.3) [12–14]. Although it has limitations, echo is highly effective in tracking RV function, RV hypertrophy and an estimate of RV volume. In addition right atrial size and surrogates of RA pressure are easily measured and can be followed throughout a pregnancy. The key to maternal outcome is RV function, and caution should be exercised in simply relying on the pulmonary stenosis gradient to monitor antenatal progress. Indeed failure of the pressure gradient to rise is not reassuring but may indicate issues regarding the RV function.

18.1.6 Other Diagnostic Tests

Clinical examination, ECG and echo are usually sufficient to assess a patient either before or during a pregnancy. However, other diagnostics may be useful especially in the more complex patients. Cardiac MRI provides additional information regarding anatomy of the RVOT and pulmonary artery. It can determine the exact location of PS and so can distinguish between PS at different levels. It is also the technique of choice for quantifying pulmonary regurgitation and right heart volumes, mass and function [15]. Neurohormones, such as N-terminal pro-BNP, may be useful in pre-pregnancy risk stratification and, in high-risk patients, in tracking progress during pregnancy [16]. Preconception cardiopulmonary exercise testing with measurements of peak oxygen consumption is useful for assessing the impact of an increased haemodynamic burden and in flagging those at increased risk of adverse maternal events [17].

18.2 Pregnancy Outcomes

18.2.1 Maternal Outcomes

Isolated PS is rarely a significant impediment to a successful pregnancy. Hameed et al. reported a small study of 17 pregnancies. The majority were asymptomatic throughout pregnancy, and there were no important maternal complications, regardless of the severity of PS [24]. In a larger study of congenital heart disease pregnancies, Drenthen et al. reported the outcomes of 148 women with pulmonary stenosis. In this cohort three patients developed arrhythmia, one heart failure and three other cardiovascular complications. In the total cohort of 1,802 pregnancies, a pulmonary outflow tract gradient of greater than 50 mmHg was not associated with a significant increase in risk. The presence of cyanosis or sub-pulmonary atrioventricular valve regurgitation was, however, associated with an increased risk [20]. As mentioned above severe PR is an independent predictor of complications especially if RV-impaired function coexists.

18.2.2 Fetal Outcomes

In general fetal outcomes are very good. The only caveats to this would be if there was significant cyanosis or very impaired maternal cardiac output. The recurrence risk for isolated PS is low in the region of 2–3 %. However, in syndromic patients and those with a dysplastic valve, genetic advice should be sought prior to conception as some of these conditions have an autosomal dominant pattern of inheritance.

18.3 Management

18.3.1 Antenatal Monitoring

In patients with mild isolated PS, antenatal care will be very similar to routine antenatal care. Patients should be offered fetal echocardiography although pulmonary stenosis is often not detected until late in pregnancy or postdelivery. Patients with more severe disease or adverse risk factors will require serial assessment by a specialist cardiac-obstetric team. Regular clinical examination, ECG and echo testing will be required. The frequency of this will be proportionate to the degree of cardiac impairment. During a pregnancy one would expect the Doppler echo gradient to increase across the valve. Heart rate will start to rise from early in the first trimester, and cyanosis may worsen as the systemic vascular resistance drops.

18.3.2 Interventions

Isolated PS at valve level is often responsive to balloon dilation. However it is rare that this is required in pregnancy and should not be embarked upon lightly. An increasing gradient per se is not a good indication for an invasive procedure that may involve ionizing radiation and possible a general anaesthetic. Intervention should be reserved for situations where delivery is not ideal (due to extreme prematurity) and where there is evidence of decompensation. Worsening cyanosis, ischaemia, chest pain and ventricular arrhythmias should trigger a discussion regarding balloon dilatation. Pulmonary stenosis in association with impaired RV function would also be concerning. Bed rest and low-dose diuretics may buy some time when planning optimal care. If intervention is planned during pregnancy, an obstetric team should be available in case the procedure triggers threatened preterm delivery. Techniques to minimize fetal morbidity associated with invasive procedures are well recognized [23], and fetal monitoring should be clearly documented.

In the very rare setting of the need for cardiac surgery during pregnancy, the women should be fully counselled regarding the risk of fetal loss which is still in the region of about 10% despite protocols to optimal care and minimize fetal morbidity.

18.3.3 Delivery

In general mode and technique of delivery will be dictated by obstetric factors. Chapter 6 outlines the generic principles. In patients who are at the more severe end of the PS spectrum, especially those with associated lesions, delivery may be challenging. Optimal right heart filling pressures need to be considered, and there is a role for measuring the central venous pressure directly. Arrhythmias should be treated promptly, and meticulous care should be taken regarding fluid balance. Bleeding or drugs that cause marked venous dilatation may be poorly tolerated. If there is marked RV hypertrophy, underfilling or prolonged pushing during the second stage may destabilize the patient. In patients with significant PS, slow incremental epidural anaesthesia can be used, but again care needs to be taken to avoid a precipitous drop in the venous filling pressures. In patients with an associated intracardiac shunt, such as a PFO or small atrial septal defect, the degree of cyanosis will be dependent on the balance between the right heart pressures and the left heart pressures. Increase in right heart pressures due to, for example, a heart rate-related dynamic outflow tract gradient or a drop in left heart pressures due to systemic vasodilatation will lead to increasing cyanosis. In extreme cases this can lead to ventricular ischaemia and further worsening of haemodynamics. There is also a risk of paradoxical embolism. In the absence of previous valve surgery or complicating issues, antibiotics are not usually given peri-delivery for endocarditis prevention. For the complex patients, a detailed delivery plan should be agreed in advance with input from the multidisciplinary cardiac-obstetric team.

18.4 Impact of Physiological Changes of Pregnancy

Due to the increase in cardiac output, the gradient over the pulmonary valve may increase during pregnancy. Already during the first trimester, these changes may occur with a peak around 26–28 weeks of pregnancy.

18.5 Preconception Counselling

Risk stratification should ideally be performed preconception. However it is not uncommon for PS to be detected for the first time during pregnancy or for these patients, who are generally very well, not to be under regular follow-up. The key components determining outcome will be RV function and propensity towards arrhythmia. The well-known risk stratification tools place mild PS in WHO Class I (no detectable increased risk of mortality and no/mild increase in morbidity) [18]. The presence of cyanosis would increase this risk classification. The CARPREG and ZAHARA scores would also place patients, who have not had rhythm issues, in a low-risk group [19, 20]. Khairy et al. reported increased maternal risk associated with impaired RV function and/or severe pulmonary regurgitation but not pulmonary stenosis per se [21].

Patients should be counselled that arrhythmia may present for the first time during pregnancy especially if the PS is severe and there is RA dilatation. In addition progressive effort intolerance may occur in those with high right-sided pressures. It should be remembered that elevated right heart pressures due to PS are much more benign than elevated pressures due to pulmonary vascular disease. Care should be taken to exclude pulmonary hypertension when elevated RV pressures are detected (Chap. 17). Risk increases when patients are symptomatic, have had prior arrhythmia, have severe RV hypertrophy, have RV dysfunction or severe PR or have cyanosis. As with other patients with congenital heart disease, preconception risk stratification and counselling should be performed by an expert multidisciplinary team [22].

> **Conclusions**
>
> The majority of patients with pulmonary stenosis tolerate pregnancy very well. Patients should however be risk stratified as soon as possible – ideally prior to pregnancy. Those with risk factors require specialist multidisciplinary cardiac-obstetric care.

References

1. Van der Linde D, Konings EE, Slager MA et al (2011) Birth prevalence of congenital heart disease worldwide: a systematic review and meta analysis. J Am Coll Cardiol 58(21): 2241–2247
2. Freedom RM, Benson L (2004) Congenital pulmonary stenosis and isolated congenital pulmonary insufficiency. In: Freedom RM, Yoo SJ, Mikailian H, Williams WG (eds) The natural and

modified history of congenital heart disease, 1st edn. Blackstone Publishing, New York, pp 107–118
3. Tynan M, Anderson RH (2002) Pulmonary stenosis. In: Anderson RH, Baker EJ, MacCartthy FJ et al (eds) Paediatric cardiology, 2nd edn. Harcourt, London, pp 1461–1479
4. Freedom RM, Benson L (2004) Congenital pulmonary stenosis and isolated congenital pulmonary insufficiency. The natural and modified history of congenital heart disease. Blackwell Pub, New York, pp 107–718
5. Libby P, Bonow RO, Mann DL, Zipes DP (2007) Braunwald's heart disease; a textbook of cardiovascular medicine, 8th edn. WB. Saunders, Philadelphia
6. Bashore TM (2007) Adult congenital heart disease: right ventricular outflow tract lesions. Circulation 115:1933–1947
7. Weidman WH, Blount SG, DuShane JW et al (1977) Clinical course in ventricular septal defect. Circulation 56(1suppl):156–169
8. Pongiglione G, Freedom RM, Cook D, Rowe RD (1982) Mechanism of acquired right ventricular outflow tract obstruction in patients with ventricular septal defect: an angiocardiographic study. Am J Cardiol 50:776–780
9. Gamboa P et al (2000) Congenital multiple peripheral pulmonary artery stenosis (pulmonary branch stenosis or supravalvular pulmonary stenosis). AJR 175:856–857
10. Vermilion RP, Snider AR, Bengur R, Meliones JN (1991) Long-term assessment of right ventricular diastolic filling in patients with pulmonary valve stenosis successfully treated in childhood. Am J Cardiol 68:648–652
11. Hayes CJ, Gersony WM, Driscoll DJ, Keane JF, Kidd L, O'Fallon WM et al (1993) Second natural history study of congenital heart defects. Results of treatment of patients with pulmonary valvar stenosis. Circulation 87:I28–I37
12. Aldousany AW, DiSessa TG, Dubois R et al (1989) Doppler estimation of pressure gradient in pulmonary stenosis: maximal instantaneous vs peak-to-peak, vs mean catheter gradient. Paediatr Cardiol 10:145–149
13. Frantz EG, Silverman NH (1988) Doppler ultrasound evaluation of valvar pulmonary stenosis from multiple transducer positions in children requiring pulmonary valvuloplasty. Am J Cardiol 61:844–849
14. Silvilairat S, Cabalka AK, Cetta F et al (2005) Outpatient echocardiographic assessment of complex pulmonary outflow stenosis: doppler mean gradient is superior to the maximum instantaneous gradient. J Am Soc Echocardiogr 18:1143–1148
15. Tandri H, Daya SK, Nasir K et al (2006) Normal reference values for the adult right ventricle by magnetic resonance imaging. Am J Cardiol 98(12):1660–1664
16. Tanous D, Siu SC, Mason J et al (2010) B-type natriuretic peptide in pregnant women with heart disease. J Am Coll Cardiol 56(15):1247–1253
17. Ohuchi H, Tanabe Y, Kamiya C et al (2013) Cardiopulmonary variables during exercise predict pregnancy outcome in women with congenital heart disease. Circ J 77(2):470–476
18. Thorne S, MacGregor A, Nelson-Piercy C (2006) Risks of contraception and pregnancy in heart disease. Heart 92:1520–1525
19. Siu SC, Sermer M, Colman JM et al (2001) Prospective multicenter study of pregnancy outcomes in women with heart disease. Circulation 104:515–521
20. Drenthen W, Boersma E, Balci A (2010) Predictors of pregnancy complications on women with congenital heart disease. Eur Heart J 31:2124–2132
21. Khairy POuyang DW, Fernandes SM et al (2006) Pregnancy outcomes in women with congenital heart disease. Circulation 113:517–524
22. Kovacs AH, Harrison JL et al (2008) Pregnancy and contraception in congenital heart disease: what women are not told. J Am Coll Cardiol 52:577–578
23. Galal MO, Jadoon S, Momenah TS (2015) Pulmonary valvuloplasty in a pregnant woman using sole transthoracic echo guidance: technical considerations. Can J Cardiol 31:103, e5-7
24. Hameed AB, Goodwin TM, Elkayam U (2007) Effect of pulmonary stenosis on pregnancy outcomes – a case-control study. Am Heart J 154(5):852–854

Printed by Printforce, the Netherlands